Fundamentals of

Oral
Histology *and*
Physiology

P9-ECI-170

85

Fundamentals of
Oral Histology *and* Physiology

Arthur R. Hand
DDS
Professor, Department of Craniofacial Sciences and Cell Biology
Assistant Dean for Medical and Graduate Education
School of Dental Medicine
University of Connecticut
Farmington, Connecticut

Marion E. Frank
PhD
Professor, Department of Oral Health and Diagnostic Sciences
University of Connecticut
Farmington, Connecticut

WILEY Blackwell

Library Resource Center
Renton Technical College
3000 N.E. 4th Street
Renton, WA 98056

This edition first published 2014 © 2014 by John Wiley & Sons, Inc.

Editorial Offices

1606 Golden Aspen Drive, Suites 103 and 104, Ames, Iowa 50010, USA

The Atrium, Southern Gate, Chichester, West Sussex, PO19 8SQ, UK

9600 Garsington Road, Oxford, OX4 2DQ, UK

For details of our global editorial offices, for customer services and for information about how to apply for permission to reuse the copyright material in this book please see our website at www.wiley.com/wiley-blackwell.

Authorization to photocopy items for internal or personal use, or the internal or personal use of specific clients, is granted by Blackwell Publishing, provided that the base fee is paid directly to the Copyright Clearance Center, 222 Rosewood Drive, Danvers, MA 01923. For those organizations that have been granted a photocopy license by CCC, a separate system of payments has been arranged. The fee codes for users of the Transactional Reporting Service are ISBN-13: 978-1-1183-4291-6 / 2014.

Designations used by companies to distinguish their products are often claimed as trademarks. All brand names and product names used in this book are trade names, service marks, trademarks or registered trademarks of their respective owners. The publisher is not associated with any product or vendor mentioned in this book.

The contents of this work are intended to further general scientific research, understanding, and discussion only and are not intended and should not be relied upon as recommending or promoting a specific method, diagnosis, or treatment by health science practitioners for any particular patient. The publisher and the author make no representations or warranties with respect to the accuracy or completeness of the contents of this work and specifically disclaim all warranties, including without limitation any implied warranties of fitness for a particular purpose. In view of ongoing research, equipment modifications, changes in governmental regulations, and the constant flow of information relating to the use of medicines, equipment, and devices, the reader is urged to review and evaluate the information provided in the package insert or instructions for each medicine, equipment, or device for, among other things, any changes in the instructions or indication of usage and for added warnings and precautions. Readers should consult with a specialist where appropriate. The fact that an organization or Website is referred to in this work as a citation and/or a potential source of further information does not mean that the author or the publisher endorses the information the organization or Website may provide or recommendations it may make. Further, readers should be aware that Internet Websites listed in this work may have changed or disappeared between when this work was written and when it is read. No warranty may be created or extended by any promotional statements for this work. Neither the publisher nor the author shall be liable for any damages arising herefrom.

Library of Congress Cataloging-in-Publication Data

Hand, Arthur R., 1943–, author.
Fundamentals of oral histology and physiology / Arthur R. Hand, Marion E. Frank.
   p. ; cm.
  Includes bibliographical references and index.
  ISBN 978-1-118-34291-6 (paper)
  I. Frank, Marion E. (Marion Elizabeth), 1940–, author.   II. Title.
  [DNLM: 1. Mouth–anatomy & histology. 2. Mouth–physiology. 3. Dental Physiological Phenomena.
4. Facial Pain–physiopathology. WU 102]
  QP88.6
  612.3′11–dc23

2014036984

A catalogue record for this book is available from the British Library.

Wiley also publishes its books in a variety of electronic formats. Some content that appears in print may not be available in electronic books.

Cover image: Large histology image (bottom), book figure 10.14: From Shepherd, G.M. (1983) Chemical Senses, Chapter 12. In: Neurobiology, Oxford University Press New York, pp. 203–226. Reproduced with permission from Oxford University Press

Far left images original; Top middle image original; Top right image original

Middle right image, book figure 8.7: From Moss-Salentijn, L. 1972. Orofacial Histology and Embryology, A Visual Integration. Reproduced by permission of F.A. Davis Company, Philadelphia, PA

Cover design by Modern Alchemy, LLC.

Set in 10/12pt Minion by SPi Publisher Services, Pondicherry, India
Printed and bound in Singapore by Markono Print Media Pte Ltd

1 2014

612 .311 HAND-A   2014

Hand, Arthur R., 1943-

Fundamentals of oral
  histology and physiology

Contents

PART III TOOTH AND JAW SUPPORT

Chapter 6

Structure and Physiology of the Periodontium

Arthur R. Hand

Chapter 7

Tooth Eruption and Shedding

Arthur R. Hand

Chapter 8

Temporomandibular Joint

Felipe Porto

PART IV MUCOSAL STRUCTURE AND FUNCTION

Chapter 9

Oral Mucosa and Mucosal Sensation

*Ellen Eisenberg, Easwar Natarajan,
and Bradley K. Formaker*

Chapter 10

Chemoreception and Perception

Marion E. Frank

PART V ORAL EFFECTORS

Chapter 11

Salivary Glands, Salivary Secretion, and Saliva

Arthur R. Hand

Chapter 12

Orofacial Pain, Touch and Thermosensation, and Sensorimotor Functions

Barry J. Sessle

Chapter 13

Anatomy and Physiology of Speech Production

Janet Rovalino

Contributor List

Martyn T. Cobourne, BDS, PhD
Professor, Department of Orthodontics
Dental Institute
King's College London
London, United Kingdom

Ellen Eisenberg, DMD
Professor, Oral and Maxillofacial Pathology
Department of Oral Health and Diagnostic Sciences
University of Connecticut
Farmington, Connecticut

Bradley K. Formaker, PhD
Research Associate
Department of Oral Health and Diagnostic Sciences
Center for Chemosensory Sciences
University of Connecticut
Farmington, Connecticut

Marion E. Frank, PhD
Professor, Department of Oral Health and Diagnostic Sciences
University of Connecticut
Farmington, Connecticut

Michel Goldberg, DDS
Docteur en Sciences Odontologiques
Docteur es Sciences Naturelles
Professeur Emerite
Biomédicale des Saints Pères
Université Paris Descartes
INSERM UMR-S 1124
Paris, France

Joseph A. Grasso, PhD
Professor Emeritus
Department of Cell Biology
School of Medicine
University of Connecticut
Farmington, Connecticut

Arthur R. Hand, DDS
Professor, Department of Craniofacial Sciences and Cell Biology
Assistant Dean for Medical and Graduate Education
School of Dental Medicine
University of Connecticut
Farmington, Connecticut

Easwar Natarajan, BDS, DMSc
Assistant Professor, Oral and Maxillofacial Pathology
Department of Oral Health and Diagnostic Sciences
University of Connecticut
Farmington, Connecticut

Felipe Porto, DDS, MS
Assistant Professor
Division of Behavioral Sciences and Community Health
Department of Oral Health and Diagnostic Sciences
University of Connecticut
Farmington, Connecticut

Janet E. Rovalino, MS
Instructor, Voice and Speech Pathologist
Otolaryngology – Head and Neck Surgery
School of Medicine
University of Connecticut
Farmington, Connecticut

Barry J. Sessle, MDS, PhD, DSc(hc)
Professor and Canada Research Chair
Faculty of Dentistry
University of Toronto
Toronto, Ontario, Canada

Paul T. Sharpe, PhD
Professor, Craniofacial Development and Stem Cell Biology
Dental Institute
King's College London
Guy's Hospital
London Bridge
London, United Kingdom

Preface

Fundamentals of Oral Histology and Physiology is a textbook for dental students. The aim of the book is to integrate oral histology and physiology, presenting the concepts of these disciplines that are relevant to clinical dentistry in a thorough but concise manner. Most dental students studying oral histology and physiology will already have or are currently obtaining a background in the basic medical sciences, including cell and molecular biology, biochemistry, genetics, general histology and physiology and immunology. Thus this text focuses on the histology and physiology that students need to know to practice dentistry and to understand and evaluate the current literature, without repeating the basic information that they learn in other courses.

The book is organized into five sections, each including two or three relevant chapters:

Development, with chapters on the embryonic development of the head, face, and mouth and the development of the teeth;

The Teeth, with chapters on enamel, and dentin, pulp, and tooth pain;

Tooth and Jaw Support, with chapters on the periodontium, tooth eruption, and the temporomandibular joint;

Mucosal Structure and Function, with chapters on the oral mucosa and mucosal sensation, and chemoreception and perception; and

Oral Effectors, with chapters on salivary glands and saliva, orofacial pain, touch, thermosensation, and sensorimotor function, and speech production.

Each chapter is organized in a logical, straightforward manner, with micrographs, drawings, charts, and tables designed to illustrate and augment the concepts presented in the text. Brief summaries at key points in the text highlight the important information and concepts presented in the preceding paragraphs, and each chapter has an extensive glossary. Clinical correlations for common diseases and conditions are included in each chapter, and many chapters include case studies, so that this book will be a useful future reference. The online version of the book also includes review questions and answers.

We have assembled a diverse group of experts to contribute chapters. These include well-known research scientists (Martyn Cobourne and Paul Sharpe, Michel Goldberg, Barry Sessle, Bradley Formaker), experienced educators (Joseph Grasso), and superb clinicians (Ellen Eisenberg and Easwar Natarajan, Felipe Porto, Janet Rovalino). We are grateful to our contributors for their enthusiastic support for the book and their prompt responses to our numerous messages and questions. We also greatly appreciate the interest and support of our editors and the staff at Wiley-Blackwell.

We thank our students at the University of Connecticut School of Dental Medicine, who have inspired us to undertake this project, and Dean R. Lamont MacNeil for his continuing support. Finally, however successful our efforts may have been, they would not have been possible without the love and support of our spouses, Dr. Maija Mednieks and Dr. Thomas Hettinger.

Arthur R. Hand and Marion E. Frank

Chapter 1 Oral Structures and Tissues

Arthur R. Hand[1] and Marion E. Frank[2]

[1]Department of Craniofacial Sciences and Cell Biology, School of Dental Medicine, University of Connecticut
[2]Department of Oral Health and Diagnostic Sciences, University of Connecticut

The oral cavity and its component cells, tissues, and structures constitute a unique and complex organ system and environment. Of necessity, we study its various parts individually, but the health and function of the components of the oral cavity depend upon and influence one another. Importantly, the oral cavity relies on as well as influences the health and function of the entire body.

The oral cavity is the gateway to the body, and most of the substances that enter our bodies do so through the oral cavity. It is exposed to the physical insults of mastication, hard objects and various food substances, and extremes of temperature. A variety of chemicals, including those present in foods and drinks and produced by commensal and pathogenic organisms, affect the oral cavity. It functions in alimentation, respiration, innate and immune defense, special and general sensation, speech, and human interactions. The tissues and structures of the oral cavity are subject to unique as well as general disease processes. Diseases originating in the oral cavity can have systemic effects; likewise, systemic diseases can affect the oral cavity and the first signs and symptoms of many diseases may appear in the mouth.

The oral cavity

The readily visible components of the oral cavity include the lips (**labia**), the inside of the cheeks (**bucca**), the teeth and gums (**gingivae**), the hard and soft palates, the floor of the mouth, and the tongue (Fig. 1.1). Not visible, but clearly important, are the muscles, nerves, blood vessels, glands, joints, and especially the bones of the upper (**maxilla**) and lower (**mandible**) jaws that provide support for and function with the visible components. The oral cavity begins at the junction of the **vermilion border** of the lips and the **mucosa** lining the inside of the lips, and extends posteriorly to the **palatoglossal folds** or **arch**. Beyond the palato-glossal folds are the **palatopharyngeal folds** and the beginning of the **oropharynx**, where the digestive and respiratory tracts come together. The **palatine tonsils** are located in the **tonsillar fauces** between the palatoglossal and palatopharyngeal folds. The lymphoid tissue of the palatine tonsils, along with that of the **pharyngeal tonsil (adenoids)** and the **lingual tonsils**, guards the entrance to the oropharynx. Anteriorly, the respiratory tract (nasal cavity) is separated from the oral cavity by the **hard palate**, and posteriorly by the **soft palate**. The hard palate has an arch-like shape that varies in width and height among individuals. It also plays an important role in manipulation and mastication of food, and in speech. The soft palate functions to seal the oropharynx from the **nasopharynx** during swallowing and speech. However, during exhalation, receptor cells that detect odors in the **olfactory mucosa** are activated by oral vapors moving from the posterior oral to posterior nasal cavity through the nasopharynx, effectively expanding the mouth. It is this **retronasal** route that gives food and drink the odors that contribute much to flavor perception.

The lips and cheeks are separated from the **alveolar processes** of the maxilla and mandible that support and hold the teeth by a space called the **vestibule**. The vestibule is limited posteriorly by the **ramus** of the mandible, and superiorly and inferiorly by the **mucolabial** and **mucobuccal folds**. The mucosal lining of the vestibule is continuous with the mucosa of the lips and cheeks, and with the mucosa covering the alveolar processes (Fig. 1.2). Folds (**frena** [singular, **frenum**]) of the mucosa, located at the midline and in the canine regions, extend across the vestibule to anchor the lips and cheek to the maxilla and mandible. The secretions of the **parotid salivary gland** enter the vestibule

Fundamentals of Oral Histology and Physiology, First Edition. Arthur R. Hand and Marion E. Frank.
© 2014 John Wiley & Sons, Inc. Published 2014 by John Wiley & Sons, Inc.

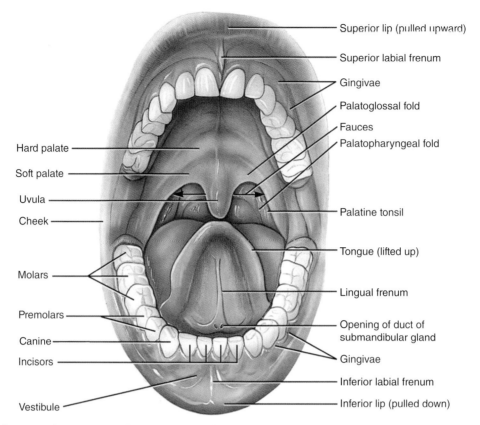

Superior lip (pulled upward)

Superior labial frenum

Gingivae

Palatoglossal fold

Fauces

Palatopharyngeal fold

Hard palate

Soft palate

Uvula

Cheek

Palatine tonsil

Tongue (lifted up)

Molars

Lingual frenum

Premolars

Canine

Incisors

Opening of duct of submandibular gland

Gingivae

Inferior labial frenum

Inferior lip (pulled down)

Vestibule

Figure 1.1   Diagram illustrating the anatomy and main structures of the oral cavity. (Modified from Tortora, G.J. & Grabowski, S.R. 2000. *Principles of Anatomy and Physiology*, 9th edition, Wiley, New York. Reproduced by permission of John Wiley & Sons.)

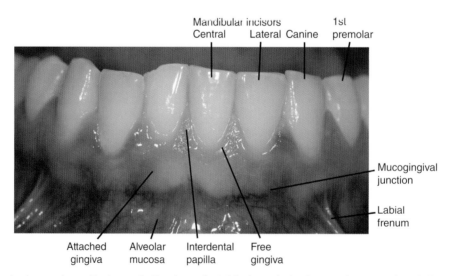

Mandibular incisors

Central   Lateral Canine

1st premolar

Mucogingival junction

Labial frenum

Attached gingiva

Alveolar mucosa

Interdental papilla

Free gingiva

Figure 1.2   Oral mucosa, gingivae and mandibular teeth. Blood vessels visible through the thin non-keratinized epithelium of the alveolar mucosa give it a redder color than the gingivae with their thicker keratinized epithelium. (From http://commons.wikimedia.org/wiki/File:Healthy_gingiva.jpg)

through its main duct, which opens at the **parotid papilla** on the buccal mucosa opposite the maxillary second molar tooth.

The mucosa surrounding the necks, or cervical regions of the teeth, is called the gingivae. The **attached gingiva** is clearly demarcated from the alveolar mucosa at the **mucogingival junction**.

The attached gingiva is firmly bound to the bone of the alveolar process, and through the **junctional epithelium** is bound to and creates a seal around each tooth. The **free gingiva** is separated from the tooth by the **gingival sulcus** or **crevice**, and forms the **interdental papilla** between adjacent teeth.

The **tongue** occupies the space within the maxillary and mandibular arches, from the floor of the mouth to the hard and soft palates. The mucosa of the dorsal surface of the tongue has several types of specialized structures called **papillae** that function in the manipulation of food and in taste. The tongue also is critical for forming proper speech sounds. The anterior portion of the tongue is anchored to the floor of the mouth by the **lingual frenum**. The ducts of the **submandibular** and **sublingual salivary glands** open on either side of the lingual frenum at the **sublingual caruncle**; smaller ducts of the sublingual gland open along the **sublingual fold** on each side of the floor of the mouth.

Oral mucosa

Mucosa is a wet, soft tissue membrane that lines an internal body space, e.g., the oral cavity, the gastrointestinal, urinary, and reproductive tracts. The oral mucosa consists of three layers: a surface **epithelium**; a supporting **lamina propria** consisting of a layer of loose connective tissue (*papillary layer*) just below the epithelium and a deeper layer of dense irregular connective tissue (*reticular layer*); and an underlying **submucosa** consisting of dense irregular connective tissue (Fig. 1.3). The submucosa frequently contains **minor salivary glands**, and in some locations may contain adipose tissue. In some regions of the oral cavity, the submucosa may be absent, and the mucosa is bound to either bone or muscle by the lamina propria.

Three subtypes of mucosa are found in the oral cavity. **Lining** or **moveable mucosa** has a **stratified squamous non-keratinized epithelium**, and is found on the inside of the lips and cheeks, in the vestibules and the floor of the mouth, and on the alveolar processes, the ventral surface of the tongue, and the soft palate. **Masticatory mucosa** has a **stratified squamous keratinized** or

parakeratinized epithelium, and is found on surfaces subjected to the stresses induced by chewing our food (mastication), the hard palate and the gingivae. **Specialized mucosa** is found on the dorsal surface of the tongue. This mucosa is considered specialized because it forms four different types of **papillae**, three of which have **taste buds** through which taste sensations are received. Multiple **fungiform papillae** dot the dorsal anterior lingual surface, whereas two series of papillae with associated trenches or troughs, the medial **circumvallate** and lateral **foliate** papillae, are found far posterior near the base of the tongue (Fig. 1.4). The walls of the trenches are lined with specialized mucosa containing taste buds. The ducts of minor salivary glands (**von Ebner's glands**) open into the trenches, and substances present in the trenches are flushed out by their secretions. Because the mucosa of the tongue has a stratified squamous keratinized epithelium, and because it plays an important role in mastication of food, this mucosa also may be classified as masticatory mucosa.

The oral mucosa has several functions. These include providing protection from physical and chemical insults through its multilayered and keratinized epithelial surface; serving as a permeability barrier to prevent passage of microorganisms and toxic materials; detecting and responding to pathogenic microorganisms and foreign antigens through its immunological components; lubricating and moistening the oral surfaces through secretion of fluid and **mucins**; and general and special sensation through free and encapsulated nerve endings and taste buds.

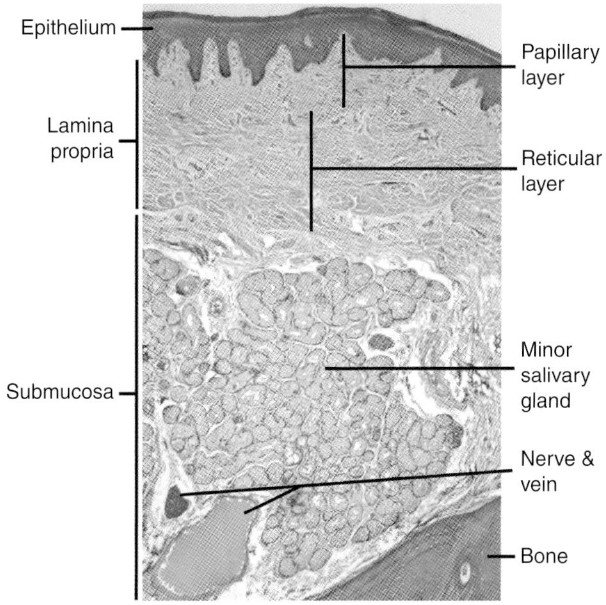

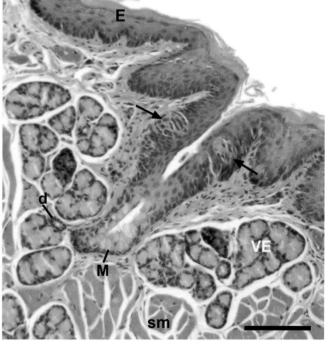

Figure 1.4   Light micrograph of a section through a foliate papillary trench of the tongue of a hamster. Arrows point to taste buds in the epithelial lining of the trench. Mucous cells (M) are present in the excretory duct of von Ebner's gland (VE) as it opens into the trench. Small duct from a VE lobule (d); skeletal muscle (sm); stratified squamous keratinized epithelium (E). Scale bar = 100 μm.

Figure 1.3   Light micrograph showing the layers and components of the oral mucosa. A submucosa is not present in all regions of the oral cavity.

Teeth

The teeth are among the most unique and complex structures of the body. Although they are designed to last a lifetime, teeth can be destroyed or lost in a relatively short time if we fail to take care of them. They consist of three different hard, or mineralized, tissues – **dentin**, **cementum**, and **enamel** – and are supported by a fourth hard tissue – **bone** (Fig. 1.5). The interface between the teeth and the gingivae is the only place in the body where a structure composed of hard tissues breaches a soft tissue covering. This unique anatomic arrangement is the site of significant pathology that can lead to the destruction of the supporting tissues of the tooth (**periodontium**) and its eventual loss.

Humans have two sets of teeth, the **primary**, or **deciduous**, teeth and the **permanent** teeth. The primary teeth are the first set to form and erupt into the oral cavity, beginning at about 6 months of age. There are a total of 20 primary teeth, 10 in the maxilla and 10 in the mandible, arranged in the form of an arch. On each side (**quadrant**) of the arch of each jaw, there is a central **incisor**, lateral incisor, **canine** (or **cuspid**), and first and second **molars**. The permanent teeth, also called **succedaneous** or **successional** teeth, which replace the primary teeth beginning at 6 to 7 years of age, develop in relation to the primary teeth. The permanent molars, or **accessional** teeth, have no primary precursors and develop posterior to the second primary molars. There are a total of 32 permanent teeth, eight in each quadrant; these include the central and lateral incisors, canine, first and second **premolars** (or **bicuspids**), and first, second, and third molars (Fig. 1.1).

A tooth consists of a **crown**, containing the **pulp chamber** and one or more **roots**, which contain the **pulp canals** (Fig. 1.5). The **anatomic crown** is covered by enamel, the hardest biological substance known; the **clinical crown** is the portion of the crown exposed in the oral cavity. One or more **cusps** and **ridges** separated by **grooves** and **sulci** are present on the **occlusal surface** (upper or grinding surface) of premolars and molars. The **incisal** surface of incisors is flatter and thinner and that of canines is more pointed; these teeth function in biting and tearing. The surfaces of the crowns of premolars and molars that face the cheeks are the **buccal** or **facial** surfaces (Fig. 1.6). The surfaces of the crowns of incisors and canines that face the lips are the **labial** or facial surfaces. The surfaces of the maxillary teeth that face the palate are the **palatal** surfaces; the surfaces of the mandibular teeth adjacent to the tongue are the **lingual** surfaces. The surfaces of the teeth in each arch that face the adjacent teeth are the **proximal** surfaces. The proximal surface of premolars and molars facing the posterior part of the oral cavity is the **distal** surface; that facing the anterior part of the oral cavity is the **mesial** (toward the midline) surface. This convention is maintained for the incisors and canines: distal, toward the adjacent tooth in the arch closer to the posterior teeth; mesial, toward the midline.

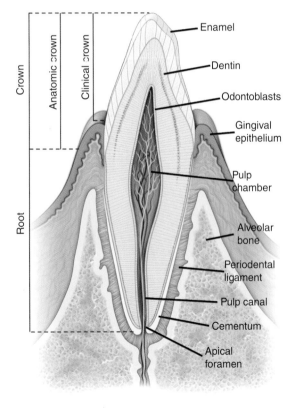

Figure 1.5   Diagram illustrating the structure of a tooth and its supporting tissues. (Modified from Ross, M.H. & Pawlina, W. 2011. *Histology: A Text and Atlas*, 6th edition, Wolters Kluwer/Lippincott Williams & Wilkins, Philadelphia. Reproduced by permission of Wolters Kluwer Health.)

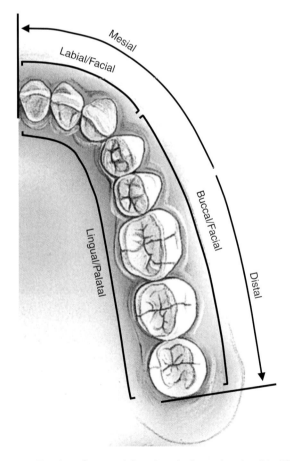

Figure 1.6   Tooth surfaces and directions in the oral cavity. (Modified from Tortora, G.J. 1995. *Principles of Human Anatomy*, 7th edition, Wiley, New York. Reproduced by permission of John Wiley & Sons.)

The main tissue of the tooth is dentin. Dentin supports the enamel, which covers the crown, and it forms the root of the tooth. Dentin encloses the **pulp**, which through its blood and nerve supply and immunologic and regenerative functions maintains the vitality of the dentin and the cells that produce it, **odontoblasts**. Odontoblasts line the periphery of the pulp and secrete and mineralize the matrix components of dentin, predominantly collagen. Each odontoblast has a long apical or distal cytoplasmic process, the **odontoblast process**, that extends partway through the dentin in a **dentinal tubule**. The dentinal tubules are created as the dentin is deposited around the odontoblast processes and the odontoblasts gradually move deeper into the pulp. Some of the dentinal tubules also contain nerve endings, which in conjunction with the odontoblasts and other nerve endings associated with the odontoblasts are responsible for the sensation of pain in dentin. Odontoblasts respond to challenges to the integrity of the tooth, such as **dental caries**, by rapidly sealing off the dentinal tubules and depositing additional dentin in an attempt to protect the pulp.

Enamel is a product of cells derived from the oral ectoderm. Thus, its composition and structure differ markedly from those of the mesenchymally derived dentin, cementum, and bone. Whereas the latter are living tissues, with collagen-based mineralized extracellular matrices, and capable of repair and regeneration (although limited in the case of dentin and cementum), enamel is non-living, has a temporary non-collagenous extracellular matrix, and is incapable of biological repair. Enamel consists of **rods**, or **prisms**, of large, elongated crystals of the mineral **hydroxyapatite**. Similar mineral crystals are located between adjacent rods, in **interrod enamel**. Enamel is formed by cells called **ameloblasts**, which progress through several morphologically and functionally distinct stages during the process of enamel matrix secretion, matrix removal, and mineralization. Upon eruption of the teeth into the oral cavity, the ameloblasts are lost, thus enamel that is damaged or worn away cannot be replaced through cellular activity.

Supporting tissues of the teeth

The teeth are supported by the **alveolar bone** of the mandible and maxilla and held in place by the collagenous **periodontal ligament** (PDL) (Fig. 1.5). The collagen fibers of the periodontal ligament insert into the cementum, which is adherent to and covers the dentin of the root, and into the alveolar bone. Although cementum is part of the tooth, its main function is to provide anchorage for the periodontal ligament fibers. Cementum is produced by cells called **cementoblasts**, and like dentin has a collagen-based mineralized matrix. However, its structure is different from that of dentin. Cementum covering the portion of the root closest to the crown is **acellular**, i.e., it is composed solely of extracellular matrix components and mineral; cells and cell processes are not present. Cementum covering the portion closer to the tip, or **apex**, of the root, and in the **furcation** area (where the roots diverge below the crown) of multirooted teeth, is **cellular**. In addition to extracellular matrix components and mineral, cellular cementum contains the cell bodies and processes of cementoblasts that have become trapped

as **cementocytes**. The continued deposition of cementum throughout life helps to maintain the attachment of the periodontal ligament as teeth reposition themselves in response to long-term functional changes.

The collagen fibers of the periodontal ligament, like collagen in other soft tissues, is produced and maintained by **fibroblasts**. Groups of fibers with different orientations help retain the tooth in the alveolus, provide resistance to intrusive forces during mastication, and hold adjacent teeth together in the dental arch. Other fibers help hold the gingival tissues against the alveolar bone and teeth. Through its blood supply, the periodontal ligament provides nourishment for the cementum and alveolar bone and the cells that form these tissues. Through its nerve supply, the periodontal ligament also functions in proprioception, so we know how hard to bite and the position of our jaw when we are chewing, and in stimulation of salivary gland secretion.

The alveolar bone of the mandible and maxilla supports the teeth. The portion of the alveolar bone lining the alveolus provides anchorage for the periodontal ligament fibers. Because of the insertion of these fibers, the bone at the surface of the alveolus is called **bundle bone**. Beneath this surface layer, typical **lamellar bone** is present. Like all bone, alveolar bone has a collagen-based, mineralized extracellular matrix that is produced by **osteoblasts**, is degraded and remodeled by **osteoclasts**, and contains **osteocytes** and their processes. Typical **Haversian systems**, or **osteons**, are found in the cortical bone of the facial and lingual (palatal) surfaces of the alveolar processes. Maintenance of the alveolar bone depends on the presence of the teeth; it forms as the teeth erupt, and it is resorbed and disappears if the teeth are lost. Alveolar bone also may be lost due to disease, e.g., **periodontitis**, with a concomitant loss of tooth support and attachment.

Salivary glands

In addition to the **minor salivary glands** present in most regions of the oral mucosa, there are three **major salivary glands**, the **parotid**, **submandibular** and **sublingual** glands (Fig. 1.7). These are paired glands located outside of the oral cavity, and connected to it by long **ducts**. The salivary glands produce and secrete the fluid, ionic and macromolecular components of **saliva**. Saliva functions to moisten and lubricate the oral tissues, clear food debris and bacterial products from the oral cavity, form a coating (**pellicle**) on all oral surfaces, buffer the acids produced by bacteria, protect the oral tissues through its content of electrolytes and antimicrobial substances, and initiate the digestion of certain food substances.

The secretory cells of the glands are arranged in spherical or tubular-shaped **endpieces**, or **acini**. Each endpiece is connected to a small **intercalated duct**, which empties into a **striated duct**. The striated ducts are a prominent component, and characteristic of the major salivary glands. They function to modify the saliva produced by the secretory cells of the endpieces by reabsorption and secretion of electrolytes. The striated ducts connect to larger ducts, the **excretory ducts**, which eventually merge to become the **main excretory duct** that empties into the oral cavity.

There are two types of secretory cells found in salivary glands, **serous cells** and **mucous cells** (Fig. 1.7). Serous cells

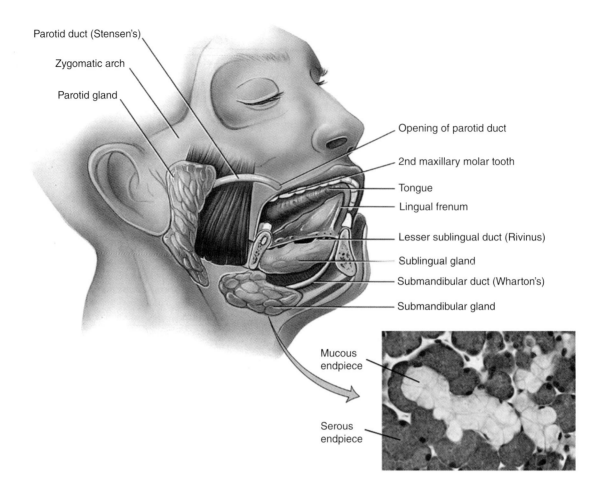

Figure 1.7   Location of the major salivary glands. (Modified from Tortora, G.J. & Grabowski, S.R. 2000. *Principles of Anatomy and Physiology*, 9th edition, Wiley, New York. Reproduced by permission of John Wiley & Sons.)

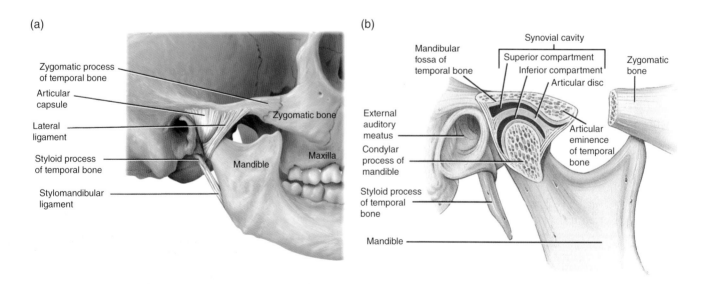

Figure 1.8   Location and structure of the temporomandibular joint. (a) Right lateral view. (Modified from Tortora, G.J. & Derrickson, B.H. 2011. *Principles of Anatomy and Physiology*, 13th edition, Wiley, New York. Reproduced by permission of John Wiley & Sons.) (b) Sagittal section. (Modified from Tortora, G.J. & Grabowski, S.R. 2000. *Principles of Anatomy and Physiology*, 9th edition, Wiley, New York. Reproduced by permission of John Wiley & Sons.)

produce a number of proteins and glycoproteins, many of which have antimicrobial or enzymatic activity or bind to various substances, including microorganisms. Mucous cells mainly produce highly glycosylated proteins called mucins. Mucins provide lubrication, allowing oral tissues to glide easily over one another, and have certain binding and antimicrobial activities. Serous cells, and to a lesser extent mucous cells, also secrete water and electrolytes. A third cell type present in the endpieces is the **myoepithelial cell**. Myoepithelial cells contract to help expel saliva from the endpieces into the duct system. They also help maintain the organization and differentiated state of the endpiece cells.

Temporomandibular joint

Although not part of the oral cavity *per se*, the health and function of the **temporomandibular joint** (TMJ) are intimately related to oral cavity function. The temporomandibular joint consists of the mandibular **condyle**, the portion of the temporal bone that includes the **mandibular fossa** and the **articular eminence**, the **articular disc**, the ligaments that hold the condyle in place, the joint capsule and associated structures, and the muscles that move the joint (Fig. 1.8).

The temporomandibular joint is a **ginglymoarthrodial synovial joint** that undergoes both translational and rotational movements. Its main function is to allow opening and closing of the mouth and movements of the mandible during mastication and speech. The unique structural and functional features of this joint can lead to specific types of dysfunction, such as displacements of the articular disc. Dysfunction of the joint, due to joint-related, muscle-related, or unknown causes, may result in pain conditions called **temporomandibular disorders**. Pathological conditions that occur in other synovial joints, such as osteoarthritis and rheumatoid arthritis, also may occur in the temporomandibular joint.

Glossary

Alveolar processes: The bony portions (*alveolar bone*) of the mandible and maxilla that support the teeth and in which their roots are embedded.

Ameloblast: The cell type that synthesizes, secretes, and mineralizes tooth enamel.

Apex: The end of the root of the tooth; *apical*:0000 of or toward the end of the root.

Articular disc: The dense connective tissue structure in the temporomandibular joint interposed between the mandibular condyle and the temporal bone.

Articular eminence: The bony prominence of the temporal bone anterior to the mandibular fossa; the articular disc slides over the eminence during mandibular function.

Bone: A mineralized, collagen-based skeletal tissue providing support and protection for internal organs and to which muscles are attached; *lamellar bone* consists of sequentially deposited sheets or lamellae of oriented collagen fibrils and mineral crystals; *bundle* or woven bone is immature bone, with a more irregular pattern of collagen fibrils, commonly found where tendons and ligaments insert into bone.

Bucca: The cheek; *buccal*: of or toward the cheek.

Canine (cuspid):   The third tooth from the midline in each arch; it has a conical shape for holding and tearing food.

Cementoblast: The cell type that synthesizes, secretes, and mineralizes cementum.

Cementocyte: Cells derived from cementoblasts that are enclosed within lacunae in cellular cementum.

Cementum: The mineralized tissue covering the roots of the teeth; cementum may contain cells present in lacunae (*cellular* cementum) or may lack cells (*acellular* cementum). Periodontal ligament fibers attach to the cementum to hold the teeth in their sockets (alveoli).

Condyle: The portion of the mandible that articulates with the temporal bone in the temporomandibular joint.

Crown: The portion of the tooth covered by enamel (*anatomic crown*); the portion of the tooth visible in the oral cavity (*clinical crown*).

Cusp: A pointed or rounded projection on the occlusal surface of a posterior tooth or canine; *ridges* are linear elevations; *grooves* or *sulci* are valleys or depressions between cusps and ridges.

Dental caries: Lesions of the tooth tissues (enamel, dentin, cementum) caused by dissolution of mineral (hydroxyapatite) by acids and destruction of organic matrix by proteolytic enzymes produced by oral bacteria.

Dentin: The main tissue of the tooth, consisting of a highly mineralized collagenous matrix produced by odontoblasts; dentin supports the enamel in the crown and forms the tooth root.

Dentinal tubules: Channels or tubules extending through the dentin from the pulpal surface to the enamel; formed by deposition of dentin matrix around the distal *odontoblast processes*.

Ducts: Epithelium-lined tubular conduits that convey secretions from salivary gland endpieces to the oral cavity and modify them in the process; they include *intercalated*, *striated*, and *excretory* ducts.

Enamel: The ectodermally derived, highly mineralized tissue covering the crowns of the teeth; produced by ameloblasts.

Endpiece (acinus):   A cluster of salivary gland secretory cells organized around a lumen and connected to an intercalated duct.

Epithelium: A layer of cells lining a body surface; the epithelium of the oral mucosa is a multilayered *stratified squamous* epithelium, either *non-keratinized*, *keratinized*, or *parakeratinized*.

Facial: Of or toward the face.

Fibroblast: The main cell type of connective tissues; responsible for secretion, maintenance, and repair of the fibrous components, glycoproteins, and proteoglycans of the extracellular matrix.

Frenum: A fold of oral mucosa that connects the alveolar process to the cheek or the ventral surface of the tongue to the floor of the mouth.

Furcation: The region on the underside of the crowns of multirooted teeth where the roots diverge.

Gingivae: The portion of the oral mucosa adjacent to the teeth, covered by stratified squamous keratinized or parakeratinized epithelium; *attached gingiva* is bound to the underlying bone or tooth surface; *free gingiva* forms the margin of the gingiva and is not bound to the tooth.

Gingival sulcus (crevice): The space between the free gingiva and the tooth surface; lined by stratified squamous, non-keratinized epithelium.

Ginglymoarthrodial synovial joint: A joint that combines hinge and gliding movements, with a joint space containing synovial fluid.

Haversian system (osteon): The basic structural unit of compact bone, consisting of a central canal containing blood vessels, nerves, and osteoblasts or bone lining (endosteal) cells, surrounded by concentric lamellae of bone with osteocytes in lacunae.

Hydroxyapatite: The crystalline calcium phosphate mineral of bones and teeth, $Ca_{10}(PO_4)_6(OH)_2$; usually present with carbonate (CO_3^-) and/or fluoride (F^-) substituting for OH^-, or CO_3^- substituting for phosphate.

Incisal Edge: The biting surface or edge of an anterior tooth; *incisal*: of or toward the incisal edge.

Incisor: Anterior teeth with a sharp edge for cutting and shearing food; each arch contains two central and two lateral incisors.

Interdental papilla: The gingival tissue located below the contact point between the proximal surfaces of adjacent teeth.

Interrod enamel: Enamel tissue surrounding enamel rods; it is produced by ameloblasts and secreted at the sides of Tomes' processes; interrod enamel crystals have a different orientation than rod enamel crystals.

Junctional epithelium: The epithelium that attaches the gingival tissues to the tooth surface; initially derived from the reduced enamel epithelium.

Labia: The lips; *labial*: of or toward the lips.

Lamina propria: The connective tissue that supports the epithelium of the oral mucosa; the *papillary layer*, consisting of loose connective tissue, is located immediately below the epithelium; the *reticular layer*, consisting of dense irregular connective tissue, is located below the papillary layer.

Lingual: Of or toward the tongue.

Mandible: The lower jaw; the *body* contains the lower teeth and the flattened *ramus* extends upward at angle, ending in the coronoid and condylar processes.

Mandibular fossa: The depression or concavity in the temporal bone that articulates with the condyle/disc complex.

Maxilla: Two maxillae form the upper jaw; each maxilla contains the upper teeth and the maxillary sinus; forms the hard palate, floor and lateral wall of the nasal cavity, and the wall of the orbit.

Molar: A multirooted posterior tooth used for grinding food; there are three molars on each side of each arch.

Mucogingival junction: The boundary between the alveolar mucosa, with non-keratinized epithelium and the attached gingivae, with thicker, keratinized epithelium.

Mucolabial, mucobuccal folds: The depth of the oral mucosa in the vestibule, from the mandible or maxilla to the lips or cheeks, respectively.

Mucosa (mucous membrane): The lining of a body cavity exposed to the external environment or of an internal organ; consists of an epithelium and supporting connective tissue; involved in secretion, absorption, and protection; mucosae of the oral cavity include *lining* or *moveable*, *masticatory*, and *specialized*.

Mucous cell: A secretory cell of the salivary glands; produces highly glycosylated proteins called mucins.

Myoepithelial cell: A contractile cell found in salivary, lacrimal, sweat, and mammary glands; its contractions force fluid from the endpieces into the ducts; also helps maintain the differentiated state of the secretory cells.

Nasopharynx: The uppermost portion of the pharynx; extends from the base of the skull to the soft palate, posterior to the nasal choanae (posterior openings of the nasal cavity).

Occlusal surface: The upper or grinding surface of premolar and molar teeth; *occlusal*: of or toward the occlusal surface.

Odontoblast: The cell type that is responsible for synthesis, secretion, and mineralization of the dentin matrix; also participates in sensory, defensive, and reparative functions; *odontoblast process*: the elongated distal portion of the odontoblast present within a dentinal tubule.

Olfactory mucosa: The mucosa of the upper portion of the nasal cavity; the epithelium contains olfactory neurons with odor receptors involved in the sense of smell.

Oropharynx: The portion of the pharynx posterior to the oral cavity, extending from the soft palate to the epiglottis.

Osteoblast: The cell type that synthesizes, secretes, and mineralizes the matrix of bone.

Osteoclast: A large multinucleated cell formed by fusion of bone-marrow-derived precursors; responsible for bone resorption through the secretion of acid and proteolytic enzymes.

Osteocytes: The cells of bone; they are derived from osteoblasts and located in lacunae surrounded by mineralized bone and function in mechanosensation and regulating bone growth and turnover.

Palate: The structure separating the oral and nasal cavities; the anterior *hard palate* consists of the bony palatal processes of the maxillae covered by masticatory muscosa orally and respiratory mucosa nasally; the posterior *soft palate* consists of muscular tissue covered by lining mucosa orally and respiratory muscosa nasally; *palatal*: of or toward the palate.

Palatoglossal fold: The arch-like fold of the oral mucosa covering the palatoglossal muscle, the anterior tonsillar pillar, and the posterior limit of the oral cavity.

Palatopharyngeal fold: The arch-like fold of the oral mucosa covering the palatopharyngeus muscle and the posterior tonsillar pillar.

Papillae: Tissue projections from the dorsal surface of the tongue filiform papillae cover most of the anterior two-thirds of the tongue; *fungiform* papillae with dorsal taste buds are present in the anterior two-thirds; *circumvallate* and *foliate* papillae with taste buds in the walls of their associated trenches are present posteriorly and laterally, respectively.

Parotid papilla: A raised area of mucosa on the inside of the cheek opposite the second maxillary molar; the site of opening of the parotid gland duct.

Pellicle: The coating on the surfaces of the teeth and oral mucosa consisting of adsorbed salivary proteins, glycoproteins, and mucins.

Periodontal ligament: The collagenous ligament attaching the cementum on the root of a tooth to the bone of the alveolus.

Periodontitis: An inflammatory disease of the periodontal tissues resulting in loss of tooth support, caused by the response to a microbial biofilm adherent to tooth surfaces.

Periodontium: The supporting tissues of the teeth, including the alveolar bone, the periodontal ligament, the cementum, and the gingivae.

Permanent (succedaneous/successional, accessional) teeth: The teeth that replace (*succedaneous or successional*) or erupt posterior to (*accessional*) the primary teeth, beginning at about 6 to 7 years of age.

Premolar (bicuspid):   A permanent tooth located between the canines and molars, shaped for grinding food; two premolars are present on each side of each arch.

Primary (deciduous) teeth: The first teeth to develop in children; four incisors, two canines, and four molars in each jaw; they are replaced by permanent teeth beginning at about 6 years of age.

Proximal (mesial, distal) surfaces: The tooth surfaces facing adjacent teeth; *mesial* surfaces face toward the midline; *distal* surfaces face toward the back of the oral cavity.

Pulp: The living tissue inside the crown and root(s) of a tooth; consists of connective tissue and connective tissue cells, and includes odontoblasts, blood and lymphatic vessels, and nerves; *pulp chamber*: the space enclosed by the dentin of the tooth crown containing pulpal tissue; *pulp canals*: narrow extensions of the pulp chamber through the length of the root containing pulpal tissue.

Quadrant: One-half of the dental arch of each jaw; contains five primary teeth or eight permanent teeth.

Retronasal: Posterior route of access to the nasal cavity and olfactory epithelium, through the oro- and nasopharynges.

Rod (prism):   The basic structural unit of enamel, extending from the dentin surface to the tooth surface; it consists of elongated enamel crystals.

Root: The portion of the tooth embedded in and attached to the alveolar bone via the periodontal ligament; consist of dentin covered by cementum; contains the pulp canal.

Saliva: The product of the salivary glands; contains water, electrolytes, proteins, glycoproteins, mucins, and small organic molecules; saliva in the mouth also contains epithelial cells, white blood cells, and microorganisms.

Salivary glands: Exocrine glands producing saliva; major glands located outside of the oral cavity are the *parotid, submandibular,* and *sublingual* glands; *minor* salivary glands are located in the submucosa in many regions of the oral cavity.

Serous cell: A secretory cell of the salivary glands; produces proteins and glycoproteins with enzymatic, antimicrobial, and other protective activities.

Sublingual caruncle: A small papilla near the base of the lingual frenum; site of opening of the submandibular gland duct and the major duct of the sublingual gland.

Sublingual fold: An elevated fold of the mucosa in the floor of the mouth, between the tongue and the body of the mandible; minor ducts of the sublingual gland open along the sublingual fold.

Submucosa: The deepest layer of the oral mucosa; it contains dense irregular connective tissue, larger blood vessels and nerves and may contain minor salivary glands and adipose tissue; it is not present in all regions of the oral cavity.

Taste buds: A small cluster of taste receptor cells, supporting cells, and nerves located within the epithelium covering fungiform papillae and lining the trenches of circumvallate and foliate papillae of the tongue.

Temporomandibular joint: The joint formed by the mandibular condyle and the temporal bone; it allows opening and closing of the mouth and lateral excursions during mastication.

Temporomandibular disorders: A group of conditions characterized by pain in the temporomandibular joint or jaw muscles, limitation of jaw movement, and clicking or crackling sounds in the joint; the cause may be joint-related, muscle-related, or unknown (idiopathic).

Tongue: The muscular organ of the oral cavity which functions in tasting, manipulating and swallowing food, and in forming speech sounds.

Tonsillar fauces: The space between the palatoglossal and palatopharyngeal folds containing the palatine tonsils.

Tonsils (palatine, pharyngeal, lingual):   Collections of lymphatic tissue located around the pharynx that guard the entrance to the digestive and respiratory tracts.

Vermilion border: The reddish-colored region of the lips, separating the skin from the oral mucosa; it is covered by a thin stratified squamous, keratinized epithelium.

Vestibule: The space between the lips or cheeks and the alveolar processes of the maxilla and mandible; lined by stratified squamous, non-keratinized epithelium.

von Ebner's glands: Minor serous salivary glands located in the tongue; their ducts open into the trenches of the circumvallate and foliate papillae of the tongue.

PART I
DEVELOPMENT

Library Resource Center
Renton Technical College
3000 N.E. 4th Street
Renton, WA 98056

Chapter 2 Development of the Head, Face, and Mouth

Joseph A. Grasso

Department of Cell Biology, School of Medicine, University of Connecticut

Introduction

Congenital facial and jaw defects represent a significant health problem worldwide, making it important for oral health professionals to understand the embryologic processes involved in facial and jaw development. While structural defects are conspicuous and gain clinical attention, developmental anomalies of the face and jaws often cause less visible functional problems, e.g., malocclusions, which challenge the oral health specialist.

The purpose of this chapter is to describe the morphological events leading to development of the face and jaws, including a brief description of early embryonic development. During the preceding decade, numerous studies have identified molecular and genetic factors involved in facial and jaw development, factors of the utmost importance to a comprehensive understanding of the development of this region. Although these factors are not addressed in this chapter, the reader is referred to several excellent reviews included in the list of references.

Early events establishing the head region

Formation of the germ layers: gastrulation

Fertilization, the union of male and female gametes, is followed by cleavage, a series of rapid cell divisions which give rise to the **blastocyst**. The blastocyst consists of an outer layer of *trophoblast* which surrounds a large cavity, or *blastocoele*, at one pole of which is located a cellular aggregation, the **inner cell mass**. (Cells of the inner cell mass of mammalian embryos, isolated and grown in culture, are called embryonic stem cells.) Early in the second week, cavitation in the inner cell mass forms a protective sac, or **amnion**. Simultaneously, delamination of the inner cell mass produces the *bilaminar disk*, which lies in and forms the floor of the amnion (Fig. 2.1). This flattened disk consists of an upper layer, the **epiblast**, which is continuous at its margins with the amnion, and a lower layer, or **hypoblast**, which grows circumferentially around the blastocoele to form the lining, or *exocoelomic membrane*, of the primitive **yolk sac** (Figs. 2.1a, 2.1b). The **epiblast**, a single layer of columnar cells, is the source of the three primary **germ layers** – **ectoderm**, **mesoderm**, and **endoderm** – which ultimately form the embryo. The trophoblast contributes to formation of the placenta.

Germ layer formation occurs during **gastrulation**, which begins early in the third week and is signaled by the appearance of the **primitive streak**. In addition to its role in formation of the germ layers, the primitive streak defines the *polarity* of the embryo: the cranial-caudal axis, the dorsal-ventral axis, medial and lateral sidedness, and the right and left axial halves of the embryo.

The **primitive streak** arises from epiblast cells which migrate toward the midline at the posterior end of the bilaminar disk, now the *embryo*. At the midline, these cells aggregate and invaginate to form a central furrow, or *primitive groove*, within the primitive streak (Fig. 2.2). As more epiblast cells move into the primitive streak, the primitive streak grows in length at its caudal end (Fig. 2.2a); at its cephalic end is a conspicuous bulge of epiblastic cells, the *primitive node*, whose center contains a depression, the *primitive pit*, which is continuous with the primitive groove (Fig. 2.2). The primitive streak and primitive node play key roles in the formation of the germ layers and the **notochord**, an axial structure of utmost importance in subsequent development.

Fundamentals of Oral Histology and Physiology, First Edition. Arthur R. Hand and Marion E. Frank.
© 2014 John Wiley & Sons, Inc. Published 2014 by John Wiley & Sons, Inc.

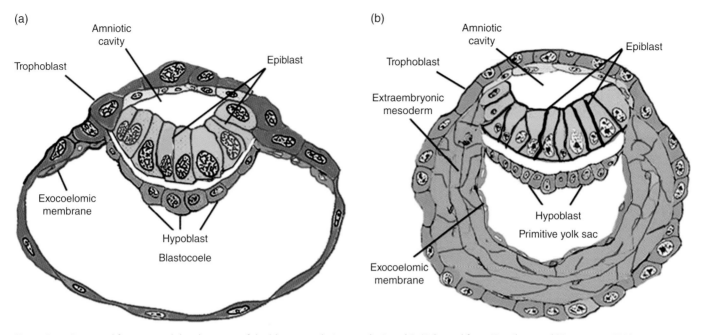

Figure 2.1   Structural features and development of the blastocyst during weeks 1 and 2. (Adapted from Hamilton and Mossman, 1972.)

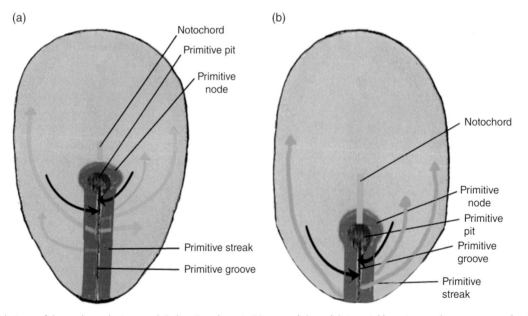

Figure 2.2   Dorsal views of the embryo during week 2 showing the primitive streak (purple), its axial location, and movements of epiblast through the primitive streak. Dark arrows denote the movement of epiblast toward the primitive streak; the gray arrows indicate directions of movement of mesenchymal epiblast from the primitive streak to form the germ layers. Note decreased length of primitive streak as germ layers and notochord (green) develop.

As formation of the germ layers and notochord progresses, the primitive streak is displaced caudally and gradually decreases in length (Figs. 2.2a, 2.2b). At the end of gastrulation, it is reduced to an insignificant aggregation of cells at the posterior end of the embryo.

The primitive streak provides a pathway through which cells of the epiblast invaginate to form *endoderm* and *mesoderm*. Dividing epiblast cells migrate to the primitive streak and sink into the primitive groove. During this migration, these epiblastic cells change shape and become motile cells, or **mesenchyme**, which detach and emerge from the primitive streak to enter the space below the epiblast.

Formation of the germ layers: the endoderm

Some of these mesenchymal cells, passing ventrally from the primitive streak, invade and intercalate between the cells of the underlying hypoblast to form endoderm, which displaces the hypoblast laterally into the extraembryonic area (Fig. 2.3). Growth of the newly formed endoderm at the expense of the

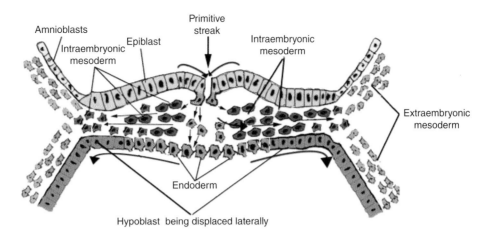

Figure 2.3   Cross-sectional view of embryo to show movements of epiblast through primitive streak to form the endoderm (orange) and intraembryonic mesoderm (red).

displaced hypoblast results in the formation of the *secondary yolk sac*, a vesicle directly attached to the ventral body of the embryo and lined entirely by endoderm.

Though displaced by endoderm, the hypoblast contributes to formation of the *extraembryonic mesoderm* (Fig. 2.1b) within which blood islands and elements of the vascular system ultimately develop. In humans, a region of the hypoblast known as *anterior visceral endoderm* participates in formation of the **prechordal plate**, an important landmark in head development. The prechordal plate appears at the cranial pole of the embryo where endoderm becomes tightly adherent to the overlying epiblast (now called ectoderm) to form a thickened bilaminar plate (Figs. 2.6; 2.7a). The prechordal plate later becomes the **oropharyngeal membrane** which separates the embryonic mouth, or **stomodeum**, from the embryonic pharynx. Although a transient structure, the prechordal plate plays a significant role in development of the head region: it induces differentiation and bilateralization of the forebrain, defines the cranial axis of the embryo, and is a useful landmark in subsequent development of the oral cavity and pharynx.

Formation of the germ layers: intraembryonic mesoderm

The major proportion of invaginating epiblast migrates laterally and cranially, filling the region between the endoderm and overlying ectoderm to form the *intraembryonic mesoderm* (Figs. 2.2a, 2.2b; Fig. 2.3). At the margins of the embryo, this mesoderm is continuous with extraembryonic mesoderm (Fig. 2.3). As the forming intraembryonic mesoderm expands toward the cranial end of the embryo, it passes in front of the prechordal plate to meet the mesoderm of the opposite side, giving rise to a concentric, horseshoe-shaped mass of mesoderm within which will appear the *cardiogenic plate* that forms the heart (Fig. 2.6).

Formation of the notochord

As the germ layers develop, mesenchymal cells detach from the cranial end of the primitive node and migrate in the midline toward the anterior end of the embryo to eventually form a solid

rod, or notochord (Fig. 2.2b). The notochord grows toward the cranial pole of the embryo where its further extension is impeded by the tightly adherent endoderm and ectoderm of the prechordal plate. Interposed between the tip of the notochord and the caudal edge of the prechordal plate is an area of mesoderm termed *prechordal mesoderm* which, augmented by **paraxial mesoderm** in the region near the midbrain, ultimately gives rise to the extraocular muscles.

The notochord provides axial support for the embryo. It interacts with the overlying ectoderm to induce differentiation of the **neural tube** which becomes the central nervous system. It influences organization of **somites** and development of the vertebral column. In an adult, it persists as the gelatinous central *nucleus pulposus* of the intervertebral disks.

At the end of gastrulation in the fourth week, the embryo consists of a trilaminar disk composed of three germ layers (Fig. 2.4a) supported by the notochord that extends forward to the prechordal plate at the cranial end of the embryo. The ectoderm lies dorsally and forms the floor of the amniotic cavity. The endoderm lies ventrally and lines the secondary yolk sac. The region between the ectoderm and endoderm is occupied by intraembryonic mesoderm which is insinuated everywhere between ectoderm and endoderm, except at the cranial and caudal poles where the prechordal and cloacal plates present impenetrable barriers and, in the midline, where the notochord is interposed between the surface ectoderm and the underlying endoderm. At the margins of the embryo, the intraembryonic mesoderm is continuous with extraembryonic mesoderm. All three primary germ layers originate from epiblast: endoderm and mesoderm from epiblast which migrates from the primitive streak, ectoderm from the overlying epiblast that remains at the outer surface of the embryo. The primitive streak is greatly reduced in length and has regressed toward the caudal pole of the embryo as the germ layers were formed. At the completion of gastrulation, it disappears, though, rarely, it may persist as a sacrococcygeal teratoma.

Regional differentiation of mesoderm: somite formation and specialization

Three specialized regions, each with different developmental fates, soon become evident within the intraembryonic mesoderm of the trunk region (Fig. 2.4a): (1) *paraxial* mesoderm, adjacent to the notochord; (2) lateral to the paraxial mesoderm, *intermediate* mesoderm, from which the kidneys, adrenal glands, and portions of the genitourinary tract are derived; and, (3) *lateral plate* mesoderm, which is continuous with the extraembryonic mesoderm at the margins of the embryo.

Beginning at 20 days, in the region of the embryo corresponding to the future occipital zone, the paraxial mesoderm undergoes segmentation to form **somites**, block-like segregated epithelioid aggregations of mesoderm (Fig. 2.4b; Fig. 2.6). Over the next 10 days, sequential segmentation of the paraxial mesoderm in a cranio-caudal wave produces 40 to 44 pairs of somites: 4 to 5 *occipital*; 8 *cervical*; 12 *thoracic*; 5 *lumbar*; 5 *sacral*; and 7 to 10 *coccygeal*. Each somite becomes associated with a specific nerve from the adjacent level of the developing spinal cord, an association responsible for the segmental pattern of the peripheral nervous system. Skeletal muscles and tissues derived from somites retain their associated spinal nerves throughout development and ultimately organize to form the body segments, or *dermatomes*, of the adult trunk. The somites and their associated nerves are responsible for the establishment of the adult metameric pattern visualized as the dermatomes of the neck and trunk.

Each somite displays three subdivisions: (1) a *ventromedial sclerotome* which will form the vertebrae and the vertebral column; (2) a *dorsolateral dermatome* which contributes to the dermis of the skin; and (3) an *intermediate myotome* which forms the skeletal muscles of the trunk and limbs.

The *occipital somites* contribute important structures to the adult head. Their sclerotome gives rise to the *occipital* bone of the skull; their myotome forms the *muscles of the tongue*.

The paraxial mesoderm cranial to the first occipital somite does not undergo segmentation or form somites. Unsegmented paraxial mesoderm constitutes the main proportion of head mesoderm. A major portion of it migrates into the embryonic pharynx to form **pharyngeal** (**branchial**) mesoderm, from which the **branchiomotor** skeletal muscles of the jaw, face, and neck are derived. It also forms certain bones of the skull: *parietal* bone, *petrous portion of temporal* bone, and *sphenoid* bones.

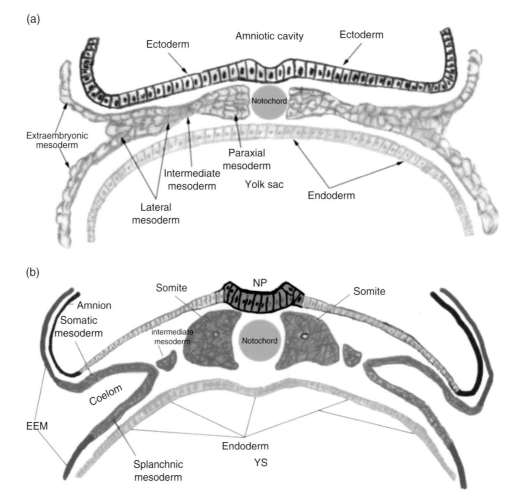

Figure 2.4　Transverse sections illustrating the organization of the three germ layers during week 4 (a) and the organization of intraembryonic mesoderm forming somites, intermediate, and lateral plate mesoderm during week 5 (b). YS, Yolk sac; NP, neural plate.

In the embryonic region destined to become the trunk, cavitation within the *lateral plate* mesoderm splits it (Fig. 2.4) into two layers: (1) a *somatic* layer that is associated with the overlying ectoderm and contributes to the formation of parietal serous membranes and connective tissue investments of trunk musculature; (2) a *splanchnic* layer that is associated with the endoderm and will form the outer layers of the digestive tract and the visceral serous membranes. The space formed by cavitation between the somatic and splanchnic layers of the lateral mesoderm coalesces to become the *intraembryonic coelom*, which eventually will be incorporated into the body of the embryo where it contributes to formation of the peritoneal, pleural, and pericardial cavities.

In the head region, the boundary between paraxial and lateral mesoderm is difficult to visualize because of the formation of the head fold (described below). Except for the lateral plate mesoderm that forms the cardiogenic plate, the lateral mesoderm of the head region probably merges with the cranial paraxial mesoderm to form the *pharyngeal* or *branchial* mesoderm (described below).

During the fourth week, the trunk paraxial mesoderm undergoes segmentation beginning in the future occipital region and extending in a cranio-caudal wave to eventually form 40–44 pairs of somites. The somites establish the body segments, or dermatomes, that characterize the adult trunk and give origin to the vertebral column, skeletal muscles of the trunk and limbs, and parts of the dermis. Cranial to the first occipital somite, there is no visible segmentation of the paraxial mesoderm. The major proportion of head mesoderm consists of unsegmented paraxial mesoderm, most of which contributes to formation of the pharyngeal (branchial) mesoderm, from which most skeletal muscles of the head are derived, and gives rise to certain bones of the skull.

Induction of the neural tube and appearance of the brain

At 17 to 18 days, before the end of gastrulation, **neurulation**, the formation of the neural tube, is initiated by molecular and chemical induction of the overlying ectoderm by the *notochord*. In response to induction by the notochord, the ectoderm in the midline and immediate flanking regions thickens and increases in height to form the *neural plate* (Figs. 2.5a, 2.5b). Growth and shifts in position of neural plate cells elevate the sides of the neural plate to form *neural folds* between which lies a furrow, the *neural groove* (Fig. 2.5b). Continued proliferation, changes in shape and size, and the cytoskeleton of the neural plate cells work in tandem to increase the length, thickness, and depth of the neural folds. Simultaneously, extrinsic forces generated by the concomitant growth of the adjacent non-neural ectoderm assist to elevate the folds and deepen the neural groove. Finally, the dorsal leading edges of the neural folds approximate one another in the midline, detach from the overlying ectoderm, and merge to form the **neural tube**, which sinks into the body of the embryo (Figs. 2.5c, 2.5d). The overlying ectoderm coalesces as a continuous sheet of *cutaneous ectoderm* over the dorsal body surface.

Fusion of the neural folds to produce the neural tube begins in the region of the embryo corresponding to the future neck and proceeds from that point in a cranial and caudal direction. Both leading edges of the forming neural tube remain temporarily open at their cranial and caudal ends as the cranial and caudal **neuropores**, respectively, but eventually they close to produce a neural tube containing a central cavity, the *neural canal*. The neural canal will become the brain ventricles and spinal canal. *Spina bifida* results from failure of the neural folds to close, leaving the spinal cord and its canal in open contact with the external environment.

The neural tube expands and enlarges at its cranial end to form the brain, but remains tapered and narrowed caudally where it forms the spinal cord. The embryonic brain initially consists of three primary divisions but subsequent subdivision of the forebrain and hindbrain produces five segments from which the adult brain develops:

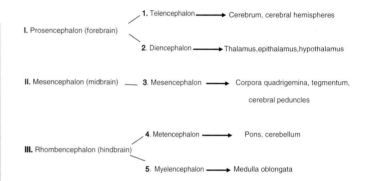

Transient segments termed neuromeres or **rhombomeres** appear in the hindbrain and are important in the subsequent formation of *cranial nerves* and the **neural crest**. In humans, seven rhombomeres appear, each designated by number (Rh1-Rh7).

Although development of the brain is beyond the scope of this chapter, growth and differentiation of the brain exert major influences on head and facial development. Its contributions to the ultimate form of the head region include the following.

1. Brain growth and expansion induce formation of the head fold (see below) which leads to the emergence of the primitive gut and embryonic pharynx, a key primordium of facial and jaw development.

2. Growth and bilateralization of the forebrain to form the cerebrum and cerebral hemispheres influences the ultimate shape and form of the head. Developmental failures affecting the forebrain can result in *holoprosencephaly*, which causes severe deformities in the shape and appearance of the head and face.

3. Evagination of the diencephalon produces the optic vesicles and cups from which originate the retina and uvea of the eye. The optic vesicles induce formation of the lens **placode** from surface ectoderm. The placode forms the lens; neural crest from the forebrain region condenses to form the cornea.

4. Establishment of appropriate central connections with the **nasal (olfactory)** and **otic placodes** whose differentiation

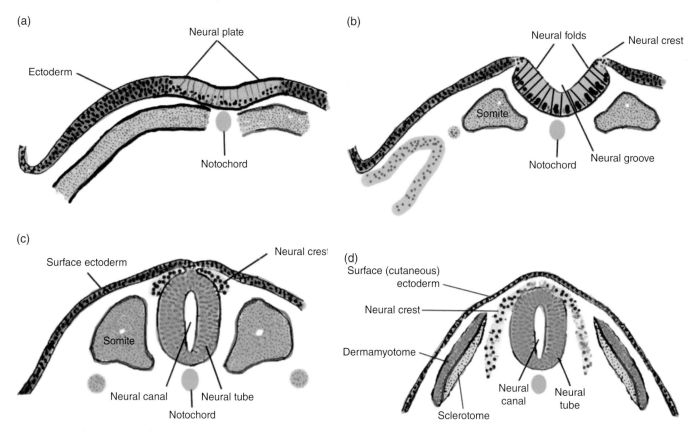

Figure 2.5 (a–d) Steps in the formation of the neural tube and neural crest. The early subdivision of somites is also depicted (d). (Modified from Hamilton and Mossman, 1972.)

from surface ectoderm elaborates the structures associated with the olfactory and auditory special senses, respectively.

5.   Formation and patterning of cranial nerves.

6.   Formation of the head neural crest, a component of primary significance in facial and jaw development.

Formation of the neural crest

Shortly before the neural folds close to form the neural tube, neuroectodermal cells at the dorsal lips of the neural folds differentiate to form the *neural crest* (Figs. 2.5b–d). Neural crest arises along the entire length of the neural tube, extending in sheets or cords along the dorsolateral margins of the neural tube, between the tube and surface ectoderm (Figs. 2.5c, 2.5d). Detaching from the neural tube, the neural crest migrates, either as individual or groups of motile cells or, more often, as sheets or clusters of contiguous cells, along specific routes which conduct it to appropriate destinations throughout the embryo.

Neural crest constitutes a *pluripotential* mesenchyme that is the source of diverse tissue types: neural, glial, skeletal, connective, pigment, and secretory. Neural crest-derived structures include craniospinal sensory and autonomic ganglia, the enteric nervous system, adrenal medulla, calcitonin-secreting cells of the thyroid, Schwann cells, dermal melanocytes, adipose cells, and the cardiac outflow tract.

In the head region, neural crest forms a major portion of the skull, maxilla, mandible, auditory ossicles, hyoid bone, and larynx. It contributes to development of the cranial sensory and parasympathetic autonomic ganglia, forms pigment retinal cells and smooth muscles of the eye, and contributes to formation of the cornea. It forms the dentin and cementum of the teeth, the periodontal ligament and alveolar bone that support the teeth, connective tissue stroma of salivary glands and of the tongue, the pia-arachnoid meninges of the brain, glial cells, and the carotid bodies and sinus. *Neural crest is a primordial tissue of fundamental importance to embryonic development, especially development of the head, face, and jaws.*

Induction of the overlying surface ectoderm by the notochord stimulates formation of the neural plate whose growth gives rise to elevated neural folds between which lies the neural groove. Fusion of the dorsal tips of the neural folds forms the neural tube, which detaches from the superficial ectoderm to sink into the body of the embryo. The neural crest forms from neuroectodermal cells at the dorsolateral free margins of the neural folds. The pluripotential neural crest cells undergo epithelial mesenchymal transformation, and migrate throughout the body, including the craniofacial region where they form important neural, skeletal, and tooth constituents.

Formation of the body folds and the head region

The formation of the head fold is a key event in the development of the face and jaws. At the beginning of the fourth week, the embryo is a flattened disk located in the floor of the amnion and forming the roof of the secondary yolk sac (Fig. 2.7a). At the cranial end, the prechordal plate and the cardiogenic plate lie in front of the leading edge of the expanding neural tube (Figs. 2.6, 2.7a). The prechordal plate consists of a dorsal layer of ectoderm tightly bound to a ventral layer of endoderm (Fig. 2.7a). The heart has begun to form and, by day 23, begins to contract to assume its life-long role as a pump that propels blood throughout the embryo and body. Over the course of several days, differential growth at the cranial and caudal ends of the neural tube, as well as expansion of the amnion, will compel folding of the embryonic disk to form the *head*, *tail*, and *lateral folds* that transform the embryo from a flat disk into a cylindrical body tube.

The cranial end of the neural tube expands to form the forebrain, which grows and extends over the prechordal plate and the developing heart (Fig. 2.7b). Coupled with the simultaneous expansion of the amnion, the growth of the forebrain causes the cephalic end of the embryo to bend ventrally, using the prechordal plate (now called the **oropharyngeal membrane**) as a hinge, to form the head fold (Fig. 2.7b). Formation of the head fold brings the heart and the trailing oropharyngeal membrane below the developing brain into the ventral region of the embryo (Figs. 2.7b, 2.7c). Expansion of the amnion simultaneous with formation and expansion of the head fold results in lateral body folds such that the embryo constricts the yolk sac like a purse-string, absorbing the proximal region of the yolk sac into the body of the embryo (Figs. 2.7b–d).

The incorporated portion of the yolk sac lined by endoderm becomes the *primitive gut* which is connected to the yolk sac lying outside the embryo by means of the **yolk stalk** (Figs. 2.7a–d). Immediately above and directly continuous with the yolk stalk is the **midgut**; behind the region of attachment of the yolk stalk lies the **hindgut**. The cranial end, or **foregut**, extends forward above the heart to terminate at and behind the oropharyngeal membrane, which closes off the anterior portion of the gut (Figs. 2.7c, 2.7c).

The formation of the head fold has inverted the position of ectoderm and endoderm in the oropharyngeal membrane relative to their initial position (compare Fig. 2.7a with Figs. 2.7c, 2.7d) so that the ectoderm is now below while the endoderm is above and directly continuous with the endoderm of the foregut. Growth of the forebrain has produced a deep depression in the surface ectoderm, the *embryonic mouth* or **stomodeum**, which lies in front of and below the oropharyngeal membrane (Fig. 2.7c). The oropharyngeal membrane separates the stomodeum from the anterior region of the foregut which will become the pharynx (Fig. 2.7c). The oropharyngeal membrane marks the boundary between *ectodermal* and *endodermal domains* in the subsequent formation of the oral cavity and pharynx (Figs. 2.7c, 2.7d). With perforation and disappearance of the oropharyngeal membrane at 24 to 25 days, the stomodeum becomes continuous with and opens directly into the embryonic pharynx (Fig. 2.7d).

Formation of the head fold and growth of the forebrain results in formation of the stomodeum. Concomitantly, lateral body folding induced by expansion of the amnion during the fourth week results in incorporation of the proximal yolk sac into the embryo to form the primitive gut. The cranial extension of the primitive gut, the foregut, terminates at the oropharyngeal membrane; its most cephalic portion becomes the embryonic pharynx, establishing the basis for subsequent appearance of primordia involved in development of the head, face, and jaws, and facilitating the initiation and completion of events leading to morphogenesis of the face and jaws.

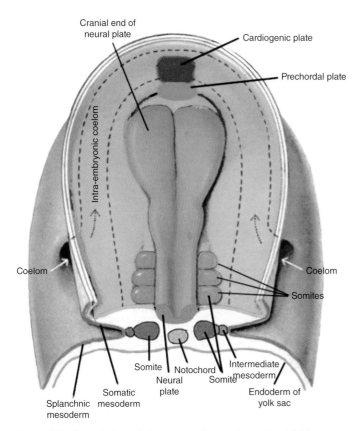

Figure 2.6 Dorsal view of a human embryo prior to head fold formation. The neural plate (blue) is expanded at its cranial end and will form the brain. The cardiogenic plate (bright red) lies anterior to the prechordal plate. Top and transverse views of the somites (light red) are shown. The course of the intraembryonic coelom, the space between the somatic and splanchnic layers of lateral plate mesoderm, is shown by the dashed lines. (Modified from Hamilton and Mossman, 1972.)

Development of the pharyngeal region and the pharyngeal arches

The developmental history of the **pharyngeal arches** is intimately linked to the formation of the face, jaws, oral cavity, and pharynx. Knowledge of the formation, organization, and fate of the

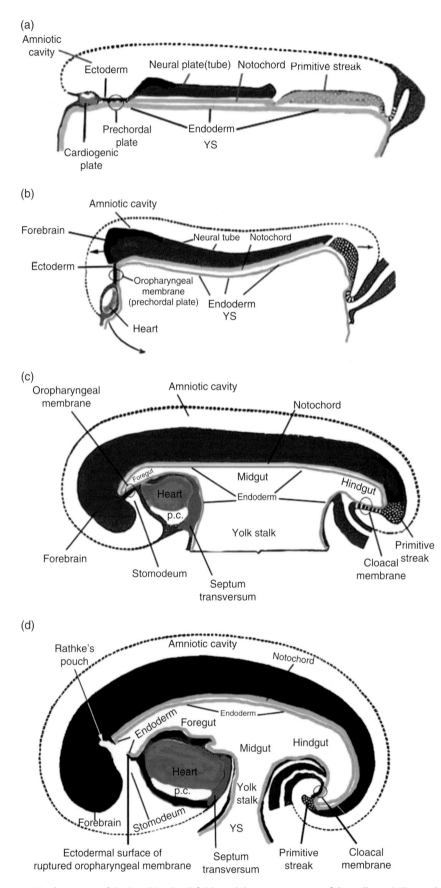

Figure 2.7   (a–d) Sagittal views showing the formation of the head (and tail) folds and the incorporation of the yolk sac (YS) into the body of the embryo to form the embryonic gut, whose subdivisions are labeled (c, d). Note the orientation of the prechordal plate (oropharyngeal membrane) as the head fold evolves; at 26-27 days, the oropharyngeal membrane ruptures to establish communication between the mouth and embryonic pharynx that arises from the foregut (c, d). (Modified from Arey, 1968.)

pharyngeal arches helps in understanding the anatomy of the adult head and the etiology of congenital defects of the jaws and oral cavity. The pharyngeal arches are responsible for the segmental distribution of cranial nerves in the adult face and jaw, a pattern of segmentation that is analogous to the dermatomes of the trunk. This segmentation or **metamerism** arises from the association of a specific cranial nerve with particular pharyngeal arches, a relationship that persists in all derivatives of the arches.

Formation and organization of the pharyngeal arches

The formation of the pharynx and the pharyngeal arches is signaled by changes in the shape of the anterior region of the foregut. As it transforms into the pharynx, this region of the foregut becomes flattened dorsoventrally and expands to form a funnel-shaped tube (Figs. 2.8a–c). It is widest immediately behind the oropharyngeal membrane and narrows as it passes posteriorly to join the caudal part of the foregut (Figs. 2.8a–c). The *pharyngeal arches* form the *lateral* walls of the pharynx, appearing as swellings or elevations that develop sequentially in a craniocaudal succession during the fourth week. The *pharyngeal endoderm* induces formation of the pharyngeal arches through its interactions with the other germ layers and with neural crest, and is the major determinant in the elaboration of the pharyngeal arch complex.

Five pairs of pharyngeal arches, numbered I–VI, ultimately appear in the human pharynx (the fifth either never appears or is rapidly absorbed into the other arches). The first and second pharyngeal arches are called the **mandibular** and **hyoid arches**, respectively, but the remaining arches are designated by number only. The boundaries of each arch are defined externally by invaginations of the surface ectoderm, the **pharyngeal clefts** or grooves, and internally by **pharyngeal pouches**, outpocketings of the endoderm lining the pharyngeal lumen (Figs. 2.8a–c). The pouches correspond precisely in position to the clefts or grooves, with the two closely approximating one another but separated by a thin membrane and never establishing continuity. The pouches and clefts separate each arch from the next and are designated by number, I-V, the first pharyngeal pouch (I) and cleft (I) separating the first from the second arch, etc. In fish and amphibians, rupture of the thin membrane separating the clefts from the pouches produces the gill slits.

The tissue mass occupying the area between the ectoderm and endoderm of each pharyngeal arch consists of a core of *pharyngeal* or *branchial mesoderm* which is surrounded by a ring of *neural crest* (Fig. 2.8b). The pharyngeal (branchial) mesoderm is derived primarily from cranial paraxial mesoderm which, together with neural crest, arise from corresponding levels adjacent to the hindbrain and migrate coordinately to their specific destination in the pharyngeal arch complex.

Coursing through the core of each pharyngeal arch is an *aortic arch* (Figs. 2.8a, 2.8b) which connects the *truncus arteriosus*, the outflow tract of the embryonic heart that is located below the pharynx (Fig. 2.8c), to the *dorsal aorta* in the dorsal body wall. Only aortic arches III, IV, and VI persist in the adult as significant vessels.

The *roof* of the pharynx consists of the dorsal body wall containing the neural tube and associated structures, while the *floor* lies directly above the forming heart (Fig. 2.8c). The floor and pharyngeal arches merge seamlessly to form ventrolateral ridges or bars whose developmental history and fate are linked and intimately coordinated during development of the jaws, oral cavity, and pharynx.

The rupture and disappearance of the oropharyngeal membrane between the pharynx and stomodeum at 25 to 26 days establishes continuity between the oral cavity and pharynx. Because of the extensive tissue migrations that occur during development of the oral cavity, tongue, and pharynx, it is difficult to delineate the original position of the oropharyngeal membrane. An imaginary line drawn from the foramen caecum and sulcus terminalis of the tongue upward toward the palate just in front of the tonsillar fossae roughly approximates its position in the adult.

Innervation of the pharyngeal arches

Each pharyngeal arch is innervated by a specific cranial nerve (Fig. 2.9), an association that is retained by all adult derivatives of the arch. Four cranial nerves provide the innervation of the pharyngeal arches: V, VII, IX, and X. These nerves contain both motor and sensory components and are, therefore, *mixed* nerves. They arise sequentially from successive levels of the mid- and hindbrain and contain functional modalities not found in other nerves. All four nerves transmit motor fibers that are designated **branchiomotor** or *special visceral motor* because the skeletal muscles they innervate are derived from pharyngeal mesoderm. In addition, cranial nerves VII, IX, and X mediate taste sensation and contain parasympathetic motor components.

The cranial nerve distribution to the pharyngeal arches is as follows.

1. Trigeminal (V) – the nerve of the first or **mandibular arch**. In addition to the first arch, the trigeminal innervates the **frontonasal process** and its derivatives, and exhibits three divisions: *ophthalmic* to the frontonasal process, *maxillary* to the **maxillary process** of the first arch, *mandibular* to the **mandibular process** of the first arch. It mediates general sensation and conveys branchiomotor fibers to muscles derived from the first arch mesoderm. It is the principal sensory nerve of the head in adults. Its sensory ganglion is the *semilunar (trigeminal) ganglion*.

2. Facial (VII) – nerve of the second or **hyoid arch**. It conveys branchiomotor and parasympathetic fibers and mediates taste from the body of the tongue. Its pretrematic branch to the mandibular arch becomes the *chorda tympani*, which conveys taste and parasympathetic fibers. Its sensory ganglion is the *geniculate ganglion*.

3. Glossopharyngeal (IX) – nerve of the third arch. It mediates general sensation from wide areas of the adult pharynx, middle ear, and root of the tongue and taste from the latter. It contains two sensory ganglia, the *superior* and *inferior (petrosal) ganglia*. It conveys parasympathetic fibers to the parotid gland and branchiomotor to a single muscle, the stylopharyngeus.

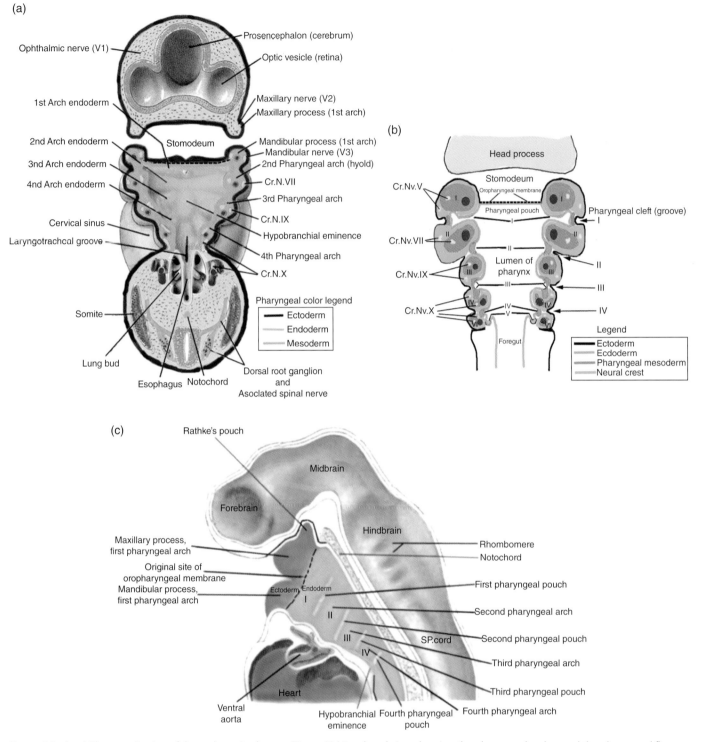

(a)

Ophthalmic nerve (V1)
Prosencephalon (cerebrum)
Optic vesicle (retina)
1st Arch endoderm
Maxillary nerve (V2)
Maxillary process (1st arch)
2nd Arch endoderm
Stomodeum
Mandibular process (1st arch)
Mandibular nerve (V3)
3rd Arch endoderm
2nd Pharyngeal arch (hyold)
4nd Arch endoderm
Cr.N.VII
3rd Pharyngeal arch
Cervical sinus
Cr.N.IX
Laryngotracheal groove
Hypobranchial eminence
4th Pharyngeal arch
Cr.N.X
Pharyngeal color legend
Somite
- Ectoderm
- Endoderm
- Mesoderm
Lung bud
Esophagus Notochord
Dorsal root ganglion and Asoclated spinal nerve

(b)

Head process
Stomodeum
Cr.Nv.V
Oropharyngeal membrane
Pharyngeal pouch
Pharyngeal cleft (groove)
Cr.Nv.VII
Lumen of pharynx
Cr.Nv.IX
Cr.Nv.X
Foregut
Legend
- Ectoderm
- Ecdoderm
- Pharyngeal mesoderm
- Neural crest

(c)

Rathke's pouch
Midbrain
Forebrain
Hindbrain
Maxillary process, first pharyngeal arch
Rhombomere
Notochord
Original site of oropharyngeal membrane
Mandibular process, first pharyngeal arch
Ectoderm Endoderm
First pharyngeal pouch
Second pharyngeal arch
Second pharyngeal pouch
SP.cord
Third pharyngeal arch
Third pharyngeal pouch
Heart
Ventral aorta
Hypobranchial eminence
Fourth pharyngeal pouch
Fourth pharyngeal arch

Figure 2.8   (a–c) The organization of the embryonic pharynx. Figure 8(a) is a dorsal view showing the pharyngeal arches and the pharyngeal floor. A schematic diagram of the pharyngeal arches shown in 8(a) is depicted in Figure 8(b). Figure 8(c) shows a sagittal section of the embryonic pharynx. Dashed lines indicate the original location of the oropharyngeal membrane. Germ layer composition is color coded. (Panels (a) and (c) modified from Hamilton and Mossman, 1972.)

4. <u>Vagus (X)</u> – nerve of arches IV and VI. It mediates general sensation from the pharynx, larynx, and many thoracic and abdominal viscera. It provides some taste sensation from the root of the tongue and taste buds in the neonate pharynx. It conveys branchiomotor fibers to laryngeal and pharyngeal musculature and parasympathetic fibers to many viscera. It contains two sensory ganglia, the *superior (jugular)* and *inferior (nodosal) ganglia.*

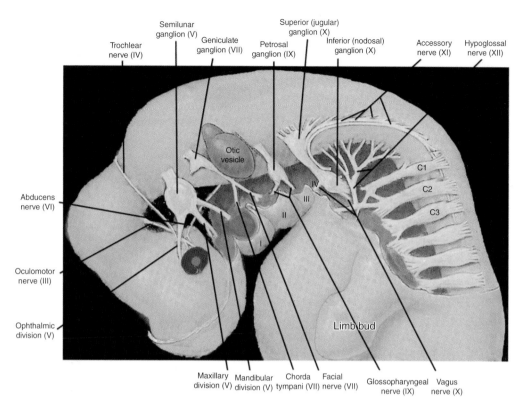

Figure 2.9   Innervation of the pharyngeal arches and the neck region in the 4 to 5 week embryo. (Modified from Hamilton and Mossman, 1972).

Factors responsible for innervation pattern of the pharyngeal arches

The association between a pharyngeal arch and its cranial nerve supply is established early in development. As the cranial paraxial mesoderm forms alongside the hindbrain, it is innervated by nerve fibers emanating from corresponding levels of the adjacent hindbrain. When this paraxial mesoderm migrates to its specified pharyngeal arch to form pharyngeal mesoderm, it carries along its innervation. These nerve fibers become *motor* fibers which provide motor innervation to the skeletal muscles derived from the pharyngeal mesoderm.

Sensory innervation of each pharyngeal arch and its derivatives is derived from distinct streams of neural crest and the **epibranchial (epipharyngeal) placodes**. The latter are specializations of surface ectoderm that are induced by the pharyngeal endoderm and are located above and behind the pharyngeal clefts of the second, third, and fourth arches. Together with the **epibranchial placodes**, the *neural crest* streams establish the *sensory* innervation of the pharyngeal arches and form the *cranial sensory ganglia*. The more proximal ganglia, or segments of ganglia, arise from *neural crest*, the more distal ganglia, or segments, from *epibranchial placodes*. Cranial neural crest is also responsible for elaboration of the *autonomic ganglia* and autonomic connections that occur in the adult head region.

Each arch receives a separate, distinct stream of neural crest that arises from the hindbrain at the same level as the nerve fibers which innervate the paraxial mesoderm (Fig. 2.10). The neural crest stream that migrates into the first arch is the *trigeminal* *crest* which originates from the first and second rhombomeres (Rh1, Rh2) of the hindbrain, close to the origin of the trigeminal nerve (V). The *mesencephalic crest*, considered part of the trigeminal crest, migrates as frontonasal mesenchyme into the frontonasal region where it forms skeletal and neural elements of the frontal and nasal regions. The mesencephalic crest also contributes the main proportion of the trigeminal or semilunar ganglion and the ophthalmic division (V). The maxillary and mandibular divisions (V) are derived from trigeminal crest.

Separate streams of neural crest course into the other pharyngeal arches (Fig. 2.10). The *hyoid* or *facial crest* originates from the fourth rhombomere (Rh4) of the hindbrain and migrates into the second arch. Behind the otic placode, the *glossopharyngeal* (Rh6) *crest* is directed into the third arch, and a part of the *vagal* (Rh7; C1–C5) *crest* stream passes into the fourth and fifth arch (Fig. 2.10). The neural crest streams create routes along which the cranial nerves to and from a specific pharyngeal arch establish their connections to the brain, resulting in the structural association between pharyngeal arch and cranial nerve.

In addition to the neural crest destined for the pharyngeal arches, other streams of neural crest contribute to the head region. The *hypoglossal stream* migrates to the tongue forming in the pharyngeal floor and contains not only neural crest cells, which form the connective tissue of the tongue, but also myoblasts from the occipital somites, which form the intrinsic muscles of the tongue. Other streams of head neural crest, e.g., the *cardiac* (Rh6, Rh7; C1–C5) and a major portion of the *vagal crest*, migrate into the trunk to give rise to the cardiac outflow tract and the enteric nervous system, respectively.

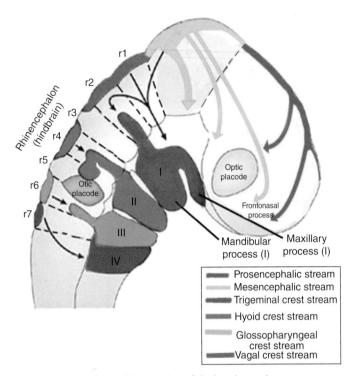

Figure 2.10   Origins and destination of the head neural crest streams. (Adapted from Carlson, *Human Embryology and Developmental Biology*, 2009.)

The pharyngeal arch complex is fundamental to the development of the adult face, jaws, and neck. Five paired pharyngeal arches appear during the third week of human development, numbered I-VI. Each arch is composed of an outer lining of surface ectoderm, an inner layer of endoderm lining the pharyngeal lumen, and a central core of mesoderm surrounded by neural crest (Fig. 2.8a, 2.8b). The arches are separated externally by pharyngeal clefts or grooves and internally by pharyngeal pouches. Each arch is innervated by a specific cranial nerve and contains an aortic arch which connects the cardiac outflow path with the dorsal aorta. The central core of pharyngeal (branchial) mesoderm is derived mainly from cranial paraxial mesoderm and is surrounded by a ring of neural crest that originates from a specific level of the hindbrain. A cardinal principle of development is that the adult derivatives of a given arch retain the innervation with which that arch was endowed during embryonic development. The metameric (segmental) pattern of innervation of the adult head region is established by the developmental properties and fates of the pharyngeal arches.

Fates of the arch neural crest and branchial mesoderm

In addition to the sensory innervation of the arches, the neural crest within the pharyngeal arches gives rise to connective tissue investments of skeletal muscles, portions of the dermis, and the **viscerocranium**, that part of the skull which includes the *skeleton* of the *upper* and *lower jaw*, the *hyoid bone*, and the *laryngeal cartilages*. The skeletal derivatives of the pharyngeal arch neural crest are listed in Table 2.1 and described below, in "Skull and Jaw Formation."

The pharyngeal mesoderm of the pharyngeal arches gives rise to most of the voluntary skeletal muscles of the head and neck region (Table 2.1). These are designated as **branchiomotor** muscles because they originate from pharyngeal (branchial) mesoderm. The adult muscles arising from pharyngeal mesoderm retain the innervation associated with the arch from which they are derived; e.g., the muscles of mastication which arise from mesoderm of the first or mandibular arch are innervated by the mandibular (motor) division of the trigeminal (V) nerve.

Fate of the pharyngeal clefts: development of the external ear

Except for the first pharyngeal cleft (groove) which forms the *external auditory meatus*, the remaining clefts (II–V) disappear and play no further role in subsequent development (Table 2.1). The occlusion of clefts II–V occurs during weeks 5 to 6 and is due to the rapid growth of the second (hyoid) arch relative to the retrohyoid arches (III–VI), causing them to sink into a deep depression, the *cervical sinus* (Fig. 2.11). Continued growth of the hyoid arch leads to closure of the cervical sinus, involution of pharyngeal clefts II–V, and occlusion of the ectodermal surfaces of the retrohyoid arches.

An alternative view attributes formation of the cervical sinus to growth of an ectodermal flap from the posterior end of the second (hyoid) arch (Fig. 2.12), similar to the operculum covering the gill slits in bony fish. The backward extension of this ectodermal flap forms a space, the cervical sinus, between the inside face of the flap and the external surfaces of the retrohyoid arches (Fig. 2.12). The pharyngeal clefts of these arches elongate to form branchial ducts that communicate with the cervical sinus. By the end of week 6, the flap fuses with the underlying arches to obliterate the cervical sinus and the branchial ducts derived from the clefts (Fig. 2-12).

Incomplete involution of the retrohyoid clefts and/or cervical sinus may produce *branchial cysts* or *fistulae*, the most common arising from the second pharyngeal cleft. The cysts occur as solitary, benign lesions along the anterior surface of the sternocleidomastoid muscle. Fistulae arise when the clefts retain their communication with the skin or internally with the pharynx.

At the level of the first cleft, events occur to form the *middle* and *external ear*. The *inner ear* develops from an ectodermal thickening, the **otic placode**, which appears during the third week on the external surface of the embryo, dorsal to the first cleft (Fig. 2.13a). The otic placode sinks into the body of the embryo, becoming the *otic vesicle*, which subsequently forms the *cochlea* and *vestibular apparatus* of the inner ear. During week 6, the *first pharyngeal cleft* becomes the *external auditory meatus* while the *first pharyngeal pouch* forms the *Eustachian tube* and

Table 2.1   Derivatives of pharyngeal arch components

Arch	Mesoderm	Neural crest[1]	Cleft	Pouch
I (Mandibular)	Muscles of mastication: masseter, temporal, lateral and medial pterygoids; anterior digastric, mylohyoid, tensor veli palatini, tensor tympani	maxilla, vomer, pterygoid plate, premaxilla, incus, mandible; malleus, anterior ligament of malleus, spheno-mandibular ligament (from Meckel's cartilage)	External auditory meatus; outer layer of tympanic membrane	Eustachian tube (auditory tube); tympanic cavity (cavity of middle ear); inner layer of tympanic membrane
II (Hyoid)	Muscles of facial expression: platysma, frontalis, orbicularis oris, orbicularis oculi, etc.; posterior digastric, stylohyoid, stapedius	stapes, styloid process, stylohyoid ligament, lesser horns of hyoid, upper rim of hyoid bone	Disappears	Stroma of palatine tonsils
III	stylopharyngeus	lower portion of hyoid bone, greater horns of the hyoid	Disappears	Thymus (dorsal wing) Inferior parathyroid glands (ventral wing)
IV	Pharyngeal constrictors: superior, middle, upper part of inferior; levator veli palatini	cuneiform, thyroid cartilages of larynx	Disappears	Superior parathyroid glands
VI	Intrinsic laryngeal muscles: cricothyroid, thyroarytenoid, vocalis, cricoarytenoids, etc.	arytenoid, corniculate, cricoid cartilages of larynx	Disappears	Parafollicular cells (C cells) of thyroid gland

[1]Skeletal derivatives only.

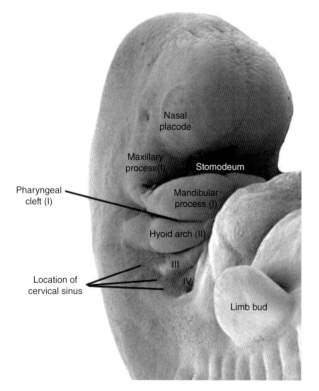

Figure 2.11   Scanning electron micrograph of a 32-day human embryo showing the retrohyoid arches (III,IV) deep in the site of the future cervical sinus. Subsequent rapid growth of the hyoid arch will close the cervical sinus and occlude the ectodermal surfaces and pharyngeal clefts of the retrohyoid arches. (Used by permission of Kathy Sulik, University of North Carolina.)

the *tympanic cavity*. The thin membrane of mesenchyme that separates the first cleft and pouch becomes the *tympanic membrane* or eardrum (Fig. 2.12b).

The *auricle* or *pinna of the ear* begins as a series of elevations or hillocks that surround the opening of first cleft (Fig. 2.13) as it is transformed into the external auditory meatus. These hillocks arise from both the first and second arch but predominantly from the latter. The auricle is initially located ventromedially (Fig. 2.13) but growth of the face and jaw gradually displaces it dorsally to the lateral side of the head (Fig. 2.13e).

The growth of the face and jaws that causes displacement of the pinna is associated with the forward migration of the *pharyngeal mesoderm* of the **hyoid arch** into the face and submandibular region. There, it forms the *muscles of facial expression* and several submandibular muscles, e.g., *posterior digastric, stylohyoid*. Elements of the hyoid arch also migrate forward to form *taste buds* in the body of the tongue (see below).

Between the ear and the forelimb, the neck will eventually form and elongate, characterized by differentiation of the trapezius and sternocleidomastoid muscles, which attach the head and skull to the pectoral girdle and shoulder and act to move the head. The innervation of the adult auricle and neck by the trigeminal, facial, and cervical nerves is an indication of the extensive migrations that take place during the development of the auricle and morphogenesis of the neck.

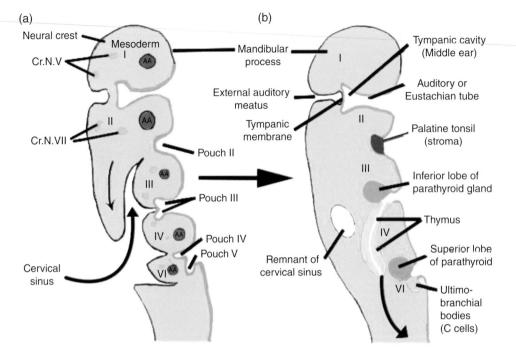

Figure 2.12 Diagram illustrating the classical view of formation of the cervical sinus and occlusion of the retrohyoid pharyngeal clefts (III–V). The backward growth of an ectodermal flap forms the cervical sinus (a). Aortic arch, AA. Fusion of the flap with the external surfaces of the retrohyoid arches (b) occludes the cervical sinus and the pharyngeal clefts. Adult derivatives of the pharyngeal pouches are indicated in (b). (Modified from Sadler, *Langman's Medical Embryology*, 6th edn. Lippincott, Williams, & Wilkins, 1990.)

> The external auditory meatus is derived from the first pharyngeal cleft. The first pharyngeal pouch gives rise to the tubotympanic recess (Eustachian tube) and middle ear cavity while the thin membrane which separates the first pharyngeal cleft from the pouch forms the tympanic membrane. Ectodermal elevations or hillocks form around the opening of the external auditory meatus and eventually give rise to the auricle of the ear. The hillocks originate mainly from the first and second pharyngeal arches, with contributions from the forming cervical region or neck. The multiple sources involved in formation of the auricle explain its innervation by the trigeminal and facial nerves and nerves from the cervical plexus.

Fate of the pharyngeal pouches

The *first pharyngeal pouch* expands to form the tympanic cavity and the Eustachian tube (tubotympanic recess) (Table 2.1 and Fig. 2.12).

The *second pharyngeal pouch* gives rise to the connective tissue stroma of the *palatine tonsils* and the *tonsillar fossa*. Subsequent seeding of the stroma by hematologic stem cells accounts for the lymphocyte populations typical of these organs.

The *third pharyngeal pouch* has a dual fate. Its dorsal wing forms a major part of the *thymic stroma* while its ventral wing differentiates to form the *inferior parathyroid glands*.

The *fourth pouch* forms the *superior parathyroid glands*. As the thymic stroma develops in the dorsal wing of the third pouch, it begins to extend and migrate from the neck region into the thorax, dragging along the parathyroid derivative of the ventral wings. Like the tonsil, seeding of the presumptive thymic stroma by hematologic stem cells leads to the appearance and elaboration of the thymocyte populations characteristic of the definitive thymus. Ultimately, due to this migration, the thymus occupies a midline position in the chest while the parathyroid derivative of the third pouch comes to lie below the parathyroid derivatives formed by the fourth pouch, thus, becoming the inferior pair of parathyroids located behind and in the capsule of the thyroid gland.

The *fifth pouch*, called the *ultimobranchial bodies*, forms the *parafollicular* or *calcitonin-secreting cells* of the *thyroid*.

Development of the face and jaws

The development of the face and jaws occurs during the fourth to sixth weeks, with the definitive form of the face and jaws clearly recognizable and established before the end of the second month. The primordia that form the face and jaws (Figs. 2.14a–e) are the:

1. median, unpaired **frontonasal process** above the stomodeum
2. paired **maxillary processes** on each side of the stomodeum
3. paired **mandibular processes** below the stomodeum.

The frontonasal process is a visible external prominence (Fig. 2.14), due to the rapid growth of the underlying forebrain. Growth and movements of the mesenchyme of the first or mandibular arch enlarge and divide the arch into a dorsolateral maxillary process and a ventromedial mandibular process.

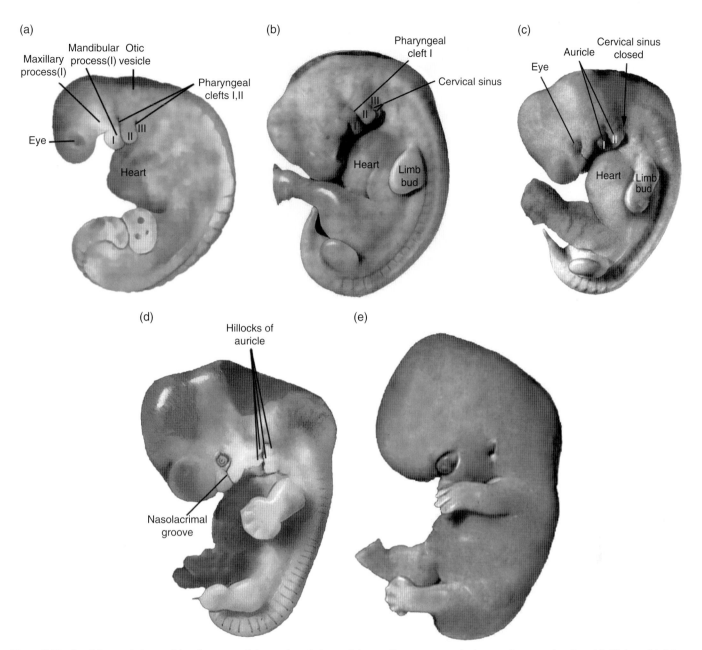

Figure 2.13   (a–e) External views of development of the neck and pinna of the ear. Roman numerals denote pharyngeal arches. (a), 30 days. (b), 33 days. The region behind the hyoid arch (II) has sunk into a depression, the cervical sinus. (c), 37 days. The pinna (auricle) of the external ear forms as hillocks bordering the first pharyngeal cleft. The cervical sinus has closed and the ectodermal surfaces of the retrohyoid arches are no longer externally visible. (d), 40 days. Note the hillocks forming the pinna. (e), 46 days. (Revised from Hamilton and Mossman, 1972.)

Early Events in Face and Jaw Development

Prior to events that establish the definitive form of the face and jaws, specializations involved in development of the eyes and nose appear in the frontonasal process as a harbinger of subsequent jaw and face development. The ectoderm on the lateral surfaces of the frontonasal process thickens to form the *optic* or *lens placodes*, the precursors of the lens. The position of the lens placodes defines the area of the frontonasal process as the region above and between the eyes (Figs. 2.14c, 2.14d).

In addition to forebrain growth, growth and expansion of the mesencephalic neural crest as frontonasal mesenchyme contributes to differentiation and shaping of the frontonasal process. Proliferation and aggregation of this mesenchyme causes thickening of surface ectoderm in the inferolateral areas of the frontonasal process to produce the *nasal (olfactory) placodes* (Fig. 2.14b). Differential growth of the placodal mesenchyme elevates the margins of the placodes to form a horseshoe-shaped ridge that surrounds a central depression, or *nasal pit*. The nasal pit deepens to become a blind sac, the *nasal sac*, which is bounded on its lateral and medial aspects by prominent elevations, the **lateral** and **medial nasal processes**

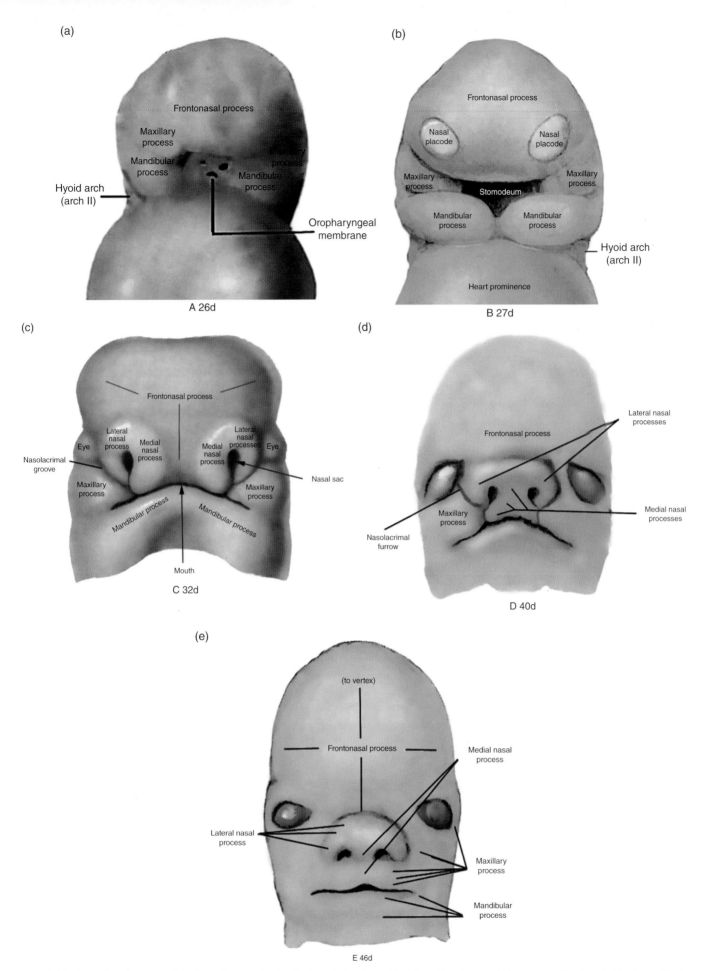

Figure 2.14   (a–e) Development of the face. See text for details. (Panels (a–c) modified from Hamilton and Mossman, 1972; Panels (d–e), modified from Arey, 1968.)

(**folds**), respectively (Figs. 2.14c, 2.14d). The nasal sac grows dorsally and backward toward the stomodeal (oral) cavity to form the *nares* (nostrils) and *nasal cavity*. Each sac expands above the confluent medial nasal processes to reach the roof of the primitive oral cavity. A thin *oronasal membrane* separating the nasal cavities from the stomodeal cavity ruptures to establish continuity of the nasal cavities with the oral cavity.

With the appearance of the medial and lateral nasal processes, all elements required for facial and jaw development are in place: the frontonasal process, including its bilateral medial and lateral nasal processes, the paired maxillary processes, and the paired mandibular processes (Figs. 2.14, a–e).

External Form of the Face and Jaws

The lower jaw appears early in facial development and is formed by fusion of the paired *mandibular processes*. Rapid growth of mesenchyme within each mandibular process causes gradual movement of each process toward the midline where they eventually merge and unite to establish the *lower lip, chin*, and *mandible* (Fig. 2.14a–e).

The upper jaw arises from the *maxillary* and *medial nasal processes* (Figs. 2.14a–e). Growth of the maxillary processes moves these processes ventrally and medially, simultaneously forcing the medial and lateral nasal processes toward the midline (Figs. 2.14c, 2.14d). Eventually both medial nasal processes converge and become confluent in the median plane. Their fusion produces the *philtrum* (the external depression immediately below the nasal septum), the *median part* of the *upper lip*, and the *intermaxillary segment*, which consists of the *premaxilla*, the *primary (primitive) palate*, and the anteroinferior segment of the *nasal septum*. Subsequently, the maxillary processes fuse with the medial nasal processes to complete the formation of the upper lip and jaw, the median portion of the upper lip arising from the medial nasal processes and the lateral portions from the maxillary processes.

As the maxillary processes move medially, they also encounter the lateral nasal processes from which they are briefly separated by an external furrow, the *nasolacrimal groove* (Figs. 2.14c, 2.14d). The ectoderm deep in the nasolacrimal groove forms a plug, which is eventually hollowed out to form the *nasolacrimal duct*. Subsequent fusion of the maxillary and lateral nasal processes obliterates all external signs of the nasolacrimal groove. The nasolacrimal duct, now enclosed within the nasolacrimal groove, extends from the lower orbital rim to the nasal cavity and expands at its orbital end to form the *lacrimal sac*. The fusion of the maxillary and lateral nasal processes establishes the *cheeks, upper jaw*, and *nose*; the cheek and upper jaw are derived from the maxillary process, the *alar wings* of the *nose* from the lateral nasal process.

The area of frontonasal process located between the eyes forms the *dorsum (apex)* of the *nose* within which mesenchyme derived from neural crest ultimately gives rise to the *nasal bones*. Initially, the nostrils face forward, but they eventually assume their adult downward position as growth of the frontonasal process shapes the dorsum and apex of the nose. Above the eyes, the mass of the frontonasal process forms the *forehead* and *frontal bone*.

The face is derived from the frontonasal process, the paired maxillary processes, and the paired mandibular processes. Subsequently, differential growth of the bilateral nasal placodes results in formation of the nares (nostrils) and the medial and lateral nasal processes on the inferolateral surfaces of the frontonasal process. Migration and fusions between these different primordia are responsible for the formation of the external form and shape of the face.

Formation of the Palate and Nasal Septum

During the fifth week, formation of the secondary palate and nasal septum results in anatomical separation of the oral and nasal cavities, and formation of right and left nasal cavities. The development of these structures involves specializations on the deep or inner aspects of the same primordia that are responsible for the external form of the face and jaws. The primordia of the palate and nasal septum (Fig. 2.15) are:

1. the median **palatal process**, or *primary palate*
2. the lateral **palatal folds** of *maxillary process*
3. the *frontonasal process*.

Union of the paired medial nasal processes in the midline gives rise to the *intermaxillary segment*, and the *primary palate* (median palatal process), a triangular wedge extending backward from the intermaxillary segment into the primitive oral cavity (Figs. 2.15b, 2.15c; Fig. 2.16). The primary palate is also known as the *premaxilla*, within which the four incisor teeth ultimately appear. At this stage, the nasal cavities communicate directly with the oral cavity through openings, the *posterior nares* or *choanae*, which lie above the lateral surfaces of the primary palate (Figs. 2.15b, 2.15c; Fig. 2.16a; Fig. 2.17).

The *secondary palate* arises from shelf-like extensions, the *lateral palatal folds*, which project from the medial surfaces of the maxillary processes. These folds move medially toward each other and the primary palate and eventually fuse to form the secondary palate (Figs. 2.15; 2.16; 2.17; 2.18c, 2.18d). Initially, the medial movement of the palatal folds is prevented by the tongue, which, though forming in the floor of the pharynx, extends upward into the nasal cavity (Figs. 2.18a, 2.18b). During this period, the leading edges of the lateral palatal folds are directed downward (Figs. 2.18a, 2.18b). Eventually the tongue descends, allowing the palatal folds to elevate and move horizontally toward the midline (Figs. 2.18c, 2.18d). They first encounter the primary palate with which they become confluent and then fuse with each other in an anterior-posterior gradient (Figs. 2.16; 2.17). The line of fusion between the primary palate and lateral palatal folds is marked in the adult by the *median incisive foramen*, which transmits the nasopalatine nerves and branches of the sphenopalatine artery.

The fusion of the lateral palatal folds with each other and the primary palate forms the secondary palate (Figs. 2.16; 2.17), which separates the oral and nasal cavities (Figs. 2.18c, 2.18d). In

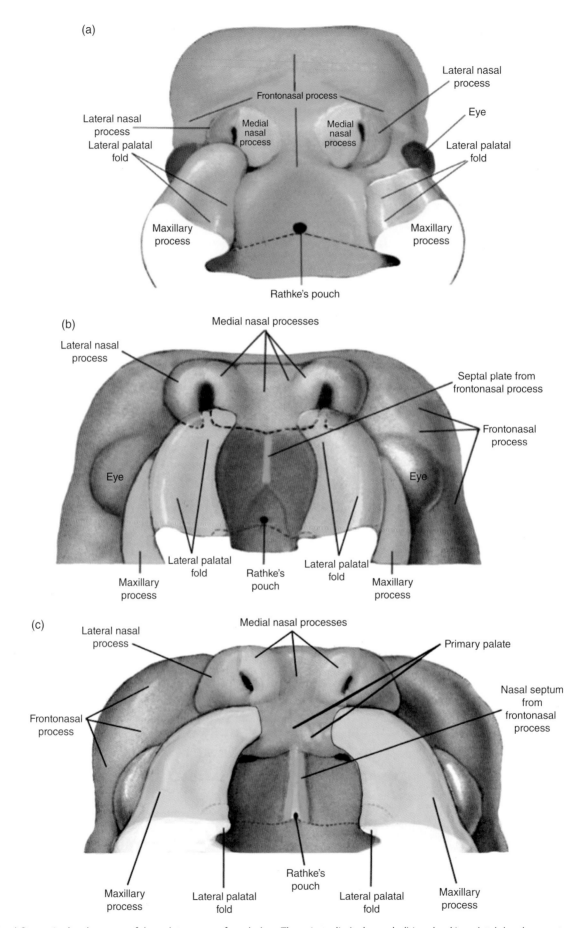

Figure 2.15   (a–c) Stages in development of the palate as seen from below. The primordia (color coded) involved in palatal development are shown at 6 weeks (a), during week 7 (b), and at the end of week 7 (c). (Modified after Hamilton and Mossman, 1972.)

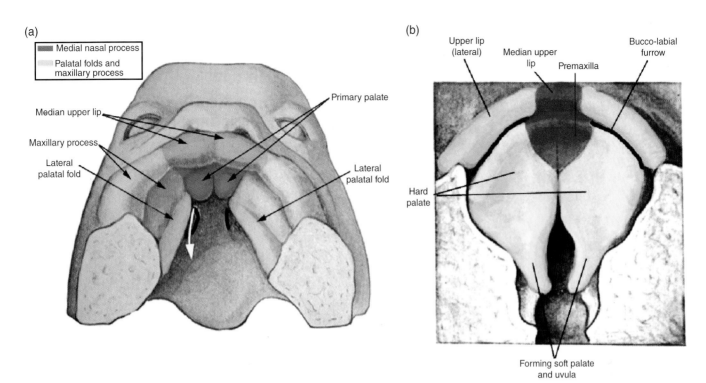

Figure 2.16   Formation of the palate at 6.5 weeks (a) and nearing completion at week 8 (b). Origins of various components are indicated by the color code shown in (a). White arrow indicates position of the posterior nares. (Modified from Arey, 1968.)

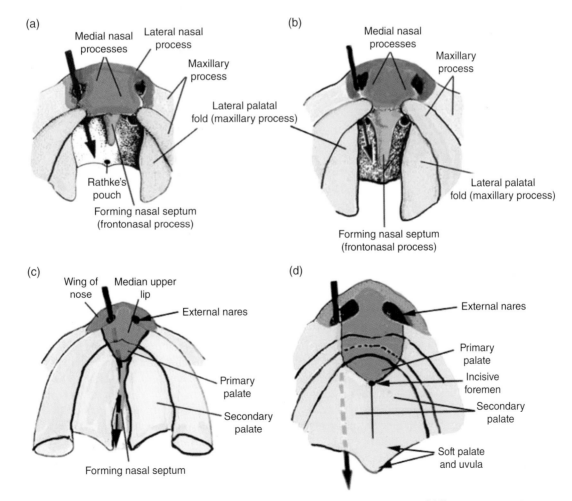

Figure 2.17   Diagram of development of the palate and adjacent structures during weeks 6–7. Origin of different structures is represented by color. Heavy arrow shows change in position of posterior nares. (Modified after Hamilton and Mossman, 1972.)

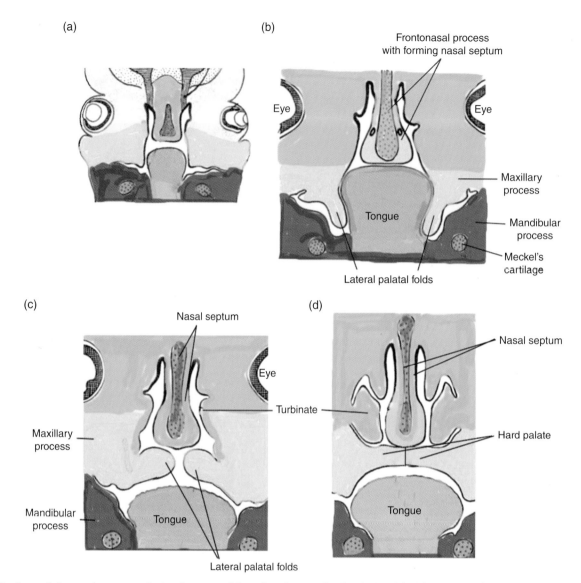

Figure 2.18   Coronal view to show stages in development of the palate. See text for details. (Modified from Hamilton and Mossman, 1972.)

the process, the posterior openings of the nasal cavities, the *choanae*, are translocated posteriorly to communicate directly with the nasopharynx (Fig. 2.17), and separation of oral and nasal cavities is complete.

The *nasal septum* originates from the *frontonasal process*, except for its anteroinferior segment immediately above the philtrum and median lip, which is derived from the confluent medial nasal processes. The septum begins as a vertical shelf which grows downward from the undersurface of the frontonasal process, extending toward the developing palate to divide the nasal cavity into right and left sides. This shelf fuses with the anterior portion of the palate, and joins the anteroinferior portion of the septum that was formed by the medial nasal processes, thus establishing a complete nasal septum between the right and left nasal cavities. Neural crest-derived mesenchyme in the forming septum differentiates to form the *ethmoid bone* and the *septal cartilage*. This mesenchyme also migrates into the wings or alae of the nose to form the *turbinates* (conchae).

Merger of the nasal septum with the anterior segment of the palate induces ossification in that segment and thus contributes to formation of the *hard palate*. The posterior segment of the palate that does not contact the nasal septum remains unossified as the *soft palate* and *uvula*; it is invaded by branchial mesoderm which gives rise to the *palatal muscles*, all of which (except the tensor veli palatini) are innervated by the *vagus nerve*. Incomplete fusion of the posterior portions of the paired lateral palatal folds produces a bifid soft palate and/or uvula.

In the early phases of palatal and nasoseptal formation, *Rathke's pouch*, an ectodermal pocket, appears in the roof of the stomodeum or oral cavity, just in front of the original location of the oropharyngeal membrane (Fig. 2.15). Rathke's pouch grows upward toward the base of the diencephalon to form the *adenohypophysis* or *anterior lobe* of the *pituitary gland*. Destined to be an endocrine gland, it eventually loses its connection to the oral cavity, though infrequently remnants of the original duct may persist to give rise to **craniopharyngiomas**.

The secondary (definitive) palate is formed from: (1) the medial palatal process or primary palate derived from the median nasal processes, (2) the lateral palatal folds of the maxillary processes and, (3) the portion of the fronto-nasal septum giving rise to the main mass of the nasal septum. Fusion of the lateral palatal folds begins anteriorly where they meet and fuse with each other and with the median palatal fold, gradually coursing posteriorly to separate the oral and nasal cavities. The anterior two-thirds of the forming palate is joined by the forming nasal septum derived from the frontonasal process, an association which induces ossification and formation of the hard palate. The posterior one-third that does not contact the forming nasal septum gives rise to the soft palate and uvula.

Development of the Tongue

The *tongue* is a muscular organ composed of skeletal muscle covered by a mucous membrane, or *mucosa*, within which taste buds are distributed and localized. It is especially sensitive to temperature, pain, and tactile stimuli and is the major gustatory organ mediating taste (see Chapters 9 and 10). The tongue consists of the *body*, or anterior two-thirds, and the *root*, the posterior one-third. The *mucosa* of the tongue originates from elements of four pharyngeal arches: major contributions from the *first* and *third* arches and lesser but important contributions from the *second* and *fourth* arches. Since adult derivatives retain the innervation of their embryonic precursors, four cranial nerves, V, VII, IX, and X, provide sensory innervation of the tongue mucosa.

The central mass of the tongue contains extensive arrays of intrinsic skeletal muscle invested with a fibrous connective tissue stroma, which enable it to play a major role in eating, swallowing, and speech (see Chapters 12 and 13). Additionally, extrinsic muscles attach and fix the tongue to the lower jaw and hyoid bone. The origins of the stroma and skeletal muscle are distinct from those of the mucosa of the body and root, adding further complexity to innervation of the tongue.

The tongue develops in the floor of the pharynx during the fifth to seventh weeks. Its formation begins with the appearance of a median swelling, the **tuberculum impar**, in the area of the pharyngeal floor that is located between the first (mandibular) pharyngeal arches (Figs. 2.19a, 2.19b). Soon, the

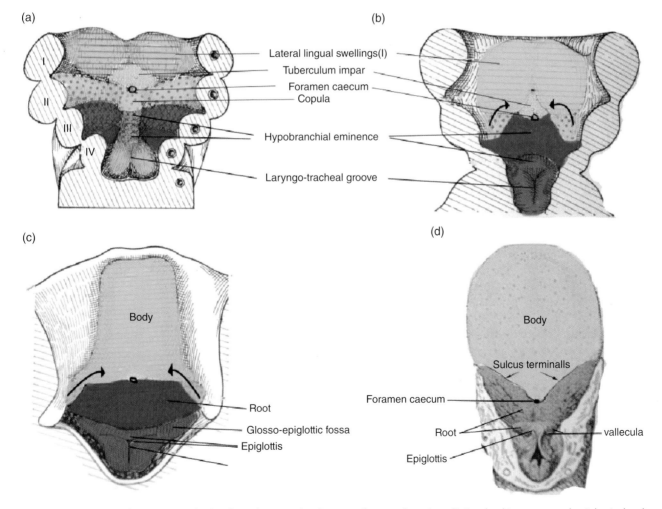

(a)

Lateral lingual swellings(I)
Tuberculum impar
Foramen caecum
Copula

Hypobranchial eminence

Laryngo-tracheal groove

(b)

(c)

Body

Root
Glosso-epiglottic fossa
Epiglottis

(d)

Body

Sulcus terminalls

Foramen caecum

Root

Epiglottis

vallecula

Figure 2.19 Development of the tongue. The first four pharyngeal arches contribute to the primordia involved in tongue and epiglottis development, shown in color for each arch (a). The subsequent changes and their pharyngeal arch relationships can be seen (b, c), leading to the definitive form of the tongue and adjacent region (d). The curved arrows in (b) and (c) indicate the migration of elements of the hyoid arch into the forming body of the tongue to form taste buds. (Modified from Arey, 1968.)

immediately adjacent ventromedial regions of the *first pharyngeal arch* enlarge to form the paired **lateral lingual swellings** (Figs. 2.19a, 2.19b). The latter grow and swing toward the median plane where they merge to form the body of the tongue. In the process, the tuberculum impar is obliterated or absorbed into the body of the tongue and can no longer be recognized (Figs. 2.19c, 2.19d). The region of confluence between the lateral lingual swellings is marked by the *lingual septum* and *median sulcus* in the adult tongue. Since the first (mandibular) arch is innervated by the trigeminal nerve (V), sensory innervation of the body of the tongue is provided by the *lingual nerve*, a branch of the mandibular division of the trigeminal (V) nerve.

Immediately behind the tuberculum impar, the endoderm in the midline invaginates and grows downward through the tongue. This invagination forms a duct, the *thyroglossal duct*, which expands at its distal end to give rise to the thyroid gland. It grows inferiorly into the neck and eventually the duct degenerates, leaving behind a depression on the surface of the tongue, the foramen caecum (Figs. 2.19a–c). Remnants of the thyroglossal duct may persist as cysts that can be located at various positions along the path of the original duct.

The *second (hyoid)* arch plays a less prominent role in tongue development. Its branchial mesoderm migrates into the face and submandibular region to become the muscles of facial expression and deeper muscles of the jaw. Nonetheless, the *hyoid arch* contributes significantly to differentiation of taste buds and elaboration of the skeletal support of the tongue. A median swelling, the **copula**, appears in the pharyngeal floor between the second or hyoid arch (Fig. 2.19a). Endoderm from the *second arch* migrates forward into the body of the tongue to form *taste buds* (Figs. 2.19b, 2.19c). Since these taste buds originate from the *second* or *hyoid arch* which is innervated by the *facial nerve (VII)*, taste in the body of the tongue is mediated by the facial nerve (VII), via the *chorda tympani*. The neural crest-derived mesenchyme of the second arch forms the skeletal support of the tongue: the *lesser wings* and the *upper rim* of the *hyoid bone* to which the tongue is attached by various extrinsic muscles. The *greater wings* and *lower half* of the *hyoid* form from the neural crest-derived mesenchyme of the *third arch*.

The root of the tongue arises mainly from the *third arch*. Behind the copula lies a midline elevation called the **hypobranchial eminence** which is flanked by the ventromedial regions of the *third* and *fourth pharyngeal arches* (Figs. 2.19a–c). The endoderm and underlying mesenchyme of the ventromedial regions of the third arch and the adjacent anterior extension of the hypobranchial eminence migrate forward as a unit, occluding the copula in the process, and forming the root of the tongue (Figs. 2.19, b–d). These elements meet and fuse with the body along a line marked in the adult by the *sulcus terminalis*. Since the root is formed by the third arch and adjacent extension of the hypobranchial eminence, the *glossopharyngeal (IX) nerve* supplies sensory innervation of the root, including both general and taste sensation.

The forward movement of the third arch to form the root creates a sulcus or depression between the root and the posterior part of the hypobranchial eminence that remains adjacent to the fourth arch (Figs. 2.19c, 2.19d). This posterior segment of the hypobranchial eminence elevates to form the *epiglottis*, which remains separated from the root of the tongue by the sulcus formed during the forward movement of the third arch. This sulcus becomes the *glossoepiglottic fossa* within which the *glossoepiglottic fold* and the *vallecula* develop (Figs. 2.19C, 2.19d). A small area of the root bordering the vallecula originates from part of the fourth arch and thus is innervated by the *vagus (X)* nerve, as are the vallecula and epiglottis.

The muscles of the tongue arise from the *myotome* of the posterior occipital somites. Myoblasts from these somites join the *hypoglossal neural crest stream* to intermingle with neural crest cells. This mixed stream of neural crest and myoblasts joins the *circumpharyngeal* neural crest stream, which passes above, behind, and around the pharynx to gain access to the region below the pharynx. Eventually the hypoglossal stream diverges from the circumpharyngeal crest to pass forward into the forming tongue, where the myoblasts give rise to the *intrinsic* and *extrinsic tongue muscles* and neural crest forms the connective tissue investments of the tongue muscles. The myoblasts originating from posterior occipital somites retain their innervation by the future hypoglossal nerve as they course to their destination, accounting for the innervation of the tongue musculature by the *hypoglossal (XII) nerve* and its designation as a *somatic motor* nerve.

> The tongue develops in the floor of the pharynx and originates from several pharyngeal arches. The paired lingual swellings from the first pharyngeal arch give rise to the body or anterior two-thirds of the tongue. The root or posterior one-third arises largely from the third pharyngeal arch with contributions from the fourth arch. Between the body and root of the tongue, the foramen caecum marks the origin of the thyroglossal duct which subsequently forms the thyroid gland. Taste buds in the body of the tongue are derived from the second pharyngeal arch; taste buds in the root arise from the third arch. The involvement of four pharyngeal arches in development of the lingual mucosa is responsible for the sensory innervation of the tongue: general sensation in the body mediated by the lingual branch of the trigeminal (V) nerve, with taste mediated by the facial nerve (VII); both general sensation and taste in the root provided by the glossopharyngeal (IX) nerve with that minor part of the root that forms from the fourth arch being supplied by sensory vagal nerves. The muscles of the tongue arise from myotomes of occipital somites and are innervated by the hypoglossal nerve (XII).

Skull and Jaw Formation

The skull consists of the **neurocranium**, the protective case enclosing the brain and special sense organs, and the **viscerocranium**, the skeleton of the face and jaw. The human skull has a complex developmental and evolutionary history. Some bones have a "hybrid" origin; they are derived from both *endochondral* and *intramembranous centers of ossification*, e.g., temporal and occipital bones. In jawless fish, the viscerocranium consists entirely of the skeleton of the gill arches. In most fish and amphibians, elements of the first gill arch have been co-opted to form the skeleton of the primitive jaw, while in mammals these same elements become the *auditory ossicles* and "new" bones form the skeleton of the jaw.

Development of the neurocranium

The neurocranium has a dual origin from *paraxial mesoderm* and *neural crest*. Many of its components are endochondral-derived bones, that is, they form initially as cartilage which is subsequently replaced by bone, while others are intramembranous or dermal bones which arise directly within mesenchyme <u>without</u> a cartilaginous precursor.

The neurocranium initially appears as the *chondrocranium*, a series of paired cartilaginous plates that ultimately merge to form the *base of the skull*. These cartilaginous plates (Fig. 2.20) arise from paraxial mesoderm or neural crest (Fig. 2.20) and include the following.

1. The *parachordal plates*, which are derived from mesoderm and are located adjacent to the notochord, extending cranially to the level of the notochordal tip.

2. The *hypophyseal plates*, also mesoderm derived, which straddle the *craniopharyngeal canal* that contains the developing adenohypophysis.

3. The *prechordal plates (trabeculae cranii)*, which are neural crest derived and located in the interorbital and nasal regions.

In addition to these median plates, a cartilaginous capsule, the *otic capsule*, encircles the developing inner ear (Fig. 2.20a) while similar capsules form in association with the nasal pits (*olfactory capsule*) and optic cups. The otic capsule originates from *paraxial mesoderm*, while recent evidence suggests a neural crest origin for the *olfactory* and *optic capsules*.

Development of the base of the skull involves the expansion and union of these cartilage plates to form a continuous mass of skeletal tissue, extending from the occipital region forward to the perinasal and periorbital regions (Figs. 2.20b, 2.20c). Fusion of the parachordal plates posteriorly with cartilage derived from sclerotome of the occipital somites produces the *basioccipital* bone, which extends from the area surrounding the *foramen magnum* forward to the *superior nuchal line*. The otic capsule joins the parachordal plate to form a *petromastoid* shelf, which eventually forms the *petrous* bone and the *mastoid process*. The petromastoid shelf encircles the incipient carotid artery to meet the hypophyseal cartilage, thus forming the *carotid canal*. Union of the parachordal and hypophyseal plates forms the *body of the sphenoid* and its *sella turcica*. Laterally, the *orbitosphenoid cartilage*, arising from neural crest-derived mesenchyme, merges with the hypophyseal plate to form the *lesser wing of the sphenoid* and the *orbital plate*, encircling the optic nerve in the optic canal. More posteriorly, the *alisphenoid cartilage*, originating from paraxial mesoderm, grows around the ophthalmic division of the trigeminal nerve (V) and cranial nerves III, IV, and VI to form the *superior orbital fissure* and the *greater wing of the sphenoid*, which encloses the maxillary and mandibular divisions in their

respective foramina. The prechordal plates form the *cartilaginous nasal septum*, the *perpendicular plate of the ethmoid*, and the *nasal* bones.

The bones of the *calvarium (vault)* and the sides of the skull are intramembranous bones, some of which are neural crest-derived and some mesodermal in origin (Figs. 2.21; 2.22). The *squamous portion* of the temporal bone arises from neural crest and contributes to formation of the *temporomandibular joint* (Fig. 2.22). The *frontal, nasal,* and *lacrimal* bones arise from a common mesenchymal mass that is neural crest derived (Fig. 2.22). The *parietal* bones and that portion of the occipital bone between the *superior nuchal line* and *lambdal suture* are intramembranous bones derived from mesoderm. The articulations between the bones of the vault remain as membranous sutures or *fontanelles*, located at the *interparietal, parietofrontal,* and *parieto-occipital* joints. As the brain grows and expands, so too do the various regions of the skull, increasing the width of the cranial base as well as that of the vault. The fontanelles provide leeway for continued expansion of the brain concomitant with skull growth, a process that is not complete until the second year after birth.

> The neurocranium, that part of the skull which encloses the brain and special sense organs, initially appears as the chondrocranium, a series of paired cartilaginous plates which arise from paraxial mesoderm or neural crest and unite to form the base of the skull. Also contributing to the neurocranium are the sclerotomes of occipital somites which form the basioccipital bone. Most of these bones are endochondral bones, bones that replace a preexisting cartilaginous model. The bones of the calvarium or vault of the skull are intramembranous or dermal bones derived from mesoderm or neural crest.

Development of the viscerocranium

The **viscerocranium**, the skeleton of the face and jaws (Figs. 2.21; 2.22) arises from neural crest of the first three pharyngeal arches (Fig. 2.22). Soon after its appearance, the first (mandibular) arch bifurcates into the dorsolateral maxillary process, the precursor of the upper jaw and cheek, and the ventromedial mandibular process, which forms the lower jaw. During week 4, each process acquires a supporting cartilage. The cartilage of the maxillary process is the **pterygoquadrate bar**, and that of the mandibular process is **Meckel's cartilage** (Fig. 2.21). In fish and amphibians, endochondral ossification of these respective cartilages forms the *pterygoquadrate bone* in the maxillary process and, in the lower jaw, the *articular bone*. The joint between these two bones constitutes the definitive jaw in these species and is designated as a "*quadrato-articular*" articulation (Fig. 2.21).

With evolutionary specialization of the middle ear in humans, the cartilages that initially appear within the maxillary and mandibular processes are co-opted to form *auditory ossicles* (Fig. 2.22) and "new" bones form the skeleton of both jaws. Centers of intramembranous ossification within neural crest

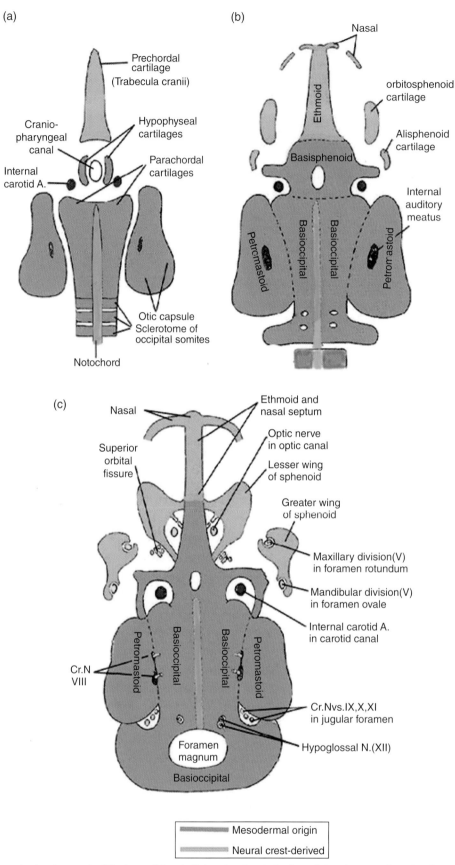

Figure 2.20 Various stages in development of the base of the skull showing the derivation of the elements that give rise to the definitive bones. (Modified after Hamilton and Mossman, 1972.)

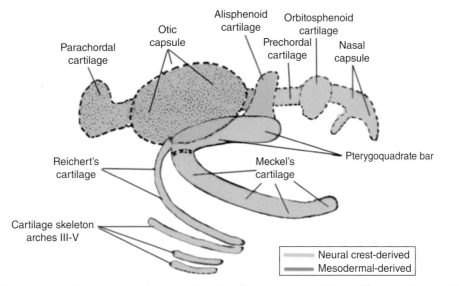

Figure 2.21   Diagram of the primitive skull of lower vertebrates and origins of its components. (Adapted from Hamilton and Mossman, 1972.)

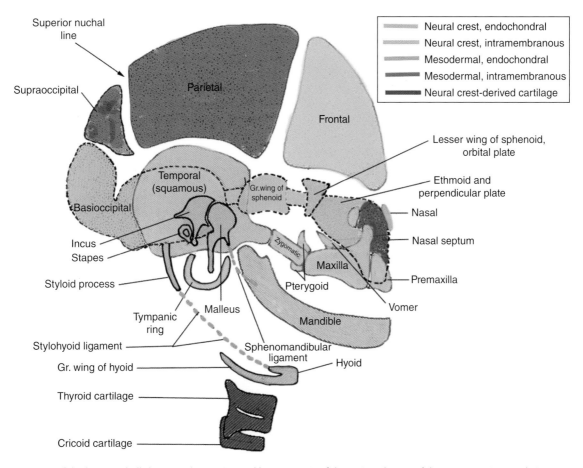

Figure 2.22   Diagram of the human skull showing the origins and histogenesis of the various bones of the neurocranium and viscerocranium. (Modified from Hamilton and Mossman, 1972.)

mesenchyme of the maxillary process produce the *maxilla, premaxilla, palatal, vomer, and zygomatic* bones (Fig. 2.22). The *pterygoquadrate bar* disappears, except for its *dorsal* portion, which becomes the *incus* in the middle ear.

In the lower jaw, *Meckel's cartilage* provides a temporary template around which the mandible develops. During week 6, intramembranous ossification begins in mesenchyme lateral to Meckel's cartilage, at the point where the *inferior alveolar nerve* divides into its *mental* and *incisive* branches. This ossification center expands dorsally and ventrally along the entire length of the mandibular process. Ossification spreads ventrally to encircle the inferior alveolar nerve and its branches, forming the *body* of the mandible. The right and left ventral halves of the mandible meet anteriorly in the midline at the *mandibular symphysis* where a fibrocartilaginous joint develops during the first postnatal year. This joint disappears with union of the two halves of the mandible in the second year after birth.

The dorsal wave of ossification extends lateral to the inferior alveolar nerve to form the *ramus* of the mandible, with the nerve and its accompanying artery medial to the ramus, entering the body through the *mandibular foramen* at the level of the *lingula*. The proximal (dorsal) portion of Meckel's cartilage becomes the *malleus* of the middle ear, the *anterior ligament of the malleus*, and the *sphenomandibular ligament* (Fig. 2.22); its distal (ventral) portion disappears and contributes nothing to the adult mandible.

The hyoid bone and the horns of the hyoid bone are derived from neural crest of the second and third pharyngeal arches. During weeks 4 to 5, neural crest differentiates to form the cartilaginous support of the *second* arch, **Reichert's cartilage**. The dorsal segment of this cartilage meets the otic capsule and is enveloped by the forming petrous bone, giving rise to the *stapes*, an auditory ossicle, within the middle ear. Outside the otic capsule, Reichert's cartilage becomes the *styloid process*, the *stylohyoid ligament*, the *lesser horns of the hyoid bone*, and the *upper rim of the hyoid bone* (Fig. 2.22). The neural crest of the third arch forms the greater horns of the hyoid and the lower half of the hyoid bone (Fig. 2.21), thus completing the skeletal support of the tongue and submandibular region.

The neural crest of the fourth and sixth arches forms the *laryngeal* cartilages: the *cuneiform* and *thyroid* cartilages arise from the <u>fourth</u> arch while the *corniculate*, *arytenoid*, and *cricoid* cartilages are derived from the <u>fifth</u> arch (Fig. 2.22).

> The viscerocranium, the skeleton of the face and jaws, arises from neural crest of the first three pharyngeal arches. Meckel's cartilage and the pterygoquadrate bar, the initial cartilage supports of the mandibular and maxillary processes of the first pharyngeal arch, recede into the middle ear cavity where they form auditory ossicles, the malleus and incus, respectively. Mesenchymal condensations in the first arch give rise to the maxilla and mandible, which develop as intramembranous or dermal bones. Reichert's cartilage of the second arch forms the stapes, the styloid process, the stylohyoid ligament, and the lesser horns and upper rim of the hyoid bone. The remainder of the hyoid bone is derived from neural-crest-derived cartilages of the third pharyngeal arch. The larynx and associated cartilages are derivatives of the fourth and sixth pharyngeal arches.

Development of the temporomandibular joint (TMJ)

In contrast to the *"quadrato-articular"* articulation of non-mammalian vertebrates (Fig. 2.21), the human jaw is phylogenetically a new joint between the tooth-bearing mandible and the squamous portion of the temporal bone (Fig. 2.22) and is designated as a *"dentary-squamosal"* or *"temporomandibular"* articulation. The *temporomandibular joint* (TMJ) develops in intimate relationship to the middle ear, a structural and developmental association that underlies the otologic symptoms often associated

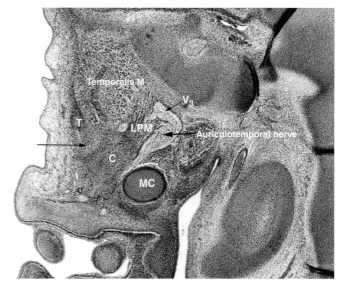

Figure 2.23   Coronal view of the temporomandibular joint at week 7 showing two mesenchymal condensations, the condylar (C) and temporal (T) blastemata. Between and separating the two blastemata is an area of loose mesenchyme (unlabeled arrow). The condylar blastema is located above and lateral to Meckel's cartilage (MC). The auriculotemporal nerve branching from the mandibular division of the trigeminal nerve (V_3) is seen coursing between them. The temporalis and lateral pterygoid (LPM) muscles are also indicated. Photograph provided by and used with the kind permission of Prof. Dr. J.R. Merida-Velasco, Facultad de Medicina, Universidad Complutense, Madrid (Spain).

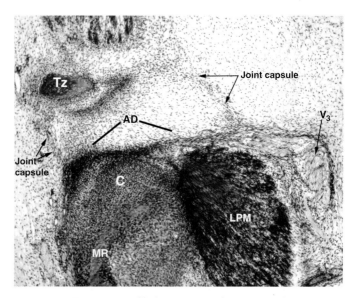

Figure 2.24   Temporomandibular joint at week 8. Intramembranous ossification has begun to form the zygomatic process of the temporal bone (Tz, blue area). The condylar blastema (C) forms a distinctive mass on the ramus of the mandible (MR). The condyle and temporal bone are separated by the anlage of the articular disk (AD), whose extent is marked. Fibers of the forming lateral pterygoid muscle (LPM) insert into the medial aspect of the condyle. Condensations representing the presumptive joint (articular) capsule are shown on the medial and lateral aspects of the forming joint. Mandibular division of trigeminal nerve (V_3). Photograph provided by and used with the kind permission of Prof. Dr. J.R. Merida-Velasco, Facultad de Medicina, Universidad Complutense, Madrid (Spain).

with TMJ dysfunction. TMJ development begins in week 7 of gestation and occurs in three stages that are complete only in the second decade of adult life.

The initial or *blastemal* stage of temporomandibular joint development during weeks 7 to 8 is characterized by the appearance of two separate mesenchymal condensations, or **blastemata** (Figs. 2.23; 2.24), each derived from neural crest. The *condylar blastema*, the precursor of the *mandibular condyle*, appears above the dorsal end of the forming mandible (Fig. 2.24), lateral to Meckel's cartilage (Fig. 2.23). Behind and lateral to the condylar blastema is the *temporal (glenoid) blastema* (Figs. 2.23; 2.24), which will form the *glenoid (mandibular) fossa, articular eminence*, and *zygomatic process* of the *temporal squama*. A third mesenchymal condensation, the anlage of the *articular disk*, is interposed between and continuous with the two blastemata (Fig. 2.24). Fibers of the *lateral pterygoid muscle* originating from first arch mesoderm merge with the medial aspects of the articular disk anlage and condylar blastema (Fig. 2.24).

During week 8, intramembranous ossification occurs within the temporal blastema, beginning the formation and shaping of the articular portion of the temporal squama. The condylar blastema differentiates to form the *condylar cartilage*, a wedge-shaped mass of cartilage attached to the dorsal surface of the ramus of the mandible (Fig. 2.24).

During weeks 9-11, the second or *cavitational* stage of TMJ development begins which results in the appearance of the *upper (superior)* and *lower (inferior) synovial cavities* and demarcation of the articular disk. During this period, the condylar cartilage grows extensively, becoming a conical or carrot-shaped mass that extends from the site of the future joint to the level of the lingula and mandibular foramen of the developing mandible (Fig. 2.25).

During week 9, apoptosis between the condylar cartilage and the articular disk anlage gives rise to the inferior joint cavity (Fig. 2.26). Subsequently, apoptosis between the articular disk

anlage and the temporal squama forms the superior joint cavity and delineates the articular disk (Fig. 2.27). The mesenchyme external to the forming joint gives rise to the joint capsule which surrounds and encloses the forming joint. Thus, the essential features of the TMJ are established during this critical period of weeks 7 to 11 and clearly visible by week 12 (Fig. 2.27).

Structures in close topographical relationship to the TMJ in the adult are readily evident during these two critical stages of TMJ development. The *auriculotemporal nerve*, which will provide sensory innervation to the adult joint and ear, courses close to the condylar cartilage (Figs. 2.23; 2.24; 2.26; 2.27). Meckel's cartilage, which serves as a template for development of the mandible, remains until mid-fetal life as a stabilizer of TMJ development. Its distal portion then degenerates and disappears while its proximal portion gives rise to the malleus and the *anterior malleolar* and *sphenomandibular ligaments*, which interconnect the mandible and TMJ with the middle ear (Fig. 2.25). The forming *lateral pterygoid* muscle inserts into the articular disk anlage and subsequently into the medial aspect of the disk and the condyle (Figs. 2.24; 2.26; 2.27). Some of its mesenchyme gives rise to the *discomalleolar ligament*, which, in the adult, runs between the malleus and articular disk.

The *maturation* stage begins at week 12 and continues into the postnatal period. During this stage, the condylar cartilage and the mandible grow extensively to keep pace with the expansion of the base of the skull. Growth and expansion of the condylar cartilage occurs by endochondral ossification, which extends from the apex of the condyle where it meets the ramus of the mandible toward the site of the joint. Mesenchymal septa invested by blood vessels invaginate the articular surface of the condyle forming "crampons," which are thought to provide nutrition of the cartilage. At birth, a significant portion of the condyle consists of bone, except over the articular surface of the condyle which is covered by a cap of cartilage. The condyle acquires its definitive histological composition during the first two decades after birth. The

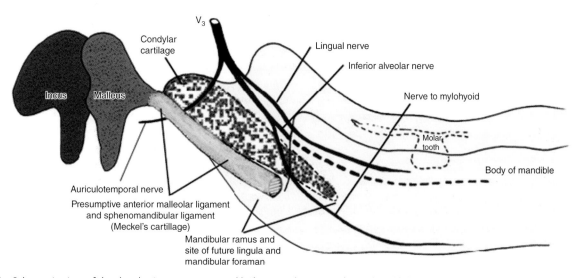

Figure 2.25   Schematic view of the developing temporomandibular joint during week 10. The condylar cartilage forms a conical or carrot-shaped structure extending from the site of the joint to the ramus of the mandible. The proximal part of Meckel's cartilage is forming the malleus within the middle ear from which extends the portion of that cartilage which will form the sphenomandibular and anterior malleolar ligaments. Mandibular division of trigeminal nerve (V$_3$). Diagram provided by and used with the kind permission of Prof. Dr. J.R. Merida-Velasco, Facultad de Medicina, Universidad Complutense, Madrid (Spain).

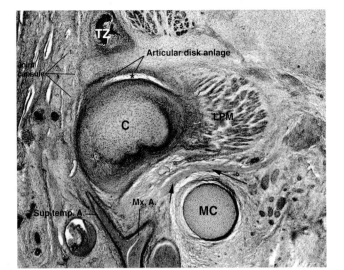

Figure 2.26 Coronal view of the temporomandibular joint during week 10. The inferior or lower synovial joint cavity is now present (*) above the condylar cartilage (C) which has formed from the condylar blastema. Fibers of the lateral pterygoid muscle (LPM) are seen merging into the medial aspect of the condylar cartilage. Intramembranous ossification is seen (red area) within the temporal blastema (TZ) but there is no indication of the superior or upper synovial joint cavity, so the temporal blastema remains continuous with the articular disk anlage. The auriculotemporal nerve (arrows) is seen between the condylar cartilage (C) and Meckel's cartilage (MC). The superficial temporal and maxillary branches of the external carotid artery are indicated. Photograph provided by and used with the kind permission of Prof. Dr. J.R. Merida-Velasco, Facultad de Medicina, Universidad Complutense, Madrid (Spain).

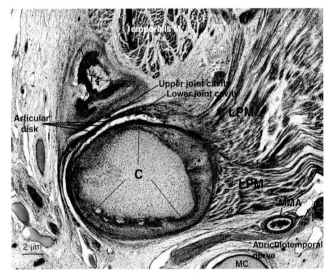

Figure 2.27 The temporomandibular joint during week 11. Intramembranous ossification continues within the temporal blastema (Tz) to produce and extend the temporal squama. The condylar cartilage (C) is shown above and lateral to Meckel's cartilage (MC) with the auriculotemporal nerve and middle meningeal artery (MMA) located between them. Inserting into the medial aspect of the condylar cartilage are fibers of the inferior portion of the lateral pterygoid muscle (LPM). Both the upper and lower synovial joint cavities have now formed and the articular disk is well defined. Inserting into the medial aspect of the articular disk are the superior fibers of the lateral pterygoid muscle (LPM). Photograph provided by and used with the kind permission of Prof. Dr. J.R. Merida-Velasco, Facultad de Medicina, Universidad Complutense, Madrid (Spain).

temporal articular surface is flat or slightly concave at birth and the articular eminence does not form completely until postnatal life. The articular disk consists of dense fibrous tissue and, during the postnatal period, acquires its fibrocartilage and biconcave shape. The development and shaping of various components of the TMJ, which occur during the maturation stage, are not completed until after birth, some as late as the second decade of life.

Jaw movements during the fetal period are essential for normal development and growth of various TMJ components, including growth and endochondral ossification of the condylar cartilage, development of masticatory muscles, and the size and normal cellularity of the articular disk. Initially, it is the movements of the "primitive" jaw between Meckel's cartilage (malleus) and the pterygoquadrate bar (incus) that provide this stimulatory mobility. By mid-fetal life, these skeletal elements have been transformed into auditory ossicles in the middle ear, and movements of the definitive jaw then sustain normal development of the TMJ.

> Formation of the temporomandibular joint (TMJ) occurs in three stages: first, the blastemal stage, marked by the appearance of the neural-crest-derived condylar blastema and temporal blastema. Between and continuous with the two blastemata lies the anlage of the articular disk. The cavitational stage is characterized by the appearance of the lower and upper joint cavities and demarcation of the articular disk. The maturational stage begins during the twelfth week and continues into postnatal life, marked by extensive growth of the various TMJ components, including expansion and endochondral ossification of the condyle, development of the masticatory muscles, and growth of the articular disk.

Clinical correlations

Congenital disorders

Developmental disorders of the face and jaws are among some of the most common anomalies and represent potential tragedy for the afflicted, especially in poorly developed countries where resources and facilities for surgical repair are limited. The causes of most craniofacial defects are unclear, but both genetic factors and environmental toxicity are involved. The most common defect is *cleft lip* and/or *cleft palate* (Figs. 2.28, a–e),which occur in 1 in 700 births. Cleft lip results from failure or deficient fusion of the *maxillary* and *median nasal processes*, and cleft palate from failure of the *lateral palatal folds* to fuse, either with each other or with the *primary palate (median palatal process)*. These can be *unilateral* or *bilateral*, with the former being more common. Cleft lip and palate often occur simultaneously. *Oblique facial cleft*, a rare anomaly, arises from absence of or abnormal fusion between the *maxillary* and *lateral nasal processes*. Frontonasal dysplasias such as *hypertelorism* (excess interocular separation) or an excessively broad, flattened nasal bridge, are associated with abnormal development of the *frontonasal process*. *Cleft mandible* arising from abnormal union of the paired *mandibular*

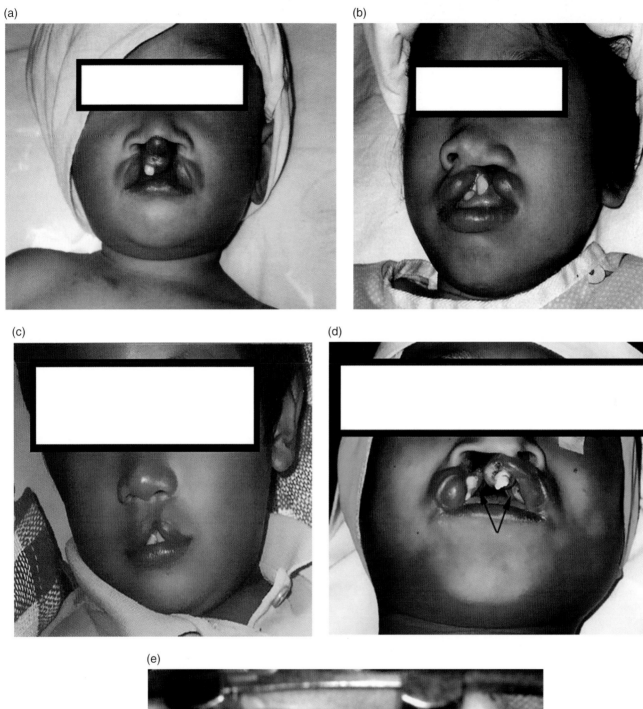

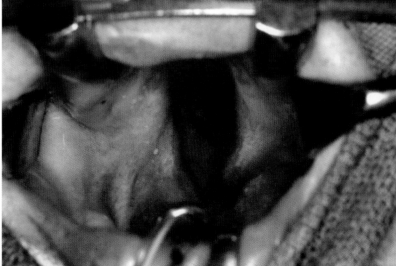

Figure 2.28 Examples of congenital facial defects. (a), bilateral cleft lip; (b), unilateral cleft lip; (c), partial or incomplete unilateral cleft lip; (d), unilateral cleft lip with cleft palate (arrows); (e), cleft palate. (Photos courtesy of Dr. Richard Topazian and Dr. David Shafer, University of Connecticut School of Dental Medicine.)

processes is very rare, though *chin clefts*, which result from incomplete fusion, are more common but still infrequent. When genes regulating neural crest development are affected, facial and jaw anomalies, such as *hemifacial microsomia* and *Treacher Collins syndrome*, can occur. In some cases neural crest-associated craniofacial defects may occur together with heart defects, especially of the cardiac outflow pathway, such as in *DiGeorge* and *velocardiofacial* syndromes. *Fetal Alcohol Syndrome*, which includes craniofacial and heart defects, along with growth deficiency, microcephaly, developmental delay, and fine motor dysfunction, is an example of environmental disruption of neural crest cell development and function.

References

1. Arey, L.B. (1965) Developmental Anatomy, 7th edn., W.B. Saunders Co., Philadelphia and London.
2. Bush, J.O., & Jiang, R. (2012) Palatogenesis: morphogenetic and molecular mechanisms of secondary palate development. *Development*, 139, 231–243.
3. Carlson, B.M. (2009) *Human Embryology and Developmental Biology*, 4th edn. Mosby-Elsevier, Philadelphia.
4. Cobourne, M.T., (ed.) (2012) Cleft lip and palate: epidemiology, aetiology and treatment. *Frontiers of Oral Biology*, 16, 1–154.
5. Cordero, D.R., Brugmann, S., Chu, Y., Bajpai, R., Jame, M., & Helms, J.A. (2011) Cranial neural crest cells on the move: their roles in craniofacial development. *American Journal of Medical Genetics*, Part A, 155, 270–279.
6. Graham, A. (2008) Deconstructing the pharyngeal metamere. *Journal of Experimental Zoology Part B: Molecular & Developmental Evolution*, 310B, 336–344.
7. Grevellec, A., & Tucker, A.S. (2010) The pharyngeal pouches and clefts: development, evolution, structure and derivatives. *Seminars in Cell & Developmental Biology*, 21, 325–332.
8. Hamilton, W.J., & Mossman, H.W (1972) *Hamilton, Boyd, and Mossman's Human Embryology; Prenatal Development of Form and Function*, 4th edn. W.Heffer & Sons, Ltd, Cambridge.
9. Keith, D.A. (1982) Development of the human temporomandibular joint. *British Journal of Oral Surgery*, 20, 217–224.
10. Merida-Velasco, J.R., Rodriguez-Vasquez, J.F., Merida-Velasco, J.A., Sanchez-Montesinos, I., Espin-Ferra, J., & Jimenez-Collado, J. (1999) Development of the human temporomandibular joint. *The Anatomical Record.*, 255, 20–33.
11. Minoux, M., & Rijli, F.M. (2010) Molecular mechanisms of cranial neural crest cell migration and patterning in craniofacial development. *Development*, 137, 2605–2621.
12. Moore, K.L., & Persaud, T.V.N. (2003) *The Developing Human, Clinically Oriented Embryology*, 7th edn. Saunders Elsevier, Philadelphia.
13. Noden, D.M., & Trainor, P.A. (2005) Relations and interactions between cranial mesoderm and neural crest populations. *Journal of Anatomy*, 207, 575–601.
14. O'Rahilly, R., & Muller, F. (2007) The development of the neural crest in the human. *Journal of Anatomy*, 211, 335–351.
15. Parada, C., Han, D., & Chai, Y.(2012) Molecular and cellular regulatory mechanisms of tongue myogenesis. *Journal of Dental Research*, 91, 528-535.
16. Schoenwolf, G.C., Bleyl, S.B., Brauer, P.R., & Francis-West, P.H. (2009) *Larsen's Human Embryology*, 4th edn. Churchill-Livingstone Elsevier, Philadelphia.

Glossary

Amnion: One of the fetal membranes which act to protect the embryo from mechanical damage.

Blastema: An aggregate or cluster of cells that has the ability to develop into or regenerate specific tissues, parts of tissue, or organs. Plural *blastemata.*

Blastocyst: Early embryonic stage produced by cleavage.

Branchial: Related to, or designating homologous derivatives of, the gills of fish and amphibians.

Branchiomotor: Term designating the motor fibers of cranial nerves V, VII, IX, X, and XI, which innervate skeletal muscles derived from pharyngeal arch mesoderm. Also called special visceral motor.

Copula: A swelling that occurs, early in formation of the tongue, in the floor of the pharynx located between the ventral extensions of the hyoid arch. Its subsequent fate is unclear.

Craniopharyngioma: A benign tumor occurring mainly in children that arises from epithelium of persistent remnants of Rathke's pouch.

Ectoderm: Dorsal or external germ layer derived from the epiblast. It gives rise to the epidermis and the nervous system.

Endoderm: Ventral or internal germ layer which will form lining epithelia of the gastrointestinal and respiratory tracts and various visceral organs.

Epiblast: Dorsal layer formed by splitting the inner cell mass. The epiblast is the source of the three germ layers and, ultimately, the embryo.

Epibranchial placode: Ectodermal aggregates that occur above the dorsal extremities of the pharyngeal arches which participate in formation of several cranial nerve components.

Foregut: The portion of the primitive gut that lies anterior to the yolk stalk.

Frontonasal process: A prominence that appears on the superoanterior region of the forming embryonic head and is destined to form the forehead, nose, and nasal septum.

Gastrulation: Developmental stage during which the notochord and three germ layers are formed.

Germ layers: Primary tissue layers from which the embryo and its tissues are derived.

Hindgut: The portion of the primitive gut that lies posterior to the yolk stalk.

Hyoid arch: The second pharyngeal arch.

Hypoblast: Ventral layer formed by splitting of inner cell mass. It contributes to formation of the yolk sac.

Hypobranchial eminence: A median prominence in the pharyngeal floor located between the third and fourth pharyngeal arches and involved in the formation of the epiglottis.

Inner cell mass: Cellular aggregate within the blastocyst that forms the embryo and its associated tissues.

Lateral lingual swellings: Prominences derived from the ventral portion of the first pharyngeal arch which give rise to the body of the tongue.

Mandibular arch: The first pharyngeal arch.

Mandibular process: Ventromedial division of the first or mandibular arch which forms the adult mandible (lower jaw).

Maxillary process: Dorsolateral division of the mandibular or first pharyngeal arch that gives rise to the adult upper jaw and its components.

Meckel's cartilage: Initial skeletal support of the mandibular process and precursor to various adult structures, including the malleus of the middle ear in mammals.

Mesenchyme: Embryonic connective tissue. Also, migrating cells formed from mesoderm and neural crest that travel in the embryo to form various tissue types and organs.

Mesoderm: Middle germ layer which gives rise to muscle, connective tissue, and various organs.

Metamerism: Body segmentation.

Midgut: The portion of the primitive gut directly continuous with the yolk sac within the yolk stalk.

Nasal process: A prominence produced by invagination of the nasal placode consisting of the *medial* and *lateral* nasal processes destined to participate in formation of the upper lip and jaw..

Nasal (olfactory) placode: Ectodermal aggregations that appear on the lateral surface of the frontonasal process whose invagination leads to formation of the nasal processes and the nares (nostrils).

Neural crest: Cells and cellular aggregates derived from the dorsal lip of the neural tube which possess the capacity to form multiple tissue types.

Neural tube: Dorsal midline cylindrical structure formed from invagination and fusion of the neural plate which gives rise to the central nervous system, i.e., brain and spinal cord.

Neurocranium: That part of the skull enclosing the brain and forming the cranial case.

Neuropores: Transient openings at the anterior (cephalic) and posterior (caudal) poles of the forming neural tube.

Neurulation: Process which gives rise to the neural plate and neural tube.

Notochord: Longitudinal central rod of tissue arising from the primitive node and extending cranially in the midplane of the embryo. It provides axial support of the early embryo, induces development of the neural tube, and influences somite organization and development of the vertebral column.

Oropharyngeal membrane: Name applied to the prechordal plate after formation of the head fold. This is a transient structure that separates the embryonic mouth (stomodeum) from the pharynx.

Otic placode: Ectodermal surface aggregation that appears above the second pharyngeal cleft which ultimately forms the inner ear and its components.

Palatal fold or process: A prominence that participates in formation of the palate.

Paraxial mesoderm: Germ layer that forms during gastrulation that lies intermediate between outer ectoderm and inner endoderm and lateral to the neural tube and notochord.

Pharyngeal arches: Complex of segmental structures that form the ventrolateral walls of the embryonic pharynx. Five paired arches occur in human embryos, each of which gives rise to definitive adult structures found in the head and neck.

Pharyngeal cleft (groove): An ectodermal invagination that separates each pharyngeal arch externally.

Pharyngeal pouch: An evagination or outpocketing of the pharyngeal endodermal lining and lumen that separates each pharyngeal arch internally.

Placode: Ectodermal aggregates involved in development of the special sense organs and certain cranial nerve components.

Prechordal plate: Bilaminar plaque-like unit of adherent ectoderm and endoderm that marks the anterior pole of the embryo and site of the future embryonic mouth or stomodeum.

Primitive streak: Dorsal midline, axial structure that is a conduit for formation of the mesoderm, endoderm, and notochord.

Pterygoquadrate cartilage or bar: Initial skeletal support of the maxillary process and precursor to the incus of the middle ear in mammals.

Reichert's cartilage: Initial skeletal support of the hyoid or second pharyngeal arch which forms various adult structures, including the stapes of the middle ear.

Rhombomeres: Segments formed in the embryonic hind brain (rhombencephalon) that are associated with the formation of several cranial nerves and the neural crest.

Somites: Dorsal segments of the paraxial mesoderm which give rise to skeletal muscle, the vertebral column, and parts of the dermis.

Stomodeum: The embryonic mouth that forms anterior to the prechordal plate (oropharyngeal membrane).

Tuberculum impar: A midline swelling in the floor of the pharynx located between the paired lingual swellings.

Viscerocranium: That part of the skull associated with the jaws, hyoid apparatus, and larynx.

Yolk sac: A fetal membrane whose proximal portion is absorbed into the body of the embryo to form the primitive gut.

Yolk stalk: The connection between the yolk sac and the ventral body of the embryo.

Chapter 3 Tooth Development

Martyn T. Cobourne[1] and Paul T. Sharpe[2]

[1]Department of Orthodontics, Dental Institute, King's College London
[2]Department of Craniofacial Development and Stem Cell Biology, Dental Institute, King's College London; Guy's Hospital

Teeth are unique and unusual organs in many respects. In humans, they are nonessential, but in all other animal species they are absolutely required for survival. In addition, their preservation in the fossil record makes them indispensable for understanding mammalian and in particular human evolution. Most interestingly, however, is the fact that teeth do not function as independent organs but only together, as a multi-organ unit or dentition, which is characteristic for each particular species. The essential processes underlying early tooth formation have been understood for some years; however, more recently scientists have begun to elucidate how teeth are formed at the molecular level.

This chapter will describe the essential histological processes associated with development of the tooth and provide some background with regard to the molecular mechanisms that control these processes. In addition, anomalies associated with tooth number that can occur in the human dentition are described.

The histology of tooth development

The first morphological evidence of tooth development occurs at around six weeks *in utero*, with the formation of a localized thickening or **primary epithelial band** in the epithelium of the putative upper and lower jaws. This thickening forms a continuous horseshoe-shaped sheet of epithelium around the lateral margins of the developing oral cavity. During the next week of development, the free margin of this band gives rise to two processes, which proliferate and invaginate into the underlying mesenchyme (Figure 3.1).

- The outer process or **vestibular lamina** is destined to degenerate and form the vestibule that demarcates the cheeks and lips from the tooth-bearing regions.

- The inner process or **dental lamina** will form the **tooth buds**.

Development of the coronal tissues

Rapid proliferation of discrete regions within the dental lamina produces a series of bud-like invaginations into the mesenchyme of the early jaws, with localized condensations of **neural crest-derived ectomesenchymal** cells appearing around the tips of these buds (Figure 3.2). During the late bud stage, the epithelium begins the process of folding, which is marked by formation of the **primary enamel knot**, a group of epithelial cells initially situated at the tip of the bud that act as a discrete, nonproliferating and transient signaling center, intimately involved with the regulation of tooth shape. Folding results in the formation of a cap-shaped **enamel organ** ultimately sitting over the **dental papilla**, which is a condensation of ectomesenchymal cells situated directly below the enamel organ. Further condensation of the papilla produces the **dental follicle**, which begins to encapsulate the epithelial cap-shaped enamel organ. Together, the enamel organ, dental papilla, and dental follicle constitute the **tooth germ** and will give rise to the essential structures of the tooth: the **enamel, dentin-pulp complex,** and **periodontium**, respectively. In multi-cusped teeth, such as premolars and molars, following the disappearance of the primary enamel knot, new **secondary enamel knots** form at the sites of the future cusp tips. These secondary enamel knots mark the first signs of a species-specific

Fundamentals of Oral Histology and Physiology, First Edition. Arthur R. Hand and Marion E. Frank.
© 2014 John Wiley & Sons, Inc. Published 2014 by John Wiley & Sons, Inc.

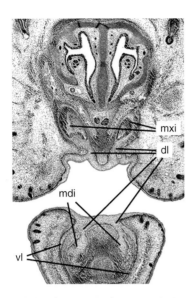

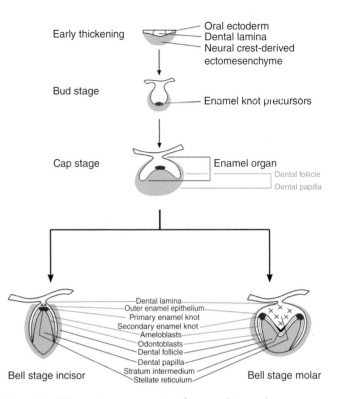

Figure 3.1   Early tooth development in the mouse incisor region. The maxillary and mandibular incisor tooth buds have formed (mxi and mdi, respectively) and are connected to the oral epithelium by the dental lamina (dl). In the lower jaw, the vestibular lamina (vl) is also clearly visible lateral to the tooth bud (hematoxylin and eosin).

Figure 3.2   Schematic representation of mammalian tooth development. An early thickening of the oral epithelium gives rise to the tooth bud, which, following signaling mediated by the enamel knot, subsequently folds to form a cap stage tooth germ. The tooth germ consists of (1) the enamel organ, which is derived from ectoderm and will form the enamel of the tooth crown and (2) the dental papilla and follicle, which are derived from neural crest cells and will form the remainder of the tooth, including the dentin, root, and periodontal tissues. At the late cap stage, further folding of the enamel organ establishes future cusp shape as the tooth enters the bell stage. During the bell stage, specific populations of cells differentiate prior to hard tissue formation.

cusp pattern and herald the bell stage of tooth development. During this stage, the tooth germ undergoes a period of differential proliferation and histodifferentiation, whereby cells begin to differentiate into discrete regional structures (Figures 3.2 and 3.3). At the same time, the dental lamina begins to break down, separating the developing tooth from the oral epithelium.

At the late bell stage, cells of the innermost layer of the enamel organ, the **inner enamel epithelium**, stop dividing and elongate. These changes preempt a reversal of polarity in these cells, and they very rapidly induce adjacent neural crest-derived cells of the dental papilla to differentiate into **odontoblasts**. Odontoblasts first appear at the sites of the future cusp tips and are responsible for secretion and mineralization of the **dentin** matrix as they differentiate along the length of the dental papilla adjacent to the internal enamel epithelium. Dentin formation is preceded by the formation of **predentin**, with this first layer acting as a signal to the overlying inner enamel epithelial cells to differentiate into **ameloblasts** and begin secreting the enamel matrix. The odontoblasts migrate in an apical direction and lay down coronal dentin, while ameloblasts migrate in a coronal direction and deposit enamel of the tooth crown (Figure 3.4).

Teeth develop from two fundamental tissue populations, the oral epithelium and neural crest-derived ectomesenchyme. In the mature tooth, enamel is derived from epithelium, whereas the dentin, pulp, and periodontium are derived from the neural crest.

While these changes are taking place in the inner enamel epithelium, other regions of cellular differentiation also become apparent within the enamel organ. Around the periphery and confluent with the inner enamel epithelium at the cervical loop are the cuboidal cells of the **outer enamel epithelium**, which are thought to provide support to the tooth germ during hard tissue formation. Within the

enamel organ, the star-shaped cells of the **stellate reticulum** are also thought to provide support and turgor to the enamel organ during amelogenesis. The maintenance of cell-cell contacts and presence of large fluid-filled spaces between these cells would seem to play a role in maintenance of coronal shape. In addition, situated adjacent to the inner enamel epithelium and stellate reticulum are the flattened cells of the **stratum intermedium**, which are thought to facilitate amelogenesis, although their precise function is unknown.

Development of the root

At the margins of the enamel organ the cells of the inner enamel epithelium are confluent with the outer enamel epithelium at the **cervical loop**. Growth of these cells in an apical direction between the dental papilla internally and the dental follicle externally forms a skirt-like sheet of cells known as **Hertwig's epithelial root sheath**, which maps out the future root morphology of the developing tooth and induces the further differentiation of odontoblasts within adjacent regions of the dental papilla. In single-rooted teeth, the sheath forms a simple skirt; however, in multi-rooted teeth such as the molars, the sheath contains horizontal extensions which

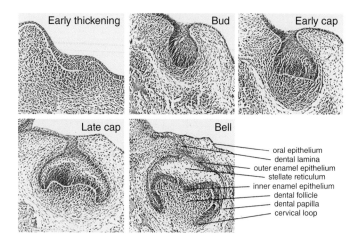

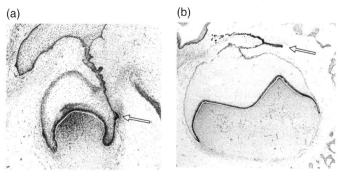

Figure 3.5   Successional teeth form via localized proliferation within the dental lamina associated with each primary tooth germ (a, arrow). Accessional teeth form as a posterior extension of the dental lamina (b, arrow) (hematoxylin and eosin). (Courtesy of Dr. Barry Berkovitz.)

Figure 3.3   The essential histology of early tooth development. The first morphological sign occurs with the appearance of a localized thickening or early dental lamina within the oral epithelium. Rapid proliferation of this region results in formation of the tooth bud, with localized condensation of neural-crest-derived ectomesenchymal cells forming the dental papilla. Folding of the early bud results in first the cap and then bell stages, with progressive histodifferentiation within the bell ultimately producing the various cell populations that are required to generate the specific hard tissues that are found in the mature tooth. These sections show molar tooth development in the mouse, taking place between embryonic days 12 (early thickening) through to 15.5 (bell stage) (hematoxylin and eosin).

partition off regions within the dental papilla and map out the individual roots. Rapid degeneration of the root sheath leads to the exposure of cells within the dental follicle to newly formed root dentin and differentiation of these mesenchymal cells into **cementoblasts**, which begin to deposit cementum onto the root surface. Surrounding the enamel organ, the outer cells of the dental follicle begin to produce the alveolar bone and collagen fibers of the periodontium, which ultimately will anchor the tooth into its bony socket within the jaw. The developing tooth remains housed in this cavity of alveolar bone until the process of eruption begins (Figure 3.4).

Successional and accessional tooth development

Humans have a primary, or deciduous, dentition, which begins eruption at around 6 months of age and is usually complete by 2-1/2 years of age. This is replaced by the secondary, or permanent, dentition, which begins with eruption of the first molars at 6 years of age and is not complete until the third molars erupt (if they are present) during the late teenage years. Within the secondary dentition there are two types of teeth, successional and accessional.

- Successional teeth have primary predecessors and consist of the incisors, canines, and premolars.
- Accessional teeth have no primary precursors and consist of the three secondary molar teeth.

During development of the secondary dentition, successional teeth form on the lingual (or palatal) side of the primary tooth germ as a result of localized proliferation within the dental lamina associated with each primary tooth germ. The accessional teeth form from a backward extension of the original dental lamina (Figure 3.5).

Chronology of human tooth development

Tooth development begins in the human embryo at around 6 weeks of development, with the appearance of the primary epithelial band within the early jaw primordia. This is followed a week later by the initiation of odontogenesis and by 11 weeks, the primary tooth germs have reached the early cap stage (Figure 3.6). The bell stage is reached at around 14 weeks of

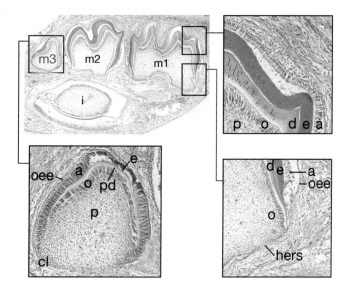

Figure 3.4   Hard tissue formation in the crown and root. During the late bell stage, cells within the inner enamel epithelium of the enamel organ differentiate into preameloblasts (a). This process, in turn, results in the differentiation of odontoblasts (o) within adjacent cells of the dental papilla (p) and the formation of, first, predentin (pd) and then dentin (d). The preameloblasts then become secretory ameloblasts and secrete enamel matrix (e). At the cervical loop (c), cells of the inner and outer enamel epithelium (oee) grow downwards as Hertwig's epithelial root sheath (hers) to map out the future root. At 10 days of postnatal life in the mouse, the incisor (i) and molar dentitions (m1-3) are at different stages of development. The first molar (m1) is at the early stage of root development, while the second molar has just completed crown development. In the third molar (m3), early hard tissue formation is occurring within the crown (hematoxylin and eosin).

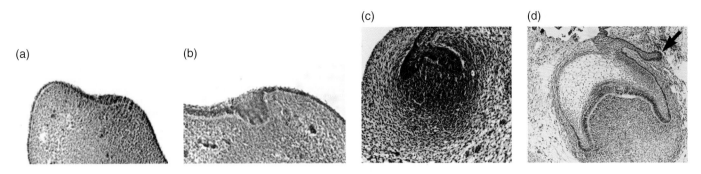

Figure 3.6 Histology of human tooth development. (a) Early thickening; (b) Bud stage; (c) Cap stage; (d) Bell stage (note early development of the successional tooth germ, arrow) (hematoxylin and eosin). (Courtesy of Dr. Ana Angelova.)

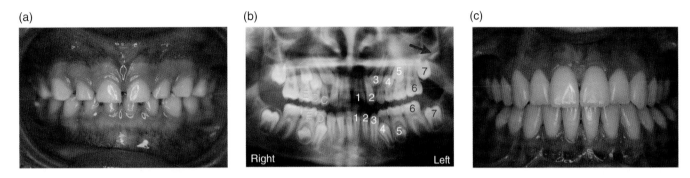

Figure 3.7 The primary (deciduous), mixed and secondary (permanent) human dentitions. (a) The primary dentition of a 4-year-old boy; (b) Panoramic radiograph of the mixed dentition in a 10-year-old girl. Arch development is symmetrical, with the exception of a solitary, early developing third molar in the upper left quadrant (red arrow). On the left, successional and accessional teeth of the secondary dentition are identified in white and red, respectively. Primary teeth are identified on the right in pale blue (note that all the premolars [4, 5], the upper permanent canines [3] and all second permanent molars [7] are unerupted and that the lower primary canines [C] have been exfoliated; (c) Permanent dentition in a 30-year-old woman.

intrauterine development, with hard tissue formation beginning at around week 16. At this stage, the first secondary tooth germs begin to appear, with the successional incisors and accessional first molars beginning their development. At birth, calcification of the primary dentition is well underway, with coronal development complete in all these teeth by the age of 1. In addition, the first evidence of secondary tooth calcification (associated with the first molars) is usually seen at birth. During the first few years of life, the primary dentition erupts, with root formation being complete by the age of 3. Thus, from this age the primary dentition is regarded as complete.

The first molars of the secondary dentition normally have completed their coronal development by 3 years of age and will erupt around the age of 6 years. Their root development is not complete until around 10 years of age, and during this time the secondary incisor dentition will have erupted and replaced the primary teeth. From the age of 10 to 12 years, the canine, premolar, and then second molar teeth will erupt, with root formation completed at around 16 years. Finally, the third molars, which began their development during postnatal life and only began their coronal calcification at around 10 years of age, will erupt during the late teenage years, although these teeth are often absent or simply fail to erupt at all. All root development in the secondary dentition is usually complete by the mid 20s (Figure 3.7).

> Development of the human dentition begins at around 6 weeks in utero with formation of the primary tooth buds and is not complete until around 20 years of age, with eruption of the third molars or wisdom teeth.

The biology of early tooth development

The development of the mammalian dentition can be considered to involve a sequence of closely related events.

- **Initiation** is the process that determines those sites along the oral axis where teeth are destined to form.

- **Patterning** of the dentition is responsible for determining the type of tooth, for example incisor or molar, that will form within a specific region.

- **Morphogenesis** ultimately generates a tooth with characteristic shape.

Initiation essentially links patterning with morphogenesis, but integral to all three of these mechanisms is **differentiation**, whereby the constituent epithelial and mesenchymal cells of the tooth germ ultimately form the specific structures of the adult tooth.

Embryonic origins of the dental tissues

The basic histology of mammalian tooth development demonstrates that this process derives from two principal cell types within the early jaws, **epithelium** and **neural crest-derived ectomesenchyme**. The epithelium is ultimately derived from the **epiblast** of the early embryo, and mammalian fate mapping studies have suggested that this component of the developing tooth is derived from ectoderm; however, in other species such as fish and reptiles teeth can develop within the pharynx from endoderm.

Mesenchyme of the early jaws is predominantly composed of cells derived from the cranial neural crest. The vertebrate neural crest is a pluripotent cell population, derived from the lateral ridges of the neural plate during early embryogenesis. Neural crest cells disperse from the dorsal surface of the neural tube and migrate extensively throughout the embryo, giving rise to a wide variety of differentiated cell types. Cranial neural crest-derived ectomesenchyme contributes to the formation of condensed dental mesenchyme at the initial bud stage and subsequently to formation of the dental papilla and follicle in the developing tooth germ. Genetic fate mapping studies have demonstrated a cranial neural crest origin for odontoblasts, dentin matrix, pulp tissue, cementum, and the periodontal ligament of mature teeth (Figure 3.8).

How the dentition is patterned

In the mammalian dentition the teeth form a series of homologous structures whose differences along the jaw axis can be described in terms of changes in shape and size. Based upon the analysis of adult dentition, two classic theories have been proposed to account for the developmental mechanisms responsible for patterning this axis (Figure 3.9).

Butler (1967) proposed that a simple morphogenetic field determined tooth shape. In this regional field theory all the tooth primordia were proposed to be initially equivalent, the shapes that the teeth ultimately develop into being controlled by substances or signals generated elsewhere in the jaw primordia. These signals would have a graded concentration along the developing jaw axis, such that each tooth primordium developed

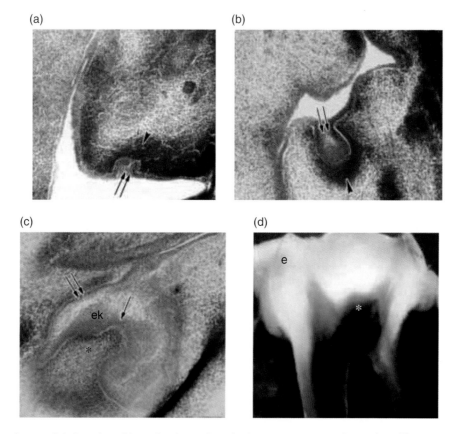

Figure 3.8   A cranial neural crest origin for odontoblasts, dentin matrix, pulp tissue, cementum and periodontal ligament. Recently, Chai and colleagues have used the expression of a *Wnt1* reporter gene as a genetic marker to follow neural crest migration and differentiation in the mouse. All cranial neural crest cells destined for the early jaws are ultimately derived from *Wnt1*-expressing cells in the central nervous system. These investigators generated mice exhibiting ubiquitous expression of a *lacZ reporter* in neural crest precursors (blue color), which allowed staining and identification of these cells at all stages of tooth development. This experiment has definitively demonstrated a cranial neural crest cell contribution to the developing dental papilla and follicle. Arrows indicate the epithelial component of the tooth germ, while the arrowheads indicate neural crest-derived cells. (a) Dental lamina (arrows) and dental mesenchyme (arrowhead); (b) Early bud stage (arrows), dental mesenchyme (arrowhead) (c) Cap stage, inner enamel epithelium (single arrow), outer enamel epithelium (double arrow), enamel knot (ek), dental papilla (*); (d) Adult maxillary molar; enamel (e), dentin and pulp (*). (Reproduced and adapted with permission from Y. Chai, X. Jiang, Y. Ito, et al. (2000) Fate of the mammalian cranial neural crest during tooth and mandibular morphogenesis. *Development* 127, 1671–1679. [http://dev.biologists.org])

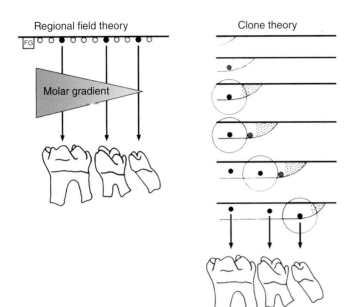

Regional field theory

Clone theory

Molar gradient

Figure 3.9 Regional field and clone theories of dental patterning. According to the regional field theory, identical tooth primordia (black dots) are acted upon by a morphogenetic substance (orange shading) generated by a field generator (FG). The substance has a graded concentration in the field, which results in each primordium (black dots) developing into a specific tooth (in this case, a molar) with a different morphology. According to the clone theory, the gradient of final tooth form is related to the times at which tooth primordia (black dots) are initiated. The stippled region represents the growing margin of the clone with an associated zone of inhibition (circle). The red dots represent tissues that have reached the critical stage to form a new primordium. (Adapted from Lumsden, 1979.)

differently according to its position relative to the source of the signal. However, within this theory the generation of the primary pattern of the dentition, or the initial primordia themselves, is not accounted for. In contrast, Osborne (1978) suggested a clone model, whereby all the teeth are suggested to develop from a single clone of mesenchymal cells. This mesenchymal clone grows to form the individual teeth in sequence. Thus, ectomesenchyme enters the jaw and, following interaction with the oral epithelium, a clone of cells is established for a specific tooth class. The clone grows forward or backward within the jaw, but surrounding each newly initiated tooth primordium is a region of inhibition, which prevents the formation of a second primordium. Once the growing clone has escaped this region of inhibition, a new primordium is initiated. Gradients of tooth shape are related to the sequence in which they are initiated, successive mitoses of the clone gradually altering the shape potential of newly initiated primordia. The fundamental principle of the clone theory, unlike the regional field theory, is that the shape of the tooth is determined from the moment its primordium has been initiated. The initiation of primordia is a prerequisite of both theories and this is a property of the oral epithelium. Isolated presumptive first molar tissue can give rise to all three molar teeth in their normal sequence when transplanted. These findings are consistent with a region of epithelium specifying a zone of ectomesenchymal cells which could subsequently spread

out posteriorly and lay down the pattern of the future molar dentition and is supportive of the clone model.

Ultimately, both the field and clone theories are fundamentally descriptive. They provide theoretical models for the mechanisms that might be involved in patterning the dentition. In recent years these mechanisms have begun to be dissected at the genetic level. With advances in the understanding of the genetics of tooth development, both the field and clone theories have become largely redundant. However, the initiation of the tooth primordia, a fundamental prerequisite of both theories, has been demonstrated to be an inherent property of the epithelium.

Signaling between tooth-forming epithelium and mesenchyme

The process of odontogenesis is characterized by numerous interactions that take place between the epithelial and connective tissue components of the developing tooth. These interactions have been elucidated by tissue recombination experiments and are reciprocal, being required at numerous stages of the developmental process. Neither tissue is able to support tooth development in isolation. The key stages include the following.

- Interaction between odontogenic epithelium and neural crest-derived ectomesenchyme of the jaws during the initiation of tooth development, which ensures that teeth form in the correct region of the jaws.
- At the bud stage of development, interactions between the epithelium and dental papilla direct the process of morphogenesis, ensuring that teeth of the correct form develop at the appropriate position within the dentition.
- At the bell stage, reciprocal interactions between the inner enamel epithelium and dental papilla direct the processes of hard tissue formation within the early crown of the tooth.

> Tooth development relies upon a series of interactions between the epithelial and mesenchymal components of the tooth germ. These interactions are mediated by molecular signaling and are reciprocal, occurring repetitively during initiation, morphogenesis and hard tissue formation.

Initiation of tooth development

A fundamental question that arises is where the instructive capacity for initiating the formation of a tooth resides. Experiments recombining oral and non-oral tissues have demonstrated that only neural crest-derived cells are able to participate in mammalian tooth development, but they only express their odontogenic potential when combined with the appropriate jaw epithelium (Figure 3.10).

- Specifically, up to the early bud stage, only oral epithelium is able to initiate tooth development, but it has to be combined with neural crest cells.
- Non-oral epithelium is unable to initiate tooth development in any neural crest cell populations.

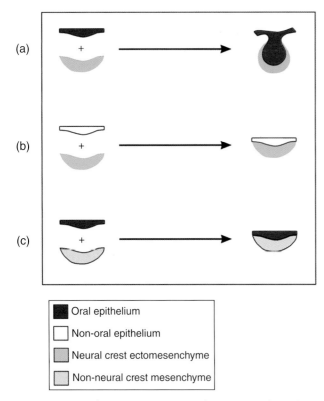

Oral epithelium

Non-oral epithelium

Neural crest ectomesenchyme

Non-neural crest mesenchyme

Figure 3.10 Recombination experiments demonstrate that prior to the bud stage oral epithelium is responsible for initiating tooth development but neural crest-derived ectomesenchyme also is needed. (a) In the embryo, oral epithelium and neural crest-derived ectomesenchyme combine to generate a tooth. (b) The recombination of non-oral epithelium with neural crest-derived ectomesenchyme does not result in tooth formation. (c) The recombination of oral epithelium with non-neural crest derived mesenchyme does not result in tooth formation.

Tooth morphogenesis

Recombination experiments also have demonstrated the dominance of neural crest-derived ectomesenchyme in the specification of tooth shape, once tooth development has been initiated (Figure 3.11).

- At the bud stage, the recombination of molar epithelium with incisor dental papilla will result in the formation of an incisor.
- Similarly, the recombination of incisor epithelium with molar dental papilla at the same stage will produce a molar tooth.

These experiments support an inductive role for dental mesenchyme from the bud stage of development and demonstrate that from this stage the ultimate shape of the tooth is a product of the mesenchymal component of the tooth germ.

Taken together, recombination experiments have indicated the following.

- Prior to the bud stage of tooth development, the capacity for tooth initiation resides within the oral epithelium.
- At the bud stage of development, odontogenic potential switches and the underlying mesenchyme then possesses the capacity to dictate shape.

It is only relatively recently that a molecular explanation for these findings has begun to be elucidated.

> Oral epithelium is responsible for initiating the process of tooth development; whereas the information required to impart shape is established in the neural crest-derived ectomesenchyme of the tooth germ from the bud stage.

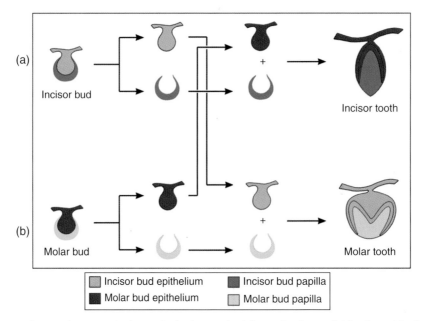

Incisor bud epithelium   Incisor bud papilla

Molar bud epithelium   Molar bud papilla

Figure 3.11 Recombination experiments demonstrate that at the bud stage the information for tooth identity resides in the dental papilla. (a) The recombination of an incisor tooth bud with a molar dental papilla results in the formation of a molar tooth. (b) The recombination of a molar tooth bud with an incisor dental papilla results in the formation of an incisor tooth.

The molecular control of early tooth development

The advent of modern molecular biology has permitted investigators to begin the process of uniting early experimental observations relating to development of the mammalian dentition with the control processes that occur at the gene level. Significant progress has been made over the last decade, and the tooth is proving to be an excellent model not only for the understanding of odontogenesis but also the general mechanisms involved in many aspects of development.

Controlling tooth shape

All teeth follow essentially the same basic developmental program; what clearly distinguishes them from all other organs is that they can form widely different shapes, which vary according to their position within the dentition. Thus, although classed as a single "organ," different tooth types (shapes) follow distinct pathways of morphogenesis. The form and function of the human (and some other mammalian) dentitions are additionally complicated by various mechanisms of tooth renewal. Humans renew their dentition once, when children's primary (or deciduous) teeth are completely replaced by adult secondary (or permanent) teeth, forming a new dentition. This is an evolutionary adaptation to changes in diet and increases in jaw size that accompany juvenile development. In some animals teeth are continuously replaced throughout life, while others have no tooth replacement. This almost infinite variety between different dentitions is directly related to evolutionary adaptation and survival, since changes in the dentition allow for different modes of feeding and diet.

Our current understanding of the molecular control of tooth development comes largely from studies of mouse first molar development. The vast majority of genes and processes identified appear common for different tooth types. However, the mechanisms of genetic regulation related to the formation of specific crown shapes (pattern formation and morphogenesis) are poorly understood.

Positional specification

Mammalian teeth develop along the margins of the oral cavity at specific positions within a thickened band of oral epithelium. What determines the position of this odontogenic-competent epithelium or dental lamina is not known; however, interactions between the **Wnt** and **Hedgehog** molecular signaling pathways appear to play a role in determining the sites of tooth bud formation, although this picture has become complicated by the discovery within the mouse dentition of rudimentary epithelial buds that do not form teeth. **Sonic hedgehog** *Shh* signaling stimulates dental epithelial cell proliferation and thus sites of localized *Shh* expression mark the positions of tooth bud formation. *Wnt7b* is expressed throughout the developing oral epithelium, but is excluded from the sites of *Shh* expression (Figure 3.12) and when experimentally mis-expressed, results in repression of *Shh* expression and arrest of tooth development. Since Wnt-Hedgehog interactions were originally discovered during insect (*Drosophila*) larval segmentation, it is tempting to equate the specification of tooth bud position as "segmentation" of the oral epithelium into regions of tooth versus non-tooth.

It is well established from studies of murine odontogenesis that Wnt signaling in the oral epithelium itself also plays an important role during the initiation of odontogenesis. Inhibition

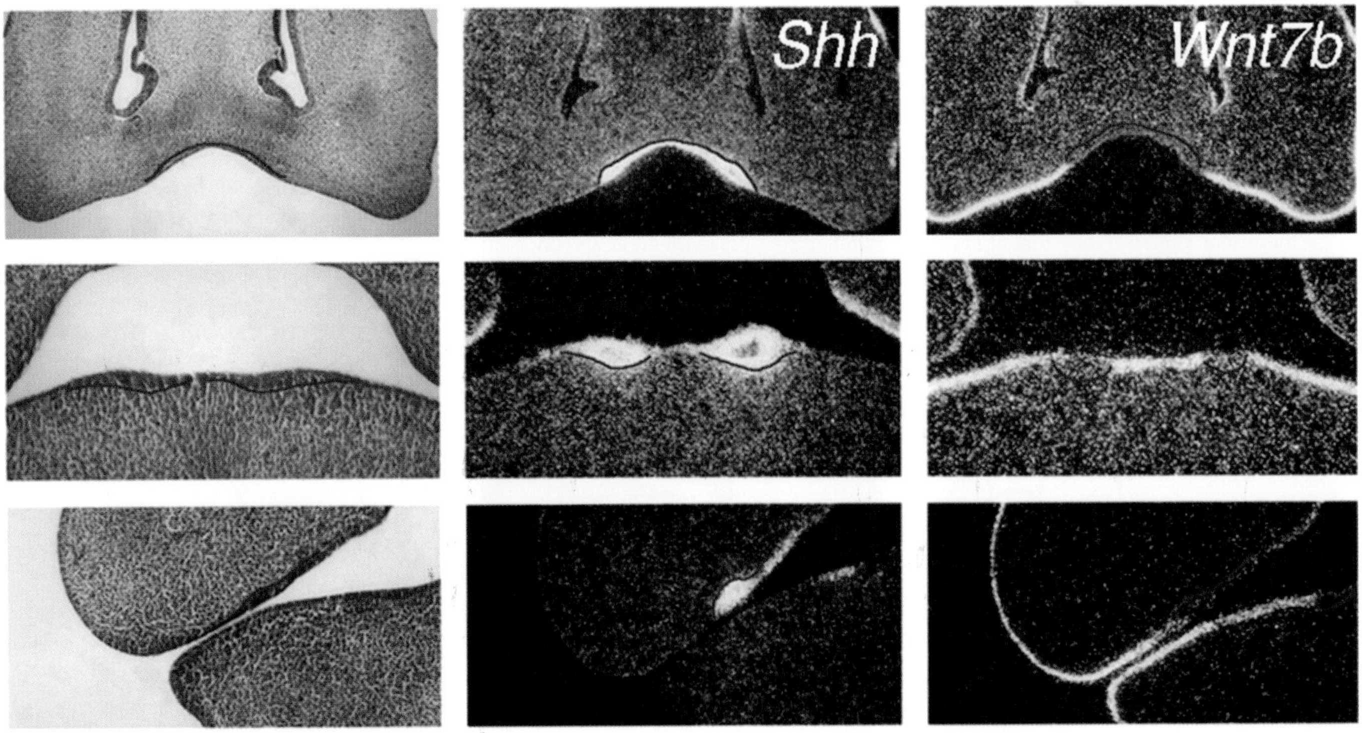

Figure 3.12   In the early mouse jaws (left panels), *Shh* is expressed in the incisor and molar tooth-forming epithelium (middle panels), while *Wnt7b* is expressed throughout the oral epithelium but absent from the tooth-forming regions (right panels). The red lines demarcate the tooth-forming epithelium from the underlying mesenchyme. (*In situ* hybridization carried out on adjacent frontal sections through the developing jaws.)

of this pathway arrests tooth development prior to the bud stage; while increased signaling, through transgenic overexpression of **β-catenin**, produces significant numbers of odontome-like supernumerary teeth.

Mice have a reduced dentition compared to the human formula (two incisors, one canine, two premolars, and three molars in the secondary dentition [I_2, C_1, PM_2, M_3]), having only one incisor and three molar teeth (I_1, M_3). Although in many respects this is fortunate in that it has made the study of tooth shape specification in mice relatively simple, the recent identification of rudimentary tooth bud formation has complicated what we understand regarding the initiation of first molar development. Rudimentary tooth buds are found on both the developing mandible and maxilla in positions that suggest they are remnants of teeth lost during mouse evolution and correspond to premolars and possibly canines. Although these rudiments never progress beyond the bud stage their initiation by expression of *Shh* and other molecules makes identification of the first molar bud complicated (Figure 3.13) and suggests that in many studies the first molar buds may have been incorrectly identified.

Recombination experiments between molar and incisor epithelium and mesenchyme identified the mesenchyme into which the epithelial buds invaginate as possessing the information that specifies crown shape. This implies that the mesenchyme in different regions of the early jaw primordia contains the positional information to specify the pathways of morphogenesis followed by individual tooth buds. Clues to the molecular basis of this positional information come from the expression of transcription factors; in particular, **homeobox genes**. Prior to epithelial invagination, several homeobox genes show spatially restricted expression patterns in jaw primordia mesenchyme (Figure 3.14). These domains have been interpreted as providing cells with a homeobox "code" that

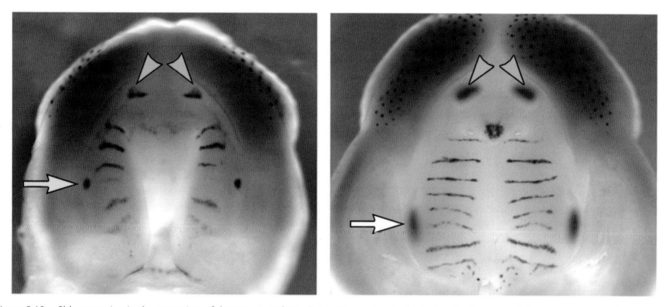

Figure 3.13   *Shh* expression in the upper jaw of the mouse embryo. Expression is seen in the incisor teeth anteriorly (green arrowheads) and initially in a vestigial molar tooth bud (yellow arrow). This expression is subsequently lost as the vestigial teeth fail to develop; however, expression is seen approximately one day later in the enamel knot of the definitive first molar (white arrow). Note *Shh* expression also in the developing palatal rugae (horizontal stripes) (Whole mount *in situ* hybridization courtesy of Dr. Andrew Economou).

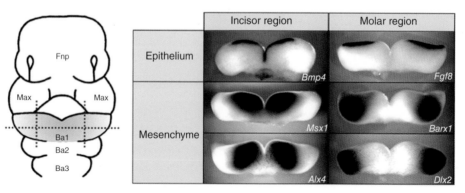

Figure 3.14   Gene expression in the early mouse mandible. Prior to any morphological sign of tooth development, *Bmp4* and *Fgf8* are transcribed in the incisor and molar epithelium, respectively. In the underlying mesenchyme, different homeobox gene combinations are switched on in these regions and these are thought to program subsequent tooth shape. In the midline incisor region at the front of the arch, *Msx1* and *Alx4* are expressed, while in the molar regions more posteriorly *Barx1* and *Dlx2* are expressed (Whole mount *in situ* hybridization.) (Courtesy of Dr. Isabelle Miletich.)

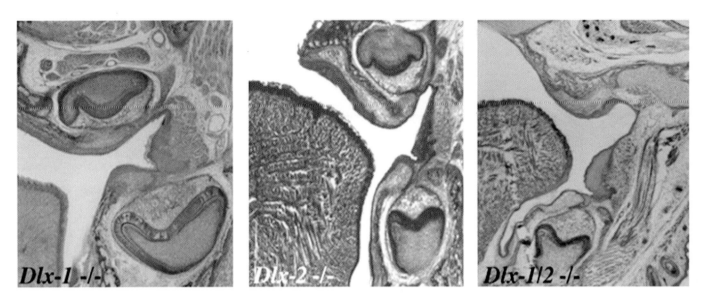

Figure 3.15   Tooth development is normal in *Dlx1* and *Dlx2* mutant mice, but loss of both genes results in a complete failure of maxillary molar development. (Courtesy of Dr. Bethan Thomas.)

determines the pathways of tooth morphogenesis. For example, *Dlx1* and *Dlx2* are co-expressed in mesenchyme at the back of the early jaws, corresponding to the positions where molar teeth will develop. *Dlx1/2* double mutant mice show a failure of maxillary molar formation, consistent with a specific role for these genes in molar development (Figure 3.15). *Barx1* is similarly expressed in mesenchymal cells corresponding to the sites of first molar development, and ectopic expression of *Barx1* in future incisor mesenchymal cells results in development of teeth with molar characteristics. The assumption from these experiments is that the expression of homeobox genes in the mesenchyme provides the instructions that direct crown morphogenesis, although nothing is currently known regarding how this happens (Figure 3.16). As tooth buds begin to form, these expression domains are lost and replaced by expression of many of the same homeobox genes in the condensing mesenchyme around the buds. Significantly, with one exception, expression is no longer confined to specific tooth types; rather these genes are expressed in the mesenchyme of all tooth buds. The one exception is *Barx1*, which is only expressed in molar tooth bud mesenchyme and is never expressed at any time during incisor development.

Morphogenesis

Morphogenesis is the process by which form is generated. In the case of teeth, this can be considered the formation of crown and root shape. The physical processes involve folding of dental epithelium, which begins from the cap stage onwards. Currently, most information is available for the mechanisms that control crown morphogenesis.

The first molecular signals involved in tooth morphogenesis are detected at the bud stage and the bud to cap transition is a key checkpoint in tooth development. This expression is induced by signals from the condensing mesenchyme, in particular *Bmp4* (Figure 3.17). The regulation of *Bmp4* expression

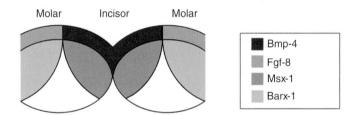
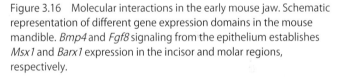

Figure 3.16   Molecular interactions in the early mouse jaw. Schematic representation of different gene expression domains in the mouse mandible. *Bmp4* and *Fgf8* signaling from the epithelium establishes *Msx1* and *Barx1* expression in the incisor and molar regions, respectively.

in the bud mesenchyme involves two homeobox transcription factors that physically interact, *Msx1* and *Pax9*. The exact mechanism of regulation of *Bmp4* transcription is not fully understood, since *Msx1* is a transcriptional repressor. However, the establishment of *Msx1* and *Pax9* expression in ectomesenchyme of the tooth bud is essential for tooth development to progress to the cap stage; mice mutant for either of these genes have arrested tooth development. In molar bud mesenchyme *Barx1* also interacts with *Msx1* and this provides a molecular difference between molar and incisor bud mesenchyme cells that may have a role in morphogenesis.

A key molecular pathway during the transition from bud to cap stage is the induction of *Msx1* expression in the mesenchyme of the tooth germ by *Bmp4* signaling from the epithelium. In turn, reciprocal induction by *Msx1* establishes *Bmp4* expression in the mesenchyme of the bud.

Epithelial folding appears to be coordinated by the enamel knots, with the primary enamel knot existing transiently as a cylindrical rod of low proliferating epithelial cells that is clearly

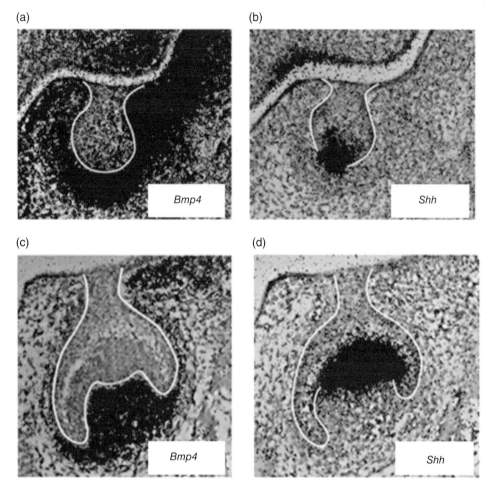

Figure 3.17   Expression of *Bmp4* and *Shh* in the bud (a and b) and cap (c and d) stage tooth germs. *Bmp4* expression becomes established within the condensing ectomesenchyme, while *Shh* is switched on in precursor cells of the enamel knot at the bud stage and becomes established in the primary enamel knot at the cap stage. (Section *in situ* hybridization.) (Courtesy of Dr. Isabelle Miletich.)

visible at the cap stage. Primary enamel knot cells express many signaling factor proteins, including *Shh*, *Wnt*, **fibroblast growth factor (FGF),** and **bone morphogenetic protein (BMP),** which coordinate the transition from bud to cap and initiation of the epithelial folding process. The primary enamel knot is short-lived and its cells are quickly removed by apoptosis. Secondary enamel knots form at the tips of the folding epithelium that marks the future cusps. Significantly, incisors only form a primary enamel knot, suggesting that the formation of secondary knots is an important process in crown morphogenesis.

At the bud stage, the future primary enamel knot cells form at the tip of the buds and can be first detected by expression of *Shh*. This expression also is induced by signals from the condensing mesenchyme, in particular *Bmp4* (Figure 3.17). The expression of *Shh* becomes localized to the enamel knots and this signaling molecule plays a further essential role during subsequent growth and development of the tooth germ.

Clinical correlations

Variation in tooth number is a common developmental anomaly in man and, while not life threatening, these conditions can represent a significant clinical problem in terms of their long-term management.

The incidence of tooth agenesis in human populations has been reported to vary from 1.6% to 9.6% excluding third molars, which are absent in around 20% of individuals. Interestingly, the incidence of missing teeth in the primary dentition is considerably lower, reported to be between 0.5 and 0.9%. Several types of tooth agenesis are recognized in humans (Figure 3.18).

- The absence of six or fewer teeth (excluding third molars) is known as **hypodontia**.
- The absence of more than six teeth (excluding third molars) is known as **oligodontia**.
- These forms of tooth agenesis occur either as an isolated (**nonsyndromic**) condition or in association with a number of clinically recognized **syndromes**.

Nonsyndromic forms of tooth agenesis are relatively common in Caucasians, particularly localized incisor-premolar hypodontia, which often affects only one or two teeth and is seen in up to 8% of the population.

In contrast, **supernumerary teeth** are those present in addition to the normal complement within the dentition. They are generally classified according to morphology (Figure 3.19).

(a)

(b)

(c)

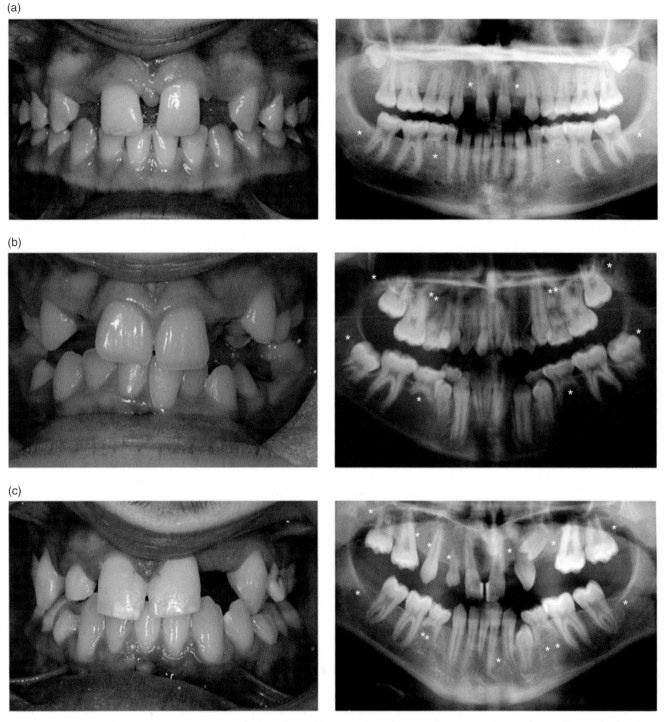

Figure 3.18   Human tooth agenesis. (a) Incisor-premolar hypodontia (the upper lateral incisors, lower second premolars, and lower third molars are absent); (b) Hypodontia (the upper first and second premolars, lower second premolars, and all third molars are absent); (c) Oligodontia (a combination of ten incisor and premolar teeth, and all third molars are absent). (* absent teeth)

- Supplemental supernumeraries have relatively normal size and shape, and resemble teeth within the dentition.
- Rudimentary supernumeraries are small and abnormally shaped, being either conical or tuberculate in their primary morphology.
- Odontomes are hamartomatous malformations containing dental hard tissues of varying levels of organization.

Within Caucasian populations, supernumerary teeth most commonly affect the permanent dentition, being seen in up to 3.2% of the population, predominantly in the anterior maxilla. In the primary dentition, they are less common, occurring in fewer than 1% of the population.

- Multiple supernumerary teeth can also occur as a localized anomaly, but more usually are associated with wider developmental disorders, such as cleft lip and palate, cleidocranial dysplasia, familial adenomatous polyposis, and some other rare syndromes.

> The human dentition can be affected by tooth agenesis or the formation of extra teeth, with these anomalies tending to affect different regions of the dentition. Both are more common in the secondary dentition; however, absent teeth tend to be lateral incisors, second premolars and third molars, whereas supernumerary teeth vary in their morphology, predominating in the anterior maxilla.

The genetics of tooth agenesis

Recent advances in our understanding of the molecular mechanisms involved in murine tooth development have led to the identification of many candidate genes that might be involved in human tooth agenesis. A number of genes and chromosomal locations have now been identified in pedigrees affected by nonsyndromic tooth agenesis (Table 3.1).

Table 3.1   Genetic loci for nonsyndromic tooth agenesis

GENE	Chromosomal location	Expression domain
MSX1	4p16.2	Mesenchyme
PAX9	14q13.3	Mesenchyme
WNT10A	2q35	Epithelium
LTBP3	11q13.1	Mesenchyme
EDA	Xq13.1	Epithelium
EDARADD	1q42-43	Epithelium
AXIN2	17q24.1	Epithelium and mesenchyme

Interestingly, mutations in some of these genes are also known to be responsible for syndromic conditions exhibiting tooth agenesis as a prominent feature. These include *EDA, EDARADD* and *MSX1*, which can all cause forms of ectodermal dysplasia, and *WNT10A*, which causes odonto-onycho-dermal dysplasia.

(a)   (b)

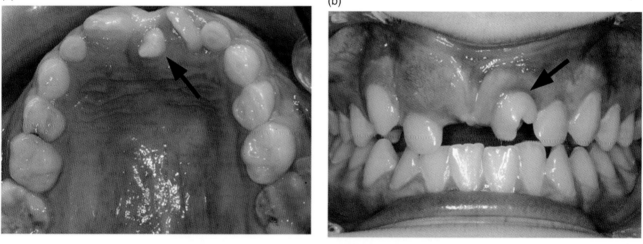

(c)

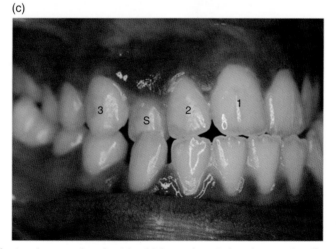

Figure 3.19   Supernumerary teeth affecting the secondary dentition (a) Erupted mesiodens (a conical midline supernumerary, arrow); (b) Erupted tuberculate supernumerary (arrow); (c) Supplemental lateral incisor tooth [S] adjacent to the normal lateral incisor [2].

Among all of the genes identified to date, *MSX1* and *PAX9* are well established as playing a key role in regulating human tooth number. The mutations in these genes that contribute to tooth agenesis are generally loss-of-function and associated with oligodontia, involving third molar agenesis combined with either premolar or molar agenesis, respectively. *MSX1* missense mutations were first identified in a family affected with oligodontia, and these led to **haploinsufficiency** of the protein. A number of mutations in the human *PAX9* gene have been identified in association with variable forms of oligodontia, particularly affecting the molar dentition. Haploinsufficiency of *PAX9* also seems to be the underlying cause of the tooth agenesis in these affected pedigrees.

The precise developmental mechanisms responsible for various forms of tooth agenesis are still only poorly understood. The findings that premolars, lateral incisors, and third molars are frequently affected invites speculation that the timing of their development, being the last teeth within each series to develop, may make them more susceptible to falling below a developmental threshold. Similarly, application of the homeobox code model may explain why some of these genes are responsible for selective tooth absence, as demonstrated in mouse models. However, it should also be remembered that while much of our current knowledge is based upon studies of mouse dentition, significant differences do exist between the two models.

The genetics of supernumerary teeth

The molecular basis of human supernumerary tooth formation also is poorly understood, although a strong genetic influence also underlies this condition. A number of theories exist regarding the developmental basis of supernumerary teeth, including excessive activity of the dental lamina, tooth germ dichotomy, and an evolutionary trend toward reduced tooth number in the mammalian dentition. In recent years a number of candidate genes for human supernumerary teeth have been identified, primarily from mouse mutants exhibiting **vestigial teeth** within their reduced dentition. Many of these mutants have supernumerary premolar or incisor teeth derived from vestigial tooth rudiments, which are initiated in the toothless region adjacent to the incisor and molar fields during normal development and then disappear around the bud stage through apoptosis. Analysis of the vestigial premolar tooth bud in mice has demonstrated complex molecular signaling interactions that ensure this tooth fails to develop beyond the bud stage.

In vestigial tooth buds, a complex molecular interplay seems to exist, acting to restrict development of these teeth primarily through repression of Wnt signaling. The principal targets of Wnt signaling appear to be the Shh and FGF pathways, with Shh in turn then acting as a potential negative mediator of Wnt, and Wnt-mediated FGF induction being tempered through activity of the FGF antagonists Sprouty2 and Sprouty4, both of which are required, at least in part, to prevent the formation of supernumerary premolar teeth in mouse. However, the mechanisms are complex. Mice mutant for Gas1, a putative Shh co-receptor, also have supernumerary premolars, all associated with increased Shh transduction in these early teeth.

> Given the large number of genes that have been identified in the developing tooth germ, it is perhaps somewhat surprising that mutations in relatively few have been identified in association with tooth agenesis or the formation of supernumerary teeth in humans.

Although the human dentition is also reduced in comparison to the ancestral mammalian dental formula of three incisors, one canine, four premolars, and three molars [I_3, C_1, PM_4, M_3], there is no direct evidence that reactivation of vestigial tooth germs is responsible for supernumerary tooth formation. Indeed, in humans the most common supernumerary teeth are associated with the successional incisor and premolar dentitions. However, the human primary maxillary lateral incisor does demonstrate a composite origin, which might go some way to explaining the vulnerability of this region of the dental lamina to supernumerary tooth formation.

References

1. Butler, P.M. (1967) Dental merism and tooth development. *J Dent Res,* 46, 845–850.
2. Chai, Y., Jiang, X., Ito, Y., et al. (2000) Fate of the mammalian cranial neural crest during tooth and mandibular morphogenesis. *Development,* 127, 1671–1679.
3. Dassule, H.R., Lewis, P., Bei, M., et al. (2000) Sonic hedgehog regulates growth and morphogenesis of the tooth. *Development,* 127, 4775–4785.
4. Gritli-Linde, A., Bei, M., Maas, R., et al. (2002) Shh signalling within the dental epithelium is necessary for cell proliferation, growth and polarization. *Development,* 129, 5323–5337.
5. Jarvinen, E., Salazar-Ciudad, I., Birchmeier, W., et al. (2006) Continuous tooth generation in mouse is induced by activated epithelial Wnt/beta-catenin signaling. *Proceedings of the National Academy of Sciences U S A,* 103, 18627–18632.
6. Jernvall, J., Åberg, T., Kettunen, P., et al. (1998) The life history of an embryonic signaling center: BMP-4 induces p21 and is associated with apoptosis in the mouse tooth enamel knot. *Development,* 125, 161–169.
7. Klein, O.D., Minowada, G., Peterkova, R., et al. (2006) Sprouty genes control diastema tooth development via bidirectional antagonism of epithelial-mesenchymal FGF signaling. *Developmental Cell,* 11, 181–190.
8. Kollar, E. J. & Baird, G.R. (1970a) Tissue interactions in embryonic mouse tooth germs: reorganization of the dental epithelium during tooth-germ reconstruction. *J Embryol Exp Morphol,* 24, 159–171.
9. Kollar, E.J. & Baird, G.R. (1970b) Tissue interactions in embryonic mouse tooth germs: the inductive role of the dental papilla. *Journal of Embryology & Experimental Morphology,* 24, 173–186.
10. Lumsden, A. (1979) Pattern formation in the lower molar dentition of the mouse. *Journal de Biologie Buccale,* 7, 77–103.

11. Ohazama, A., Haworth, K.E., Ota, M.S,. et al. (2010) Ectoderm, endoderm, and the evolution of heterodont dentitions. *Genesis*, 48, 382–389.

12. Ohazama, A., Haycraft, C.J., Seppala, M., et al. (2009) Primary cilia regulate Shh activity in the control of molar tooth number. *Development*, 136, 897–903.

13. Peterková, R., Peterka, M., Viriot, L,. et al. (2002) Development of the vestigial tooth primordia as part of mouse odontogenesis. *Connective Tissue Research*, 43, 120–128.

14. Peters, H., Neubuser, A., Kratochwil, K., et al. (1998) Pax9-deficient mice lack pharyngeal pouch derivatives and teeth and exhibit craniofacial and limb abnormalities. *Genes & Development*, 12, 2735–2747.

15. Prochazka, J., Pantalacci, S., Churava, S., et al. (2010) Patterning by heritage in mouse molar row development. *Proceedings of the National Academy of Sciences U S A*, 107, 15497–15502.

16. Rothova, M., Thompson, H., Lickert, H., et al. (2012) Lineage tracing of the endoderm during oral development. *Developmental Dynamics*, 241, 1183–1191.

17. Sarkar, L., Cobourne, M., Naylor, S., et al. (2000) Wnt/Shh interactions regulate ectodermal boundary formation during mammalian tooth development. *Proceedings of the National Academy of Sciences U S A*, 97, 4520–4524.

18. Satokata, I. & Maas, R. (1994) Msx1 deficient mice exhibit cleft palate and abnormalities of craniofacial and tooth development. *Nature Genetics*, 6, 348–356.

19. Stockton, D.W., Das, P., Goldenberg, M., et al. (2000) Mutation of PAX9 is associated with oligodontia. *Nature Genetics*, 24, 18–19.

20. Thomas, B.L., Tucker, A.S., Qui, M., et al. (1997) Role of Dlx-1 and Dlx-2 genes in patterning of the murine dentition. *Development*, 124, 4811–4818.

21. Tucker, A.S., Matthews, K.L., & Sharpe, P.T. (1998) Transformation of tooth type induced by inhibition of BMP signaling. *Science*, 282, 1136–1138.

22. Vainio, S., Karavanova, I., Jowett, A., et al. (1993) Identification of BMP-4 as a signal mediating secondary induction between epithelial and mesenchymal tissues during early tooth development. *Cell*, 75, 45–58.

23. Vastardis, H., Karimbux, N., Guthua, S.W., et al. (1996) A human MSX1 homeodomain missense mutation causes selective tooth agenesis. *Nature Genetics*, 13, 417–421.

Further reading

1. Berkovitz, B.K.B., Holland, G.R., & Moxham, B.J. (2009) Oral Anatomy, Histology and Embryology, 4th edn. Mosby Elsevier, St. Louis.

2. Cobourne, M.T. & Sharpe, P.T. (2003) Tooth and jaw: molecular mechanisms of patterning in the first branchial arch. *Arthives of Oral Biology*, 48, 1–14.

3. Cobourne, M.T. & Sharpe, P.T. (2010) Making up the numbers: The molecular control of mammalian dental formula. *Seminars in Cell & Developmental Biology*, 21, 314–24.

4. Cobourne, M.T. & Sharpe, P.T. (2012) Diseases of the tooth: the genetic and molecular basis of inherited anomalies affecting the dentition. *WIREs Developmental Biology*, 10.1002/wdev.66.

5. Fleming, P.S., Xavier, G.M., DiBiase, A.T., et al. (2010) Revisiting the supernumerary: the epidemiological and molecular basis of extra teeth. *British Dental Journal*, 208, 25–30.

6. Jernvall, J. & Thesleff, I. (2012) Tooth shape formation and tooth renewal: evolving with the same signals. *Development*, 139, 3487–3497.

7. Nanci, A. (2013) Ten Cate's Oral Histology: Development, Structure and Function, 8th edn. Elsevier Mosby, St. Louis.

8. Nieminen, P. (2009) Genetic basis of tooth agenesis. *Journal of Experimental Zoology Part B: Molecular & Developmental Evolution*, 312B, 320–42.

9. Osborne, J.W. (1978) Morphogenetic gradients: fields versus clones. In: Development, Function and Evolution of Teeth (eds. P.M. Butler & K.A. Joysey). London: Academic Press.

10. Sharpe, P.T. (1995) Homeobox genes and orofacial development. *Connective Tissue Research*, 32, 17–25.

11. Ten Cate, A.R. (1995) The experimental investigation of odontogenesis. *International Journal of Developmental Biology*, 39, 5–11.

12. Tucker, A.S. & Sharpe, P. (2004) The cutting edge of mammalian development: how the embryo makes teeth. *Nature Reviews Genetics*, 5, 499–508.

Glossary

Ameloblasts: Enamel-secreting cells derived from the inner enamel epithelium of the enamel organ.

Bone morphogenetic proteins (BMPs): A large family of biological growth factors.

β-catenin: A key protein involved in the intracellular mediation of canonical *Wnt* signaling.

Cementoblasts: Cementum-secreting cells derived from the dental follicle.

Cervical loop: Region of convergence between the inner and outer enamel epithelia, which rapidly proliferates and maps out the early tooth root.

Dental follicle: Neural crest-derived mesenchymal cells which give rise to the cementum and periodontal attachment of the mature tooth.

Dental lamina: Band of epithelial tissue which gives rise to the enamel organ.

Dental papilla: Neural crest-derived mesenchymal cells which give rise to the dentin and pulp of the mature tooth.

Dentin: Specialized mineralized tissue which supports the enamel in the crown and constitutes the bulk of the root of the mature tooth.

Dentin-pulp complex: Region within the mature tooth which includes the pulp and surrounding dentin.

Differentiation: Process whereby a cell becomes a more specialized type.

Enamel: Highly specialized hard tissue which covers the crown of the mature tooth.

Enamel organ: Epithelial component of the tooth germ, which gives rise to the enamel of the tooth crown.

Epiblast: A fundamental tissue within the very early embryo derived from the inner cell mass.

Epithelium: A basic type of tissue that lines surfaces and some cavities of the body.

Fibroblast growth factors (FGFs):   Large family of growth factors involved in multiple processes during embryonic development.

Haploinsufficiency: The presence of only one functional copy of a particular gene.

Hedgehog: Family of intercellular signaling molecules, which in vertebrates includes Sonic hedgehog (*Shh*).

Hertwig's epithelial root sheath: Epithelial derivative of the enamel organ, composed of inner and outer enamel epithelia, which maps out early root architecture.

Homeobox genes: Highly conserved family of genes that encode transcription factors.

Hypodontia: Agenesis of six or less teeth, excluding third molars.

Initiation: Start of the tooth development process.

Inner enamel epithelium: Population of epithelial cells within the enamel organ, which ultimately differentiate into ameloblasts.

LacZ reporter: A reporter gene used by biologists to map the activity of some gene of interest by placing the reporter (which can be easily visualized) under the regulation of that gene. *LacZ* is a gene derived from the bacterium *E. coli*, which encodes the beta-galactosidase enzyme. This enzyme, when present in cells or tissues expressing the gene, causes those cells or tissues to appear blue when they are incubated in a medium that contains a substrate called X-gal.

Morphogenesis: The biological process that establishes shape.

Neural crest-derived ectomesenchyme: Specialized embryonic connective tissue derived from neural crest cells.

Nonsyndromic: Familial disorder, which is not associated with any other phenotypic features.

Odontoblasts: Specialized cells derived from the dental papilla, which secrete dentin.

Oligodontia: Agenesis of six or more teeth, excluding the third molars.

Outer enamel epithelium: Population of epithelial cells extending around the periphery of the enamel organ; thought to provide support during amelogenesis. At the cervical loop they contribute to Hertwig's epithelial root sheath.

Patterning: The biological process that achieves complex cell organization in both time and space.

Periodontium: The supporting structures of the tooth, including the root (dentin and cementum), periodontal ligament, and alveolar bone.

Predentin: The first formed, unmineralized layer of dentin.

Primary enamel knot: A signaling center located within the apical region of the enamel organ responsible for generating primary coronal shape.

Primary epithelial band: Initial thickening of oral epithelium that marks out the tooth-forming regions of the jaws.

Secondary enamel knots: Signaling centers that form in multi-cusped teeth after the primary enamel knot has disappeared, located at the future cusp tips within the apical region of the enamel organ and responsible for generating multiple cusps in the tooth crown.

Sonic hedgehog (Shh):   A vertebrate member of the Hedgehog signaling family, with a key role in many aspects of development.

Stellate reticulum: A population of star-shaped epithelial cells within the enamel organ at the bell stage.

Stratum intermedium: Population of flattened epithelial cells situated adjacent to the inner enamel epithelium that appear during the bell stage.

Supernumerary teeth: Teeth that develop in excess of the normal number within the dentition.

Syndrome: The association of several clinically recognizable features, signs, symptoms, or characteristics that often occur together.

Tooth bud: Initial invagination of tooth-forming epithelium associated with localized condensation of dental papilla.

Tooth germ: The developing embryonic tooth, comprised of the enamel organ, dental papilla, and dental follicle.

Vestibular lamina: Ingrowth of oral epithelium that is destined to degenerate and produce the vestibule between cheek and jaw.

Vestigial teeth: Rudimentary tooth buds that form within the early mouse dentition whose development is destined to be arrested. They are thought to represent teeth that have been lost during evolution.

Wnt: A large network of proteins involved in cell-cell communication.

PART II
THE TEETH

Chapter 4 Enamel

Arthur R. Hand

Department of Craniofacial Sciences and Cell Biology, School of Dental Medicine, University of Connecticut

Enamel is the hard, mineralized tissue that covers the **anatomic crowns** of the teeth. Although the color of enamel generally appears to be white, enamel is relatively translucent and its appearance can be affected by the color of the underlying dentin or adjacent restorations. The formation, composition, and structure of mature enamel are unique. Unlike the other mineralized tissues of the body, bone, dentin, and cementum, which are formed by cells of mesenchymal origin, enamel is formed by epithelial cells. Whereas the formation of dentin and cementum continues after tooth eruption, enamel is completely formed before eruption. Mature enamel is acellular, and its formative cells are lost upon eruption of the tooth. This dictates that enamel repair (except in the case of initial caries lesions; see "Dental Caries" later in this chapter) or replacement, at least at present, must be achieved through the use of non-biological substances.

Enamel structure, composition, and properties

Enamel is the hardest substance in the vertebrate body. Enamel contains about 96% mineral, 2% organic material, and 2% water, by weight. The mineral component, as in all other vertebrate mineralized tissues, is **hydroxyapatite**, $Ca_{10}(PO_4)_6(OH)_2$. Like other mineralized tissues, some of the calcium, phosphate, and hydroxyl ions of the enamel hydroxyapatite crystals may be replaced by other ions. These include strontium, magnesium, carbonate, and fluoride. Technically, the mineral of enamel is a **substituted hydroxyapatite**.

Hydroxyapatite forms hexagonal crystals, thus enamel crystals have six sides when seen in cross-section (Fig. 4.1). Enamel crystals are much larger than the hydroxyapatite crystals in other tissues, whose dimensions typically are 5 to 10 nm in width, 1.5 to 3.5 nm in thickness, and 40 to 50 nm in length. Enamel crystals may be up to 70 nm in width and 30 nm in thickness, and are much longer than the crystals in bone, dentin, and cementum. Although their exact length has not been determined, some investigators believe that individual enamel crystals may extend from the **dentinoenamel junction** to the enamel surface. The difference in size of hydroxyapatite crystals found in enamel and those in other mineralized tissues most likely can be attributed to the properties of their matrix components.

> Enamel crystals are large, hexagonally shaped, very long, and composed of substituted hydroxyapatite.

The organic content of mature enamel consists mainly of residual enamel matrix proteins or fragments of these proteins, mostly coating the surfaces of the enamel crystals. These proteins are produced by **ameloblasts**, the cells that make the enamel, and they have critical functions in the formation and mineralization of the enamel. During the maturation of the enamel, most of the matrix proteins are degraded, and along with most of the water in the matrix removed to create space for the mineral. The surface layers of enamel also may contain some salivary proteins that are adsorbed to the enamel crystals or incorporated during the repair of initial caries lesions.

The enamel crystals are organized into **enamel rods** (or **prisms**) that extend from the dentinoenamel junction to the surface of the tooth (Fig. 4.2). Within the rods the crystals are oriented predominantly parallel to the rod. Each rod is about 4 to

5 µm in diameter, with a more or less circular or slightly oval cross-section. The rods may be up to 2.5 to 3 mm in length, depending on the tooth and the location on the tooth. Additional enamel crystals, located in the **interrod enamel**, surround each rod. The interrod enamel crystals are oriented at an angle to those of the rod (Fig. 4.3). Around the occlusal or incisal three-quarters of each rod, the differing orientation of the rod and interrod crystals creates a slight space. This space contains an increased amount of residual matrix proteins and is called the **rod sheath** (Fig. 4.4). Along the cervical one-fourth of each rod, the divergence of the rod and interrod crystals is more gradual, and the rod sheath is absent. In scanning electron micrographs (Fig. 4.5), or in sections cut perpendicular to the rods, the cervical interrod enamel appears to form a "tail" attached to the "body" of the rod just occlusal to it. The observation of this pattern gave rise to the initial interpretation that the enamel rods were shaped like keyholes. It is now generally accepted that the rod-interrod organization described above reflects the true structure of enamel.

> Enamel crystals are organized into rods or prisms that extend from near the dentinoenamel junction almost to the tooth surface, and interrod enamel located between adjacent rods with a differing crystal orientation. A rod sheath, with slightly greater matrix protein content, exists between the rod and interrod enamel around the occlusal three-fourths of the rod.

In **ground sections** of enamel, individual enamel rods exhibit a pattern of **cross-striations** along their length, at regular intervals of about 4 µm (Fig. 4.6). These cross-striations are thought to represent the daily rhythm of enamel formation and mineralization. Because ground sections of enamel may be up to 100 µm thick, the orientation of the rods within the section is difficult to determine. If the rods are sectioned obliquely, the interrod enamel between adjacent rods may appear as cross-striations along a single rod. Also, when viewed in the scanning electron microscope, the rods show periodic variations in diameter, which may contribute to the appearance of cross-striations in ground sections.

Additional longer-term variations in enamel formation result in **incremental lines**, or **striae of Retzius**, representing the position of the forming enamel surface at that point in time (Fig. 4.7). The striae of Retzius occur at approximately 7- to 11-day intervals during enamel formation and are thought to arise from the coincidence of two separate biological rhythms. In an erupted tooth, the intersection of the striae of Retzius with the enamel surface results in shallow horizontal grooves, **perikymata**, that encircle the crown of the tooth.

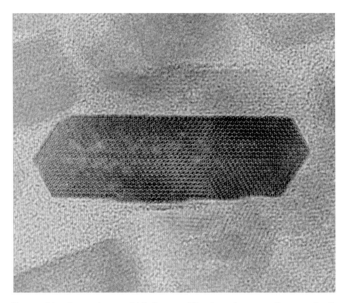

Figure 4.1   Enamel crystal. High magnification electron micrograph of a cross-sectioned hydroxyapatite enamel crystal. The separation of the lattice striations, which intersect at 60° angles, is 0.817 nanometers. (Reproduced with permission from: Yanagisawa, T. (2009) *A Color Atlas of Oral Histology and Embryology*, 3rd edn. Wakaba, Tokyo.)

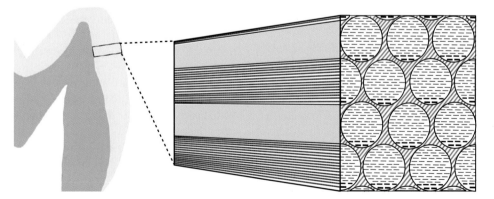

Figure 4.2   Diagram of the main structural features of enamel. Enamel consists of circular- or oval-shaped rods that extend from close to the dentinoenamel junction to the enamel surface. The rods consist of very long enamel crystals, oriented parallel to the long axes of the rods. The enamel crystals are seen in cross-section in the rod profiles in the right portion of the diagram. Interrod enamel is located between the rods. The crystals of interrod enamel, shown here as lighter diagonal lines, have a different orientation than those of the rods.

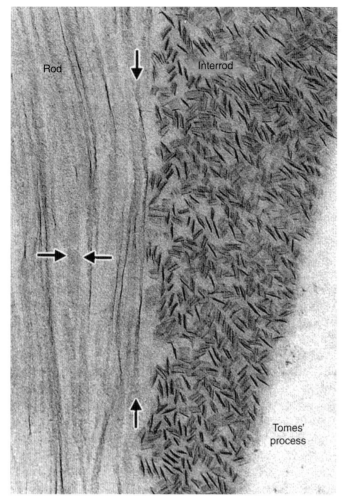

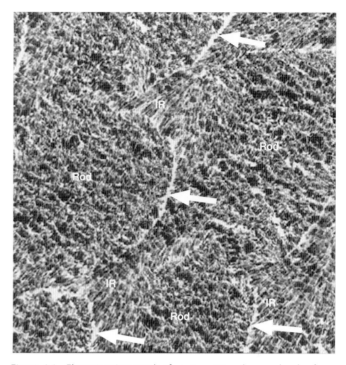

Figure 4.4   Electron micrograph of cross-sectioned enamel rods of mature enamel. Note the different orientations of the enamel crystals in the rod and interrod (IR) enamel. The rod sheathes (arrows) can be seen as increased space at the interface between the rod and interrod enamel. The residual enamel matrix proteins in between the crystals and in the rod sheathes are not visible due to the high contrast of the enamel crystals. (Courtesy of T. Yanagisawa, Tokyo Dental College.)

Figure 4.3   Transmission electron micrograph of newly formed enamel showing the differing orientations of crystals in rod and interrod enamel. The longitudinally oriented crystals in the rod are seen on edge or in face view (between the horizontal arrows). Twisting of an individual crystal is seen between the vertical arrows. The crystals of the interrod enamel are seen mainly in cross-section. (From: Warshawsky, H. (1988) The teeth. In: *Cell and Tissue Biology: A Textbook of Histology* (L. Weiss) 6th edn. pp. 595–640. Urban and Schwarzenberg, Baltimore. Reproduced by permission of Elsevier.)

Systemic disturbances that occur during tooth development, such as fevers, will cause the formation of additional incremental lines. The physiological changes that occur at birth also cause a prominent incremental line, the **neonatal line** (Fig. 4.8). Because enamel is not remodeled over its lifespan, the cross-striations and the striae of Retzius are permanent indicators of the incremental pattern of enamel growth.

> Individual enamel rods show cross-striations that represent a daily rhythm of enamel formation; a regular pattern of longer-term variations in enamel formation results in incremental lines (striae of Retzius).

The course of each rod from the dentinoenamel junction to the surface of the tooth is not straight, but shows a slight curvature. Additionally, each horizontal row of rods is oriented at a slight angle to the adjacent occlusal and cervical rows, creating an undulating pattern of rod orientations from the occlusal/incisal edge of the tooth to the cervical margin (Fig. 4.5). This pattern is evident in ground sections of mature enamel viewed in reflected light, where adjacent bright and dark bands, the **Hunter-Schreger bands**, can be seen extending from the dentinoenamel junction to the enamel surface (Fig. 4.9). This varying orientation of the rods and matrix also is visible in sections of immature enamel stained with hematoxylin and eosin. In regions of sharp surface curvature, such as cusp tips and incisal edges, the curved path of the rods is accentuated; in ground sections this results in the appearance of **gnarled enamel** (Fig. 4.10).

> The course of the enamel rods exhibits an undulating pattern, changing slightly from one horizontal row to the next, resulting in Hunter-Schreger bands when ground sections are viewed in reflected light and gnarled enamel at cusp tips.

The dentinoenamel junction is the interface between dentin and enamel. It is established when the matrices of these two

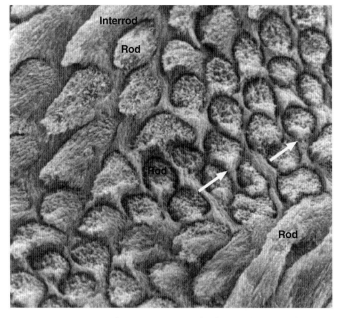

Figure 4.5   Scanning electron micrograph of enamel rods and interrod enamel of a human molar. The surface was etched with a demineralizing agent to enhance the features. The differing orientation of the rods is evident. At the top left and bottom right of the image, the rods run obliquely; in the center the rods are seen in cross-section. The interrod enamel forms a continuous phase around the rods. In the cross-sectioned rods, the cervical portion of the rod is continuous with the interrod enamel (arrows), whereas a space (rod sheath, exaggerated due to the etching) is present around the other surfaces of the rods. (From: Warshawsky, H. (1988) The teeth. In: *Cell and Tissue Biology: A Textbook of Histology* (L. Weiss) 6th edn. pp. 595–640. Urban and Schwarzenberg, Baltimore. Reproduced by permission of Elsevier.)

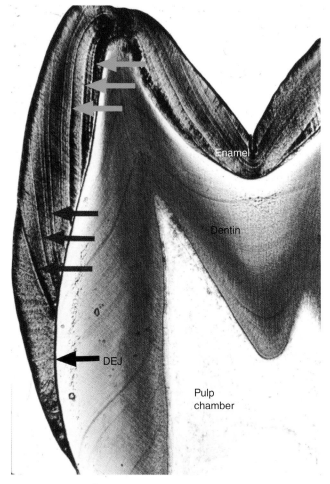

Figure 4.7   Striae of Retzius. The striae of Retzius or incremental lines (red arrows) extend from the dentinoenamel junction (DEJ) to the enamel surface. Perikymata are found where the striae of Retzius intersect the enamel surface. Because enamel formation begins at the cusp tips, striae of Rezius formed early in development (green arrows) do not intersect the tooth surface.

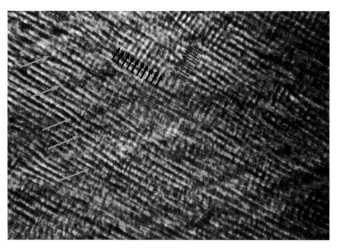

Figure 4.6   Enamel rods. High magnification light micrograph of a ground section showing enamel rods (red arrows) running from lower right to upper left. The closely spaced light and dark lines perpendicular to the rod direction are cross-striations (black arrows). Incremental lines (striae of Retzius, green arrows) run from lower left to upper right.

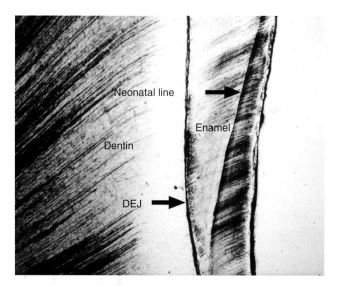

Figure 4.8   Neonatal line. The neonatal line is a prominent incremental line formed in the enamel of teeth developing at birth. Dentinoenamel junction (DEJ).

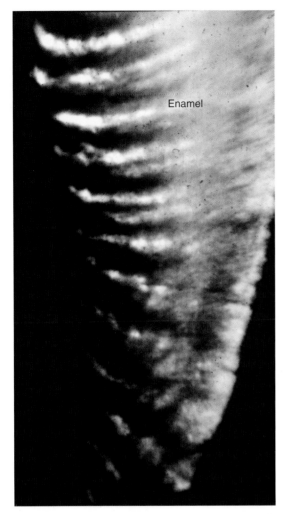

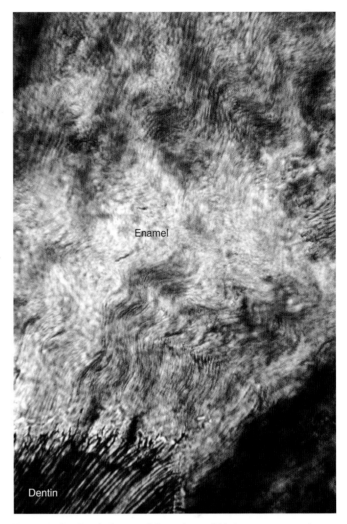

Figure 4.9   Hunter-Schreger bands. The varying direction of the enamel rods results in a group of rods with relatively similar directions adjacent to a group of rods with different directions. In a ground section examined in reflected light, the orientation of the enamel crystals in the rods in one group reflects the light back to the observer, appearing white, whereas light from the adjacent group of rods is reflected away from the observer, and that area appears dark.

Figure 4.10   Gnarled enamel. In regions of high curvature, such as cusp tips, the varying direction of the enamel rods results in an apparent twisting of the rods around one another. (From: Moss-Salentijn, L. *Orofacial Histology and Embryology: A Visual Integration*. Reproduced with permission from F.A. Davis Company, Philadelphia, PA.)

tissues are first deposited and mineralization begins. This is not a smooth interface; in sections it presents a scalloped profile (Fig. 4.11). The irregular profile of the dentinoenamel junction is thought to increase adherence of the enamel to the dentin, especially in areas of occlusal stress. The region of enamel within a few hundred micrometers of the dentinoenamel junction has a higher content of organic matter, mainly protein, and a lesser hardness than enamel further from the dentinoenamel junction. The different composition of this region results in slightly different physical properties, which are thought to be important in arresting the progression of cracks through enamel and into dentin.

Two structural features of enamel associated with the dentinoenamel junction are frequently observed in ground sections of enamel. **Enamel spindles** are short extensions of dentinal tubules across the dentinoenamel junction into the enamel

(Fig. 4.12). During early dentin formation, prior to the deposition of enamel matrix, odontoblasts may extend their distal process across the future dentinoenamel junction, between adjacent presecretory ameloblasts. When the ameloblasts begin to deposit and partially mineralize the enamel matrix, the odontoblast process is surrounded by matrix and becomes trapped, resulting in an unmineralized space, the enamel spindle. **Enamel tufts** are bush-like structures that extend from the dentinoenamel junction for a short distance into the innermost enamel (Fig. 4.13). They are hypomineralized regions containing increased residual enamel matrix proteins, thought to be due to changes in direction of adjacent enamel rods originating from different areas of the scalloped dentinoenamel junction.

Another structural feature of enamel, **enamel lamellae**, are longitudinal hypomineralized defects that originate at the enamel surface and extend part way or in some cases all the way

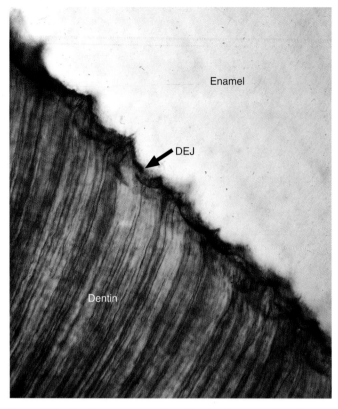

Figure 4.11 Dentinoenamel junction. The dentinoenamel junction (DEJ) exhibits a scalloped outline in sections.

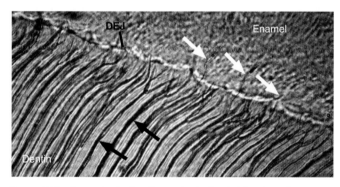

Figure 4.12 Enamel spindles. Enamel spindles (white arrows) are formed when odontoblast processes extend across the dentinoenamel junction (DEJ) and are trapped in the enamel when ameloblasts begin secreting enamel matrix. Dentinal tubules (black arrows).

> The interface between dentin and enamel, the dentino-enamel junction, has a scalloped profile and different physical and chemical properties than the rest of the enamel. Other structural features of enamel include enamel spindles, enamel tufts, and enamel lamellae.

to the dentinoenamel junction (Fig. 4.14). The lamellae contain an increased amount of organic material, either remnants of the enamel organ or connective tissue that has penetrated into the defect. No clinical significance is presently attributed to either tufts or lamellae.

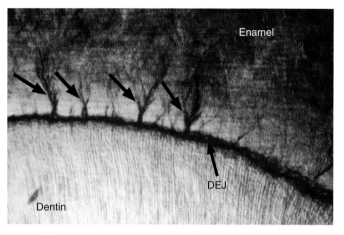

Figure 4.13 Enamel tufts. Enamel tufts are bush-like hypomineralized regions extending from the dentinoenamel junction into the innermost enamel.

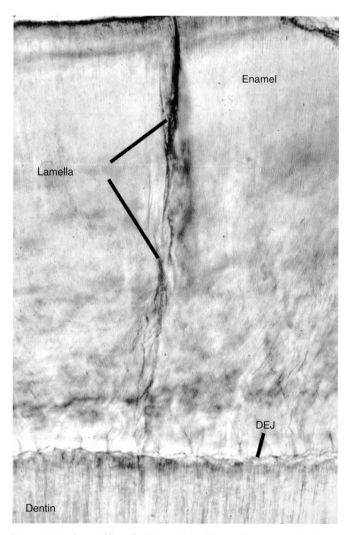

Figure 4.14 Enamel lamella. Enamel lamellae are hypomineralized defects extending from the enamel surface toward the dentinoenamel junction (DEJ).

Enamel formation

The process of enamel formation is called **amelogenesis**. The formation and mineralization of enamel occurs in stages, beginning at the cusp tips or incisal edges and progressing along the sides of the crown toward the cervical margin (Fig. 4.15). The cells that form the enamel are ameloblasts, which differentiate from the inner enamel epithelium of the enamel organ, as described in Chapter 3. The stages of amelogenesis (Fig. 4.16) are:

- presecretory, when the cells prepare to begin enamel matrix formation;
- secretory, during which the ameloblasts deposit and initially mineralize the full thickness of the enamel matrix;
- transition, a short stage in which the cells prepare to become maturation ameloblasts;
- maturation, during which the ameloblasts complete the removal of matrix proteins and the addition of mineral; and
- protective, during which the ameloblasts cover the enamel surface until the tooth erupts.

The function as well as the morphology of the ameloblasts changes as they progress through each stage.

Presecretory stage

During the presecretory stage, the inner enamel epithelial cells induce the peripheral cells of the dental papilla to differentiate into odontoblasts. Shortly after that, the inner enamel epithelial cells begin their differentiation to ameloblasts (Figs. 4.16, 4.17). The cells elongate, the nucleus relocates to what was the apical end of the cell (now called the proximal end), the Golgi complex migrates to the supranuclear cytoplasm, between the nucleus and the former basal end of the cell (now called the distal end), and the rough endoplasmic reticulum increases in amount and forms a cylindrical sleeve around the Golgi complex. The junctional complexes are maintained at the proximal end of the cell, and new junctional complexes are formed at the distal end. These cells are now called **presecretory ameloblasts**; they have not yet begun to secrete enamel matrix. The distal cell membrane of the presecretory ameloblasts has a relatively smooth outline, and the basal lamina between these cells and the early odontoblasts is still intact (Fig. 4.18a).

> The presecretory stage of amelogenesis includes the induction of odontoblast differentiation by the inner enamel epithelial cells and the elongation and reversal of polarity of these inner enamel epithelial cells to become presecretory ameloblasts.

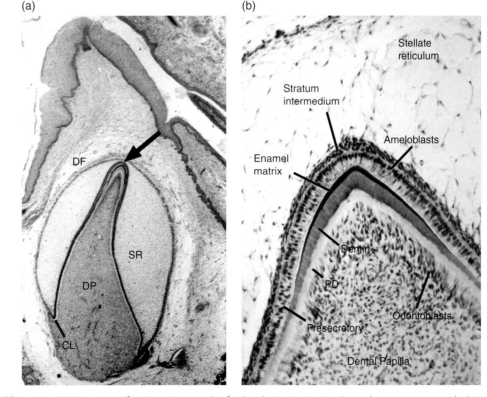

Figure 4.15 Enamel formation. (a) Low magnification micrograph of a developing incisor in the early crown stage, with deposition of enamel and dentin matrices at the cusp tip (arrow). Cervical loop (CL), dental follicle (DF), dental papilla (DP), stellate reticulum (SR). (b) Higher magnification of a similar developing cusp tip. Secretory ameloblasts have differentiated at the cusp tip and have deposited a thin layer of enamel matrix on the outer surface of the dentin. Along the sides of the cusp, closer to the cervical loop, the ameloblasts are in the presecretory stage of differentiation, and at the lower left inner enamel epithelial cells are seen. Predentin (PD).

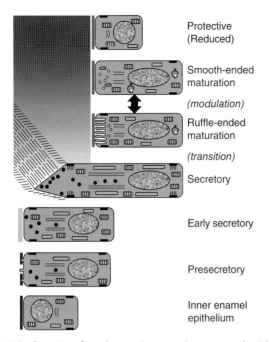

Protective
(Reduced)

Smooth-ended
maturation

(modulation)

Ruffle-ended
maturation

(transition)

Secretory

Early secretory

Presecretory

Inner enamel
epithelium

Figure 4.16   Drawing of amelogenesis stages. Inner enamel epithelial cells are separated from the dental papilla mesenchymal cells by a basal lamina (red line). Their nuclei are located basally, and apical junctional complexes hold the cells together. The inner enamel epithelial cells induce the peripheral cells of the dental papilla to differentiate into odontoblasts. Under the influence of the odontoblasts, inner enamel epithelial cells differentiate into presecretory ameloblasts. The cells elongate and the nuclei move to the former apical end of the cells, now called the proximal end. The Golgi complexes (blue lines) increase in size and relocate between the nuclei and the former basal end of the cells, now called the distal end, and the amount of rough endoplasmic reticulum (elongated beige organelles) increases. Junctional complexes develop at the new distal end of the cells, small cellular protrusions penetrate the basal lamina, and the basal lamina begins to disintegrate. As predentin begins to mineralize, the presecretory ameloblasts become early secretory ameloblasts and begin to synthesize large amounts of enamel matrix proteins and deposit them onto the newly formed mantle dentin, creating the dentino-enamel junction. Partial mineralization of the matrix occurs as it is deposited. This initial immature enamel is unstructured, lacking the typical rod-interrod structure of mature enamel. As the ameloblasts deposit and partially mineralize additional enamel matrix and retreat from the dentinoenamel junction, the cells further elongate, and Tomes' processes form at the distal end of the cells. The cells are now fully differentiated secretory ameloblasts. Tomes' processes create the rod-interrod stucture of enamel; rods form from enamel matrix released at the tip of Tomes' processes, and interrod enamel forms along the sides of Tomes' processes. After the full thickness of enamel matrix is deposited, the ameloblasts undergo a transition (not shown) to become maturation ameloblasts. The cells shorten, much of their synthetic machinery is degraded, a new basal lamina (orange line) is deposited, and about 25% of the cells die by apoptosis. Maturation ameloblasts modulate their morphology between ruffle-ended and smooth-ended forms. Ruffle-ended ameloblasts add mineral to the immature enamel, whereas smooth-ended ameloblasts allow removal of degraded matrix proteins and water. During maturation, an additional 25% of the cells die. Once mineralization is complete, the ameloblasts again shorten and become protective (reduced) ameloblasts.

Secretory stage

Prior to the initial secretion of enamel proteins, the basal lamina disintegrates and disappears, and the distal ends of the presecretory ameloblasts develop small projections (Figs. 4.16, 4.18b). The cells increase their synthesis of enamel matrix proteins, package them in small secretory granules in the Golgi complex (Fig. 4.19), and release them by exocytosis from the distal ends of the cells, adjacent to the dentin. At this point the cells are early secretory ameloblasts (Fig. 4.16). The initial enamel matrix and forming crystals are closely integrated with the matrix and mineral of dentin. As more enamel matrix is deposited, the distal membrane of the ameloblast again becomes smooth. This early enamel adjacent to the dentin is structureless, i.e., the rod-interrod structure described earlier has not yet been established. As the ameloblasts deposit more enamel matrix and continue to move away from the dentinoenamel junction, an elongated process, **Tomes' process**, is formed on the distal end of each cell. The cells are now fully differentiated **secretory ameloblasts** (Figs. 4.16, 4.20, 4.21). Release of matrix proteins from secretory granules at the tip of Tomes' process creates the enamel rod, which is oriented at an approximately 45° angle to the ameloblast cell body (Fig. 4.22). The matrix proteins of the interrod enamel are released along the sides of Tomes' processes, nearer the junctional complexes between adjacent cells. Thus, the rod is created by a single ameloblast, whereas the interrod enamel is created by that ameloblast and all of its immediate neighbors (Figs. 4.22, 4.23). As the cells retreat from the dentinoenamel junction and deposit additional enamel matrix, the interrod enamel is formed first, then the rod enamel is deposited, filling up the spaces formerly occupied by Tomes' processes (Fig. 4.24). The secretion of the rod and interrod enamel at two different sites on the ameloblast is responsible for the differing orientation of the enamel crystals in these two regions, as described earlier.

> During the secretory stage of amelogenesis, ameloblasts initiate enamel matrix secretion and partial mineralization, develop distal Tomes' processes, produce the rod and interrod structure of enamel, and deposit the full thickness of enamel matrix.

As the enamel matrix is deposited by the secretory ameloblasts, it rapidly accumulates mineral. The initial enamel matrix contains about 15% mineral, which increases to approximately 30% of the final mineral content by the end of the secretory stage. Thus, there is no unmineralized layer of enamel on the surface, as occurs during the formation of bone, dentin, and cementum. The initial mineral crystals are thin and narrow, about 1.5 nm thick and 15 nm wide, but grow in width, thickness, and length as more matrix is deposited and the ameloblasts retreat further from the dentinoenamel junction (Fig. 4.25a). As the enamel crystals elongate, the mineral added at their growing tips adjacent to Tomes' process is **amorphous calcium phosphate**, which is converted to hydroxyapatite after a short interval. The space between the crystals is occupied by intact matrix proteins as well as proteolytic fragments, which serve to initiate

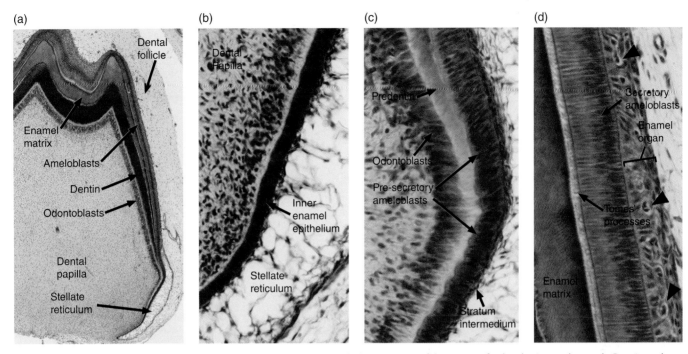

Figure 4.17   Ameloblast differentiation. (a) Low magnification micrograph showing part of the crown of a developing molar tooth. Dentin and enamel matrix formation is underway. (b) Higher magnification showing part of the dental papilla, inner enamel epithelium, and stellate reticulum. Near the top of the image, the peripheral cells of the dental papilla are just beginning to differentiate into odontoblasts, and the inner enamel epithelial cells are beginning to elongate. (c) The inner enamel epithelial cells are elongating and are now presecretory ameloblasts. Odontoblast differentiation is occurring in the lower third of the image, and just below the middle of the image predentin secretion has begun. (d) Tall secretory stage ameloblasts with Tomes' processes and nuclei located proximally or at a mid-cytoplasmic level. Evidence of the rod pattern can be seen in the enamel matrix. The stellate reticulum has collapsed and the enamel organ forms a compact layer adjacent to the ameloblasts. Blood vessels (arrowheads) from the dental follicle have penetrated the enamel organ.

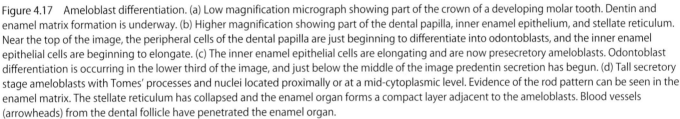

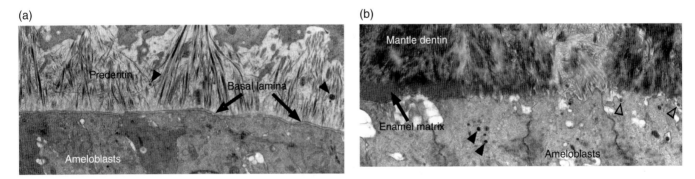

Figure 4.18   Electron micrographs of presecretory and early secretory ameloblasts. (a) Predentin of the mantle layer is deposited prior to enamel matrix secretion. The distal ends of odontoblasts are visible at the top, and matrix vesicles (arrowheads) are present in the predentin. The presecretory ameloblasts have a relatively smooth distal surface with an intact basal lamina. (b) The basal lamina has disappeared, and small projections of the distal end of the ameloblasts are seen at the right. These cells are just beginning to release enamel matrix (open arrowheads). A few secretory granules (arrowheads) containing enamel proteins are seen in the early secretory ameloblasts, and at the left a thin layer of initial enamel matrix has been deposited. (Courtesy of V.-L. Ferrer and A. Lichter, University of Connecticut School of Dental Medicine.)

and regulate crystal growth, absorb the protons released as the hydroxyapatite crystals form, and maintain the differentiation and function of the ameloblasts (Fig. 4.26).

Shortly after the initial layer of enamel matrix is deposited and mineralized, and as the dentin increases in thickness, the stellate reticulum collapses, and the three outer layers of the enamel organ, the stratum intermedium, stellate reticulum, and outer enamel epithelium form a compact, multilayered structure (see Fig. 4.17d). Blood vessels from the surrounding dental follicle penetrate into this layer, coming close to (although not in contact with) the proximal ends of the secretory ameloblasts. It is presumed that dentin and the enamel matrix create a mineralized barrier that limits diffusion of nutrients, electrolytes, and oxygen between the dental papilla and the ameloblasts. The collapse of the enamel organ and ingrowth of blood vessels from the dental follicle facilitate access of the ameloblasts to these constituents.

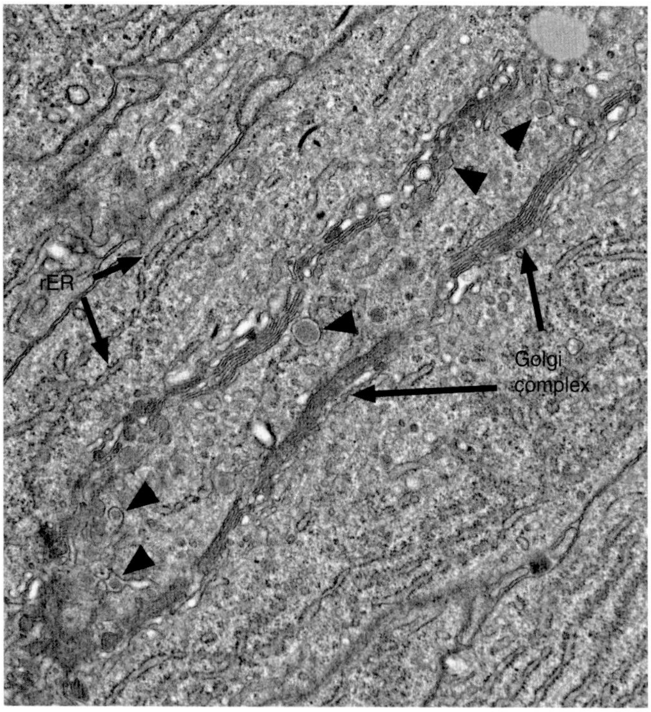

Figure 4.19 Electron micrograph of the Golgi complex of a secretory ameloblast. The Golgi complex consists of stacked membranous saccules in a cup-shaped structure in the supranuclear cytoplasm. Small secretory granules (arrowheads), with a dense content of enamel matrix proteins, form at the trans face of the Golgi complex. Cisternae of rough endoplasmic reticulum (rER) are located in the lateral cytoplasm, peripheral to the Golgi complex. (Courtesy of V.-L. Ferrer and A. Lichter, University of Connecticut School of Dental Medicine.)

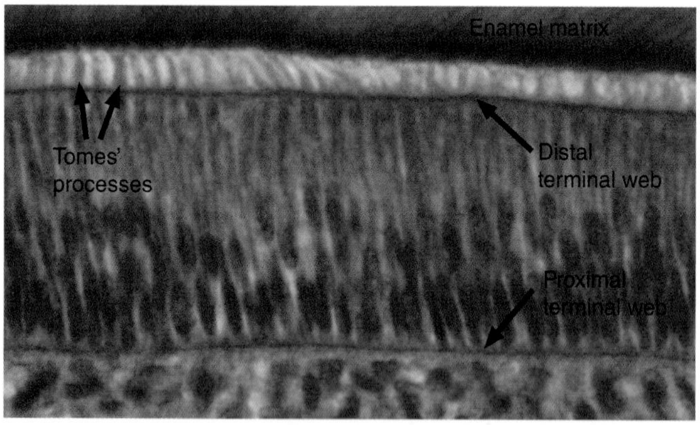

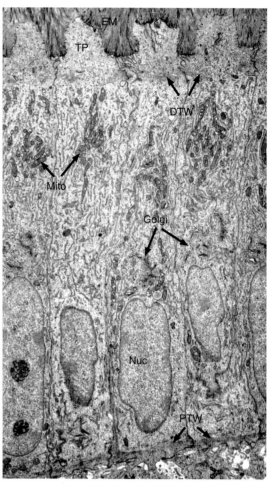

Figure 4.21 Electron micrograph of monkey secretory ameloblasts. These tall columnar cells have basally located nuclei (Nuc), and terminal webs located proximally (PTW) and distally (DTW) in association with intercellular junctions. Rough endoplasmic reticulum, the Golgi complex (Golgi) and numerous mitochondria (Mito) are present in the supranuclear cytoplasm. Tomes' processes (TP) extend into the enamel matrix (EM). (Courtesy of T. Sawada, Tokyo Dental College.)

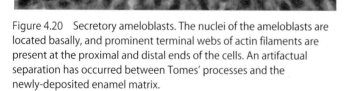

Figure 4.20 Secretory ameloblasts. The nuclei of the ameloblasts are located basally, and prominent terminal webs of actin filaments are present at the proximal and distal ends of the cells. An artifactual separation has occurred between Tomes' processes and the newly-deposited enamel matrix.

Secretory ameloblasts continue to produce and mineralize the enamel matrix until the full thickness of the enamel is deposited. As the last several micrometers of matrix is deposited, Tomes' processes are retracted and the surface enamel again lacks the rod-interrod structure, as occurs during initial enamel formation at the dentinoenamel junction.

Transition stage

During the brief transition stage, the ameloblasts shorten, and many of their synthetic organelles are degraded in autophagic vacuoles. Studies of amelogenesis in experimental animals indicate that approximately 25% of the ameloblasts undergo apoptosis during this stage; it is generally assumed that a similar phenomenon occurs in the transition stage in humans. These transitional stage ameloblasts initiate synthesis and secretion of a proteinase that breaks down the remaining matrix proteins. As these cells complete the transition stage, they also begin forming a basal lamina-like structure at their distal ends (see Fig. 4.28). This basal lamina, although similar in appearance to that at the interface between epithelium and connective tissue, contains the unique molecular components **amelotin** and **odontogenic ameloblast-associated protein (ODAM)**. The basal lamina is maintained through the remaining stages of amelogenesis and serves to attach the ameloblasts, via hemidesmosomes on their distal cell membrane, to the enamel surface.

During the transition from the secretory to the maturation stage, ameloblasts shorten, many organelles are degraded, and about one-fourth of the ameloblasts undergo apoptosis.

Maturation stage

During the maturation stage, degradation of the enamel matrix proteins is completed, water and matrix protein fragments are removed, and the bulk of the mineral is added to the enamel. The enamel crystals increase in width and thickness until they occupy almost the entire volume of the enamel (Fig. 4.25b–d). When maturation is complete, only a small amount of matrix protein and water remains, in the narrow spaces between the enamel crystals and bound to their surfaces. Maturation may take several years to complete, depending upon the particular tooth. Two distinct morphologies are exhibited by the ameloblasts during this stage. **Ruffle-ended ameloblasts** have a ruffled border adjacent to the enamel at their distal end, consisting of infolded membranes separated by irregular cytoplasmic processes (Figs. 4.16, 4.27, 4.28, 4.29). Abundant small vesicles are located in the cytoplasmic processes, and numerous mitochondria are present in the cytoplasm deep to the ruffled border. The distal ends of adjacent cells are held together by junctional complexes that include tight junctions. **Smooth-ended ameloblasts** have a relatively flat distal cell membrane, with a few shallow pits and hemidesmosomes that attach the cells to the basal lamina (Figs. 4.16, 4.27, 4.30). Numerous small vesicles and mitochondria are found close to the distal borders of the cells. Junctional complexes are present at the proximal ends of the cells, but are lacking at the distal ends. Ruffle-ended ameloblasts are involved in adding mineral to the enamel, whereas smooth-ended ameloblasts permit the removal of degraded matrix proteins and water. The ameloblasts modulate their morphology between the ruffle- and smooth-ended forms numerous times during the maturation stage. The cells are found in groups of either ruffle- or smooth-ended forms and spend about 75% of their time as ruffle-ended ameloblasts.

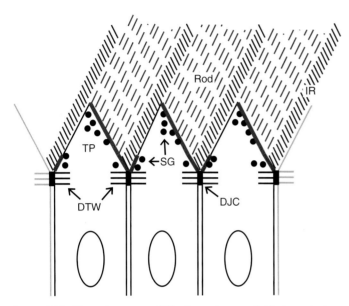

Figure 4.22   Tomes' processes (TP) of secretory ameloblasts control the formation of rod and interrod enamel. Secretion and partial mineralization of rod enamel matrix occurs at rod growth regions (blue) near the tips of Tomes' processes. Secretion of interrod (IR) enamel occurs at interrod growth regions (red) along the sides of Tomes' processes, near the distal junctional complexes (DJC). Secretion granules (SG), distal terminal web (DTW).

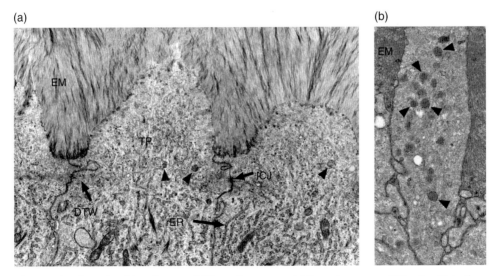

Figure 4.23   Electron micrographs of monkey (a) and mouse (b) Tomes' processes. (a) Tomes' processes (TP) extend into the enamel matrix (EM) distal to the terminal web and intercellular junctions (IJC). Thin needle-like enamel crystals are present in the matrix. Enamel proteins present in small secretory granules (arrowheads) are released by exocytosis from the tip of Tomes' process to form the enamel rod, whereas those released along the sides of Tomes' process and near the intercellular junctions contribute to interrod enamel. Rough endoplasmic reticulum (rER). (b) Numerous dense secretory granules (arrowheads) containing enamel matrix proteins are present in Tomes' process. (a: Courtesy of T. Sawada, Tokyo Dental College. b: Courtesy of V.-L. Ferrer and A. Lichter, University of Connecticut School of Dental Medicine.)

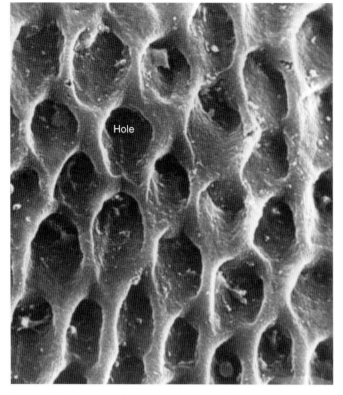

Figure 4.24   Scanning electron micrograph of the forming enamel surface after removal of the layer of secretory ameloblasts. The holes were occupied by the Tomes' processes of the ameloblasts. Interrod enamel forms the walls surrounding the holes, which are being filled by enamel rods forming from the tips of Tomes' processes at the bottom of the holes. (From: Warshawsky, H. 1988. The teeth. In: *Cell and Tissue Biology: A Textbook of Histology* (L. Weiss) 6th edn. pp. 595–640. Urban and Schwarzenberg, Baltimore. Reproduced by permission of Elsevier.)

Studies in experimental animals indicate that by the end of the maturation stage an additional 25% of the ameloblasts die by apoptosis.

During the maturation stage, the outer layers of the enamel organ, which forms a compact, multilayered structure covering the proximal ends of the secretory ameloblasts, reorganizes and increases in thickness. The blood vessels from the dental follicle penetrate deeply into this layer, creating "papillae" of enamel organ cells with intervening vessels. This layer is now called the **papillary layer**. The papillary layer is believed to function in concert with the maturation ameloblasts to create an optimal environment for mineralization of the enamel (see page 78).

> During the maturation stage, ameloblasts modulate their morphology between ruffle-ended and smooth-ended forms. Ruffle-ended ameloblasts add mineral to the enamel; smooth-ended ameloblasts allow removal of water and degraded matrix proteins. At the end of the maturation stage, almost all of the matrix protein originally deposited during the secretory stage has been degraded and lost from the enamel.

Protective stage

Following completion of enamel maturation, the ameloblasts again shorten and lose their ruffled border, to become **reduced (protective) ameloblasts**. The papillary layer is reduced in thickness; in combination with the reduced ameloblasts, this entire layer is called the **reduced enamel epithelium** (Figs. 4.16, 4.31). One function of the reduced enamel epithelium is to cover the enamel surface until the tooth erupts, potentially protecting it from exposure to connective tissue cells that could deposit cementum on the enamel. A second function of the reduced enamel epithelium is to proliferate as the tooth approaches the oral epithelium during eruption. Fusion of the now thickened enamel epithelium with the oral epithelium, followed by disruption of the fused epithelia, creates an opening through which the tooth erupts. Finally, as the tooth emerges into the oral cavity, the cervical one-third of the reduced enamel epithelium forms the **junctional epithelium** that attaches the gingiva to the tooth.

> The reduced ameloblasts cover the enamel surface until the tooth erupts, then, with the other cells of the reduced enamel epithelium, form the junctional epithelium.

Enamel matrix proteins

Because enamel is formed by epithelial cells, its matrix proteins differ from those of mesenchymally derived mineralized tissues. The enamel matrix proteins are members of the proline- and glutamine-rich group of secretory calcium-binding phosphoproteins (SCPP) and are synthesized and secreted by the ameloblasts (Table 4.1). The most abundant, accounting for about 90% of the protein in the enamel matrix, is **amelogenin**. Non-amelogenin matrix proteins include **ameloblastin**, **enamelin**, and possibly a protein called **tuftelin**. **Enamelysin (MMP-20)** (matrix metalloproteinase-20) begins the degradation of matrix proteins during the secretory stage, and **kallikrein 4 (KLK4)**, a serine proteinase, is active during the maturation stage. The non-amelogenin proteins make up only about 10% of the total enamel matrix protein, however, they have important roles in the formation and mineralization of enamel.

Amelogenin is encoded by the *AMELY* gene on the Y chromosome and by the *AMELX* gene on the X chromosome. The major isoform of amelogenin secreted by the ameloblasts is a 175-amino-acid protein. Due to alternative splicing of the amelogenin mRNA and proteolysis occurring after secretion, amelogenin molecules of several different sizes are found in the enamel matrix. After secretion by the ameloblast, amelogenin self-assembles into small, 20-nm-diameter spheres that, along with other matrix proteins, organize the mineralization front and function to direct the formation and growth of the enamel crystals. Amelogenin also serves to buffer the protons released during enamel crystal formation (see page 78). Proteolysis of the amelogenin during the secretion stage and particularly the maturation stage and removal of the amelogenin fragments along with water create space for the growth in width and thickness of the enamel crystals.

(a)

(b)

(c)

(d)

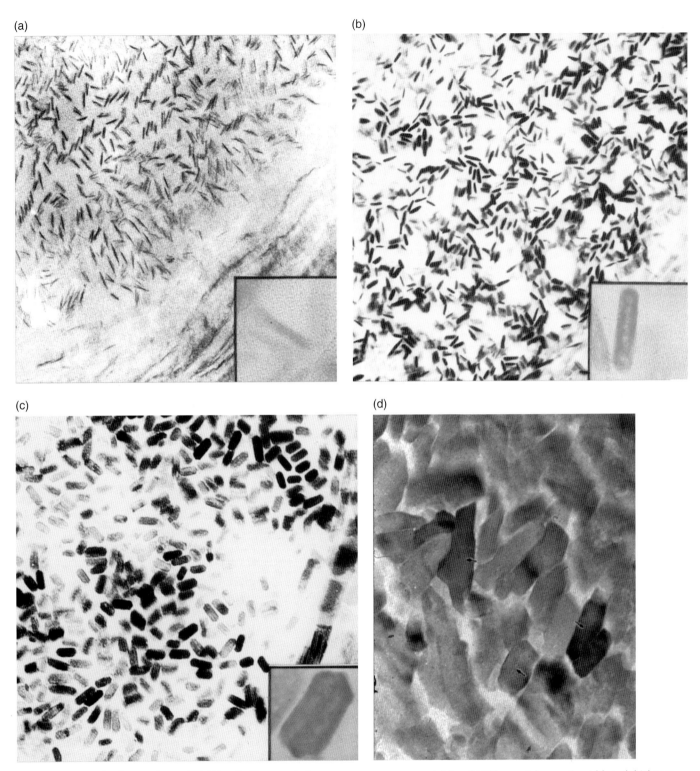

Figure 4.25   Growth of enamel crystals. (a) Needle-like crystals from secretory stage enamel. (b) and (c) The crystals grow in width and thickness during the maturation stage. (d) Mature crystals from an erupted tooth. The insets show individual immature crystals at higher magnification. (a–c reproduced with permission from: Wakita, M. et al. (2006) *Oral Histology and Embryology*. Ishiyaku, Tokyo; d reproduced with permission from: Yanagisawa, T. (2009) *A Color Atlas of Oral Histology and Embryology*, 3rd edn. Wakaba, Tokyo.)

Amelogenin is the major protein constituent of the enamel matrix; it functions to direct the formation and growth of the enamel crystals.

Ameloblastin, also called amelin or sheathlin, is encoded by the *AMBN* gene, located on chromosome 4. It is expressed at low levels compared to amelogenin, but has a critical role in enamel formation and mineralization. Ameloblastin is found predominantly

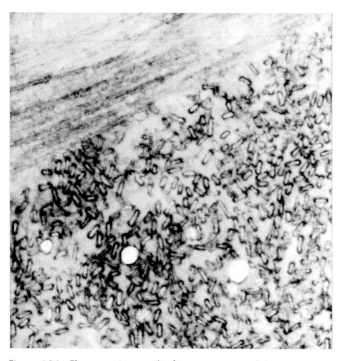

Figure 4.26   Electron micrograph of immature enamel showing the relationship of enamel matrix and enamel crystals. The enamel matrix proteins (dark ovals and lines) were stained with phosphotungstic acid, which simultaneously dissolved the mineral. The matrix proteins are closely adherent to the surfaces of the crystal "ghosts." (Reproduced with permission from: Wakita, M. et al. (2006) *Oral Histology and Embryology*. Ishiyaku, Tokyo)

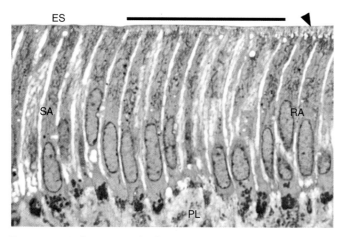

Figure 4.27   Light micrograph of maturation ameloblasts of the rat incisor, in the region of transition (black bar) from ruffle-ended ameloblasts (RA) to smooth-ended ameloblasts (SA). The distal ruffled border (arrowhead) becomes shorter, eventually forming a smooth distal surface. This sample was demineralized prior to sectioning, so there is a space (ES) where the enamel was present. Papillary layer (PL). (Reproduced with permission from: Josephsen, K. & Fejerskov, O. (1977). Ameloblast modulation in the maturation zone of the rat incisor enamel organ: a light and electron microscopic study. *Journal of Anatomy*, 124(1), 45–70.)

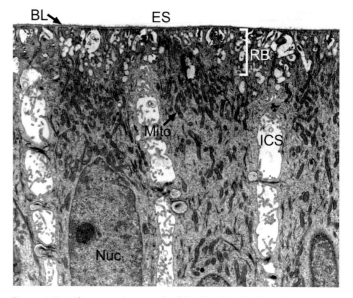

Figure 4.28   Electron micrograph of the distal ends of monkey ruffle-ended maturation ameloblasts. A basal lamina (BL), formed during transition from the secretory stage to the maturation stage, is present along the infolded distal cell membrane of the ruffled border (RB). Numerous mitochondria are located in the distal cytoplasm. Wide intercellular spaces are present between adjacent ameloblasts. Enamel space (ES). (Courtesy of T. Sawada, Tokyo Dental College.)

in newly formed enamel, mainly near the distal membranes of the ameloblasts. It also is concentrated in the rod sheath space. Along with enamelin, ameloblastin is believed to be important for the formation and maintenance of the mineralization front, as well as for the adherence of secretory ameloblasts to the surface of the forming enamel.

Enamelin is encoded by the *ENAM* gene, also located on chromosome 4. Enamelin is the largest size enamel matrix protein, but it is expressed at even lower levels than ameloblastin. The protein is present in highest concentration at the mineralization front, but a proteolytic fragment of enamelin is located among the enamel crystals throughout the secretory stage enamel matrix. Molecular interactions between enamelin and amelogenin have been shown in *in vitro* experiments and very likely are important for proper enamel crystal growth.

Tuftelin is encoded by the *TUFT1* gene, located on chromosome 1. Tuftelin was originally found in developing and mature enamel and thought to be important in the initial stages of enamel mineralization. It is concentrated at the dentinoenamel junction. However, many different cells, including those of soft tissues, express tuftelin, and its status as a true enamel matrix constituent and role in enamel formation and mineralization remain to be determined.

Amelotin and odontogenic ameloblast-associated protein are produced by the ameloblasts following the secretory stage. Both proteins are found in the basal lamina formed at the distal end of the ameloblasts, at the enamel surface. They are believed to be important for the adhesion of the ameloblasts to the enamel surface. They also are found in the (internal) basal lamina that attaches the junctional epithelium to the tooth surface.

Several non-amelogenin proteins, present in low concentrations, are important for proper enamel formation and the adhesion of ameloblasts to the forming enamel surface.

(a)

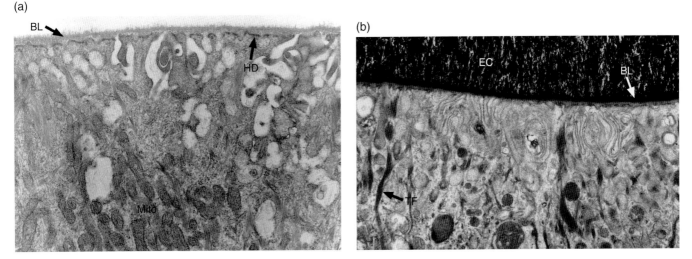

Figure 4.29   Electron micrographs of monkey ruffle-ended maturation ameloblasts. Mitochondria (Mito), bundles of tonofilaments (TF), and small vesicles are present in the distal cytoplasm, below the ruffled border. Hemidesmosomes (HD) attach the ameloblasts to the basal lamina (BL). (a) Demineralized sample. (b) Non-demineralized sample showing enamel crystals (EC) closely apposed to the basal lamina. (a) Courtesy of T. Sawada, Tokyo Dental College. (b) From: Sawada, T., and Inoue, S. (2000) Specialized basement membrane of monkey maturation stage ameloblasts mediates firm ameloblast-enamel association by its partial calcification. *Calcified Tissue International*, 66(4), 277–281. (With kind permission from Springer Science and Business Media.)

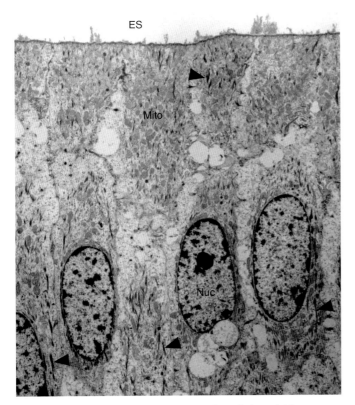

Figure 4.30   Electron micrograph of smooth-ended ameloblasts. Mitochondria (Mito) are present in the distal cytoplasm of the ameloblasts. Numerous tonofilament bundles (arrowheads) are scattered throughout the cells. Enamel space (ES); Nucleus (Nuc). (Courtesy of T. Sawada, Tokyo Dental College.)

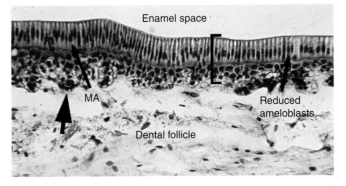

Figure 4.31   Light micrograph of the end of the maturation stage and the beginning of the protective stage of amelogenesis. The height of the maturation ameloblasts (MA) decreases as they become reduced ameloblasts. The large arrow indicates the papillary layer of the maturation stage, and the bracket indicates the reduced enamel epithelium. (From: Moss-Salentijn, L. *Orofacial Histology and Embryology: A Visual Integration.* Reproduced with permission from F.A. Davis Company, Philadelphia.)

Mineralization of enamel

The mineralization of enamel begins immediately upon secretion of the matrix by secretory ameloblasts, and continues through the secretory and maturation stages. It is well accepted that the ameloblasts control the mineralization process. Although not all of the steps are completely understood, a model for enamel mineralization is shown in Figure 4.32. The model depicts events in ruffle-ended maturation ameloblasts; similar mechanisms for mineral transport probably exist in secretory ameloblasts. Calcium enters the ameloblast at the proximal membrane via store operated calcium entry channels (SOCE)

Table 4.1 Proteins Involved in Amelogenesis

Protein	Properties and Function
Amelogenin	Major protein of enamel matrix Guides crystal formation at mineralization front Degraded by enamel proteases and removed during maturation stage
Ameloblastin	Critical for enamel mineralization and adhesion of ameloblasts to enamel surface during the secretory stage
Enamelin	Critical for enamel mineralization and adhesion of ameloblasts to enamel surface during the secretory stage
Enamelysin (MMP20)	Protease secreted by secretory ameloblasts Degrades enamel matrix proteins during secretory stage
Kallikrein 4 (KLK4)	Protease secreted by ameloblasts at end of secretory stage Bulk degradation of enamel matrix proteins during maturation stage
Tuftelin	Enriched at the dentinoenamel junction Status as enamel matrix protein uncertain
Amelotin	Present in basal lamina reformed by ameloblasts following secretory stage
Odontogenic ameloblast-associated (ODAM)	Present in basal lamina reformed by ameloblasts following secretory stage

and apical calcium entry channels (ACEC) and is sequestered in the endoplasmic reticulum. This allows much higher calcium concentrations than can be tolerated in the cytoplasm, and the cells are able to transport the large amount of calcium necessary for enamel maturation. Calcium diffuses through the endoplasmic reticulum, is released into the distal cytoplasm, and is extruded into the matrix via calcium-ATPase pumps and sodium-calcium exchangers. The mechanisms of phosphate transport into and out of the cell are currently unknown, but presumably involve sodium-phosphate cotransporters. A vacuolar proton pump (H^+-ATPase) at the apical membrane acidifies the matrix for optimum activity of enamel proteinases. Hydroxyapatite (HA) is formed from calcium, phosphate, and water in the matrix, releasing additional protons into the matrix.

> Enamel mineralization is an active process, regulated by ameloblasts, which have calcium channels and transporters, and probably phosphate transporters, in their proximal and distal membranes.

Regulation of pH in enamel

During mineralization, approximately 11 hydrogen ions are released as each unit cell of the hydroxyapatite crystal forms, resulting in a decrease in the pH of developing enamel. Because of the large amount of mineral added by ruffle-ended ameloblasts, the pH of the enamel matrix adjacent to these cells is acidic (~6.0). The presence of the H^+-ATPase in the distal membrane of ruffle-ended ameloblasts contributes to the low pH. In contrast, the pH of the enamel matrix adjacent to the smooth-ended ameloblasts is near neutral (~7.2). Because a low pH potentially could inhibit the further growth of the enamel crystals, several mechanisms exist that serve to regulate the pH in developing enamel.

In the secretory stage, amelogenin and its proteolytic fragments serve as buffers to absorb the hydrogen ions released during crystal growth, maintaining the pH of the enamel matrix at about 7.2. Additionally, both secretory and maturation ameloblasts express a number of proteins that function in pH regulation (Fig. 4.32). Whether the ameloblasts upregulate expression of these various electrolyte transporters and enzymes in response to the low pH or as a mechanism to create microenvironmental conditions favorable to enamel crystal formation is unknown. The ameloblasts produce both intracellular and secreted forms of **carbonic anhydrase** (CA2 and CA6, respectively), the enzyme that catalyzes the reversible formation of bicarbonate (HCO_3^-) and H^+ from CO_2 and H_2O. Bicarbonate produced intracellularly is exchanged for chloride ions in the matrix via $Cl^- - HCO_3^-$ anion exchangers in the distal membrane of the ameloblasts. Also located in the distal membrane is the cystic fibrosis transmembrane conductance regulator (CFTR), a chloride channel that transports Cl^- from the cytoplasm to the matrix. The secreted carbonic anhydrase catalyzes the combination of HCO_3^- and the hydrogen ions generated by crystal growth in the matrix to form CO_2 and H_2O. Finally, the hydrogen ions produced during the intracellular formation of HCO_3^- are exchanged for extracellular sodium ions, probably via a Na^+/H^+ exchanger located in the proximal cell membrane. The interstitial fluid is an additional source of bicarbonate.

Cells of the papillary layer of the enamel organ are ionically coupled to one another and to the ameloblasts by gap junctions, forming a functional syncytium. The papillary cells express $Na^+ - HCO_3^-$ cotransporters that transport extracellular HCO_3^- into the cells. The gap junctions allow the HCO_3^- to diffuse from cell to cell and into the ameloblasts. The plasma membrane $Na^+ + K^+ - $ATPase is expressed by the papillary cells but not the ameloblasts, which contributes to maintenance of the intracellular ionic environment of the ameloblast-papillary complex.

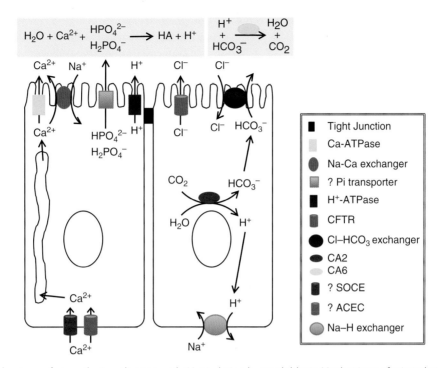

Figure 4.32 Possible mechanisms of enamel mineralization and pH regulation by ameloblasts. Mechanisms of mineral transport are shown at the left; mechanisms of pH regulation are shown at the right. The diagram depicts two ruffle-ended ameloblasts; secretory ameloblasts and smooth-ended ameloblasts may utilize some of these mechanisms for mineral transport and pH regulation. Not all of the electrolyte transporters and exchangers shown have been identified in these cells. Calcium enters the ameloblast via calcium entry channels (SOCE, ACEC) in the basolateral membrane, is sequestered in the endoplasmic reticulum, and extruded into the matrix via calcium pumps (Ca-ATPase) and sodium-calcium exchangers. Phosphate transport occurs by sodium-phosphate cotransporters, and hydrogen ions enter the matrix via a vacuolar H^+-ATPase. Formation of hydroxyapatite (HA) crystals is accompanied by the release of 11 hydrogen ions per unit cell. To regulate the extracellular pH, intracellular chloride ions are transported to the matrix by the CFTR, then exchanged for bicarbonate produced by intracellular carbonic anhydrase (CA2). Extracellular carbonic anhydrase VI (CA6), secreted by the ameloblast, catalyzes the formation of carbon dioxide and water from hydrogen ions and bicarbonate. Intracellular pH is maintained by basolateral sodium-hydrogen exchangers. See text for additional details.

> Enamel crystal formation releases protons, causing acidification of the matrix; amelogenin proteolytic fragments absorb protons during the secretory stage, and maturation ameloblasts secrete HCO_3^- and carbonic anhydrase to neutralize the acid. The cells of the papillary layer participate in maintaining the proper environment for enamel mineralization.

Clinical correlations

The Enamel Surface

When a tooth emerges into the oral cavity, the enamel surface is covered with a thin **enamel cuticle**, a remnant of the reduced enamel epithelium and the basal lamina that attaches it to the tooth surface. The enamel cuticle is quickly worn away by normal masticatory processes.

Another thin coating, the **acquired pellicle**, rapidly forms on exposed tooth surfaces after brushing or cleaning of the teeth. The acquired pellicle varies in thickness from 0.1 to 1 μm and consists of a variety of proteins, glycoproteins, and mucins, derived mainly from saliva but also from gingival crevicular fluid and from oral bacteria. The pellicle concentrates these constituents at the tooth surface, where they have different roles in maintaining the tooth surface as well as interactions with oral bacteria. Acidic proline-rich proteins, statherin, histatins, and cystatins bind calcium ions, creating a calcium-rich environment at the tooth surface. The presence of calcium, phosphate, and especially fluoride ions opposes demineralization caused by acids and promotes remineralization of enamel. Mucins provide lubrication and a slippery surface to facilitate the movement of the mucosal tissues across the tooth surface. The pellicle also provides a barrier to the diffusion of bacterial acids. In addition to their protective role, the proline-rich proteins and other salivary proteins have binding sites for oral bacteria, which allow the bacteria to adhere to the tooth surface and initiate plaque formation. Salivary amylase also binds to certain streptococcal species, which utilize its enzymatic activity to generate fermentable substrates from ingested starch.

Plaque is the bacterial coating, or biofilm, that forms on tooth surfaces exposed to saliva. The initial attachment to salivary pellicle is followed by proliferation of the bacterial cells, production of an extracellular polysaccharide matrix, and the formation of organic acids on exposure to fermentable carbohydrates, such as sucrose. As the plaque increases in thickness, interactions occur between the different bacterial species, including specific binding interactions and metabolic cooperation.

> Salivary proteins, glycoproteins, and mucins bind to the enamel surface, forming a pellicle that opposes demineralization and promotes remineralization of enamel and provides binding sites for bacteria that form plaque.

Dental caries

Dental caries is one of the most common, yet preventable, diseases experienced by humans. When bacterial plaque is allowed to remain on the tooth surface and is provided with nutrients that can be metabolized to produce acid, the local pH rapidly falls to about 5.0 to 5.5, and demineralization of enamel crystals occurs. Remineralization can occur if the nutrients are removed, if the clearance, buffering, and acid neutralizing properties of saliva are adequate, and if the local concentrations of calcium, phosphate, and fluoride ions are sufficient. With sufficient time between the demineralization and remineralization events, the resistance of the enamel to acid will increase through the dissolution of the more soluble carbonated apatite and the formation of less soluble fluoroapatite. This process is termed posteruptive enamel maturation. However, if the acidic conditions remain or recur repeatedly, the lesions will progress. Repeated bouts of demineralization followed by remineralization lead to incipient or "white spot" lesions, where a thin, relatively intact surface layer of enamel covers a deeper, more demineralized region. The interrod enamel crystals are the first to be dissolved; deeper in the lesion, crystals of the enamel rods are dissolved. If, as described above, saliva function and electrolyte concentrations are sufficient, these initial caries lesions can remineralize. However, if the surface layer collapses and cavitation occurs, plaque can form deep in the lesion where it is difficult or impossible to remove. Eventually the lesion reaches the dentin, remaining intact enamel may be undermined and fracture, and the size of the lesion further increases.

> Dental caries results from repeated demineralization events due to acid production by plaque bacteria; intermittent remineralization leads to a mineralized surface layer over a subsurface lesion; collapse of the surface layer results in cavitation.

Fluoride and fluorosis

Fluoroapatite, created when fluoride ions are incorporated into hydroxyapatite as the crystals initially form or during remineralization events, is less soluble than hydroxyapatite or hydroxyapatite substituted with carbonate ions. At low concentrations (0.7–1.2 mg/L), fluoride ingested during tooth development is incorporated into the forming enamel and imparts increased resistance to acid solubility. After tooth eruption, fluoride in drinking water or application of fluoride at higher concentrations, such as in toothpastes, mouth rinses, or professionally applied gels or varnishes, provides an even greater caries resistance effect. Topically applied fluoride increases fluoride concentration in "bioavailable" reservoirs in plaque and on enamel and mucosal surfaces. In saliva and on enamel surfaces, available fluoride is present mainly as calcium fluoride (CaF_2). In plaque, fluoride reacts with bacterial calcium to form calcium-fluoride (Ca-F) bonds. During acidic conditions, both calcium and fluoride are released from plaque and available for enamel remineralization. Locally high concentrations of fluoride in plaque inhibit glucose uptake and utilization by plaque bacteria and also may have bacteriostatic or bacteriocidal effects. Even larger amounts of fluoride are found on mucosal surfaces; it is likely that these mucosal fluoride deposits are similar in nature to plaque fluoride deposits.

If fluoride is present at any level during enamel development there is a risk of dental fluorosis, or mottled enamel. The greater the concentration of fluoride, the greater the risk. At levels of 2 mg/L or more, the risk of fluorosis is significant. The mechanism underlying dental fluorosis is believed to be an inhibition of the proteolysis of enamel matrix proteins, and/or a reduction in the rate of removal of the degradation products, resulting in subsurface hypomineralization. Depending upon the severity, the enamel of teeth affected by fluorosis may have white spots or yellow to brown stains, or exhibit surface breakdown and pitting due to post-eruptive mechanical damage. The teeth are unsightly, and cosmetic procedures are often necessary, but the teeth are generally caries free.

> Incorporation of fluoride into hydroxyapatite reduces its solubility. Topical fluoride in plaque inhibits bacterial metabolism, is released during acid conditions, and promotes enamel remineralization. Excessive fluoride concentrations during tooth development can result in enamel fluorosis.

Inherited diseases of enamel

Mutations in genes that are critical for the normal development of enamel result in **amelogenesis imperfecta**, a group of conditions with variable phenotypes (Table 4.2). Depending on the gene involved, amelogenesis imperfecta may have an X-linked, autosomal dominant or autosomal recessive mode of inheritance. Mutations in the genes for enamel matrix proteins such as amelogenin (*AMELX*) and enamelin (*ENAM*) result in varying degrees of enamel hypoplasia and hypomineralization. These include pitting and grooves, as well as generalized thin enamel, and disruption of the normal rod structure. Mutations in the genes for enamelysin (*MMP20*) and kallikrein 4 (*KLK4*) (Fig. 4.33a) result in hypomineralized enamel, although the enamel apparently is of normal thickness. Estimates of the incidence of amelogenesis imperfecta vary widely, from 1 in 700 people to 1 in 14,000 people, depending upon the region of the world.

Mutations in several other genes also have effects on the formation and mineralization of enamel. The most common and most severe form of amelogenesis imperfecta in the United

Table 4.2   Inherited Diseases Affecting Enamel

Disease	Gene
X-Linked Amelogenesis Imperfecta (AI)	Amelogenin (AMELX)
Autosomal Dominant Hypoplastic AI	Enamelin (ENAM)
Autosomal Recessive Pigmented Hypomaturation AI	Enamelysin (MMP20)
Autosomal Recessive Pigmented Hypomaturation AI	Kallikrein 4 (KLK4)
Autosomal Dominant Hypocalcified AI	FAM83H
Autosomal Recessive AI and Gingival Fibromatosis	FAM20A
Familial Proximal Renal Tubular Acidosis	Electrogenic Bicarbonate Cotransporter (SLC4A4)
Autosomal Recessive Cone-Rod Dystrophy & AI (Jalili Syndrome)	Magnesium Ion Transporter (CNNM4)
Junctional Epidermolysis Bullosa, Enamel Hypoplasia	Laminin-β3 (LAMB3), Collagen 17 (COL17A1)
Occulodentodigital Dysplasia	Connexin 43 (GJA1)
Autosomal Recessive Hypomaturation AI	WDR72
Autosomal Dominant Trichodentoosseus Syndrome; Hypoplastic-Hypomaturation Type with Taurodontism (AIHHT)	DLX3

(a)

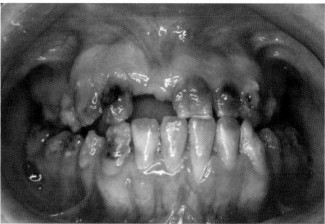

(b)

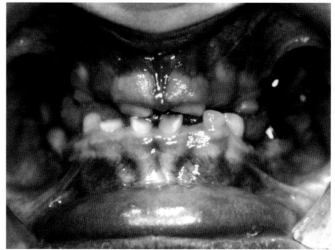

(c)

States, autosomal dominant hypocalcification amelogenesis imperfecta (Fig. 4.33b), is due to a mutation in the *FAM83H* gene, which codes for a protein involved in vesicle trafficking. Recently, it was shown that an autosomal recessive syndrome called amelogenesis imperfecta and gingival fibromatosis is caused by mutation of the *FAM20A* gene, which codes for a protein kinase associated with the Golgi complex (Fig. 4.33c). Other genes that when mutated have been shown to cause enamel defects include those for certain electrolyte transporters, cell adhesion proteins, gap junction proteins, and transcription factors involved in tooth development.

> Mutations in enamel matrix protein genes and other genes critical for proper ameloblast function result in amelogenesis imperfecta, with poorly formed and mineralized enamel.

Other enamel defects

Enamel defects may occur in individual teeth or be present in many or all of the teeth. Local factors, such as trauma or a localized infection, or systemic conditions, such as a febrile illness or ingestion of a toxic substance during tooth development, may

Figure 4.33   Clinical photographs of patients with amelogenesis imperfecta. (a) Autosomal recessive pigmented hypomaturation amelogenesis imperfecta due to a kallikrein 4 (KLK4) mutation. (b) Autosomal dominant hypocalcified amelogenesis imperfecta due to a FAM83H mutation. (c) Autosomal recessive generalized hypoplastic amelogenesis imperfecta associated with a FAM20A mutation. (Courtesy of J.T. Wright, University of North Carolina.)

lead to enamel defects. Quantitative, or hypoplastic, defects have thin or poorly formed enamel of normal hardness. Qualitative defects are hypomineralized, with relatively normal-appearing enamel that contains less than normal amounts of mineral and wears more rapidly or is more susceptible to dental caries. Hypoplastic defects typically appear as pits, grooves, or areas of missing enamel; if due to a systemic disturbance the defect may be localized to different regions of the teeth, depending on the stage of development at the time of the disturbance. Hypomineralized defects may appear as opacities, without the normally translucent appearance of enamel. Molar incisor hypomineralization is a relatively common developmental condition of unknown etiology, present in permanent molars and often involving incisors at the time of eruption. Affected molars are subject to breakdown and rapid progression of dental caries upon eruption.

Staining

Staining or discoloration of enamel can be caused by a number of factors. Staining either is extrinsic, caused after eruption by substances in contact with the enamel, or intrinsic, generally occurring during tooth formation but in some cases also in erupted teeth. Extrinsic staining, such as the brown stain that may occur with use of the antimicrobial agent chlorhexidine, usually can be removed by tooth brushing or polishing. Excessive use of tobacco products, chewing areca (betel) nut, or heavy coffee or tea drinking also may result in enamel staining. Products of chromogenic bacteria in dental plaque can cause extrinisic staining.

Intrinsic staining may be localized or generalized, depending on the cause, and may be difficult or impossible to remove. Trauma to an individual tooth during development or after eruption causing loss of tooth vitality or failure of endodontic treatment may result in discoloration. Generalized intrinsic staining may occur as a result of certain drug treatments or systemic diseases during tooth development. Tetracycline antibiotics bind to mineral as it is being deposited, resulting in yellow to gray or brown stains, depending on the particular tetracycline administered. Minocycline administered for the treatment of acne may cause green-gray to blue-gray tooth staining. Erythropoietic porphyria, in which porphyrin is deposited in many tissues, causes pink to red enamel staining that fluoresces. Neonatal hemolytic anemias or hepatitis resulting in excessive bilirubin formation or incomplete elimination may cause yellow, green, brown, gray, or black staining, principally of the primary teeth.

> Enamel defects result from disturbances during enamel development, and may be localized or generalized, hypoplastic or hypomineralized in nature. Enamel staining results from either extrinsic causes, such as excessive tobacco or coffee use, or intrinsic causes, such as tetracycline use or neonatal systemic diseases.

References

1. Aoba, T. & Fejerskov, O. (2002) Dental fluorosis: chemistry and biology. *Critical Reviews in Oral Biology and Medicine,* 13(2), 155–170.
2. Atar, M. & Körperich, E.J. (2010) Systemic disorders and their influence on the development of dental hard tissues: a literature review. *Journal of Dentistry,* 38(4), 296–306.
3. Fejerskov, O. & Kidd, E.A.M. (eds.) (2008) *Dental Caries: The Disease and its Clinical Management,* 2nd edn. Blackwell Munksgaard, Oxford.
4. Josephsen, K., Takano, Y., Frische, S., Praetorius, J., Nielsen, S., Aoba, T,. & Fejerskov, O. (2010) Ion transporters in secretory and cyclically modulating ameloblasts: a new hypothesis for cellular control of preeruptive enamel maturation. *American Journal of Physiology Cell Physiology,* 299(6), C1299–C1307.
5. Lacruz, R.S., Nanci, A., Kurtz, I., Wright, J.T., & Paine, M.L. (2010) Regulation of pH during amelogenesis. *Calcified Tissue International,* 86(2), 91–103.
6. Simmer, J.P., Papagerakis, P., Smith, C.E., Fisher, D.C., Rountrey, A N., Zheng, L., & Hu, J.C.-C. (2010) Regulation of dental enamel shape and hardness. *Journal of Dental Research,* 89(10), 1024–1038.
7. Tredwin, C.J., Scully, C., & Bagan-Sebastian, J.-V. (2005) Drug-induced disorders of teeth. *Journal of Dental Research,* 84(7), 596–602.
8. Wright, J.T. (2006) The molecular etiologies and associated phenotypes of amelogenesis imperfecta. *American Journal of Medical Genetics Part A,* 140A(23), 2547–2555.
9. Wright, J.T., Torain, M., Long, K., Seow, K., Crawford, P., Aldred, M.J., Hart, P.S., & Hart, T.C. (2011) Amelogenesis imperfecta: genotype-phenotype studies in 71 families. *Cells Tissues Organs,* 194(2–4), 279–283.

Glossary

Acquired pellicle: The thin coat on the enamel surface consisting of adsorbed salivary proteins, glycoproteins, and mucins.

Ameloblast: The enamel-forming cell that differentiates from the inner enamel epithelium of the enamel organ.

Ameloblastin: An enamel matrix protein, produced by ameloblasts; constitutes approximately 5% of the organic matrix.

Amelogenesis: The process of enamel formation, consisting of presecretory, secretory, transition, maturation, and protective stages.

Amelogenesis imperfecta: A family of inherited diseases of enamel, caused by mutations in the genes of enamel matrix proteins or proteins essential for matrix synthesis, secretion, and mineralization; results in thin and/or poorly mineralized enamel.

Amelogenin: The major protein of the enamel matrix, produced by ameloblasts; constitutes approximately 90% of the organic matrix.

Amelotin: A protein present in the basal lamina produced by ameloblasts following the secretory stage of amelogenesis; involved in the adhesion of ameloblasts to the enamel surface.

Amorphous calcium phosphate: A noncrystalline calcium phosphate mineral phase, with a Ca/PO_4 molar ratio of approximately 1.45; carbonate, magnesium, and pyrophosphate ions also may be incorporated in amorphous calcium phosphate.

Anatomic crown: The portion of the tooth covered by enamel.

Carbonic anhydrase: The enzyme catalyzing the reversible hydration of carbon dioxide to form carbonic acid.

Cross-striations: Lines seen crossing enamel rods at regular intervals in ground sections viewed in the light microscope; believed to represent daily increments of enamel formation.

Dental caries: Lesions of the enamel or dentin of teeth initiated by the dissolution of mineral crystals by acid produced during metabolism of carbohydrates by microorganisms in the microbial film (*plaque*) on the tooth surface.

Dentinoenamel junction: The interface between dentin and enamel.

Enamel: The hard, white tissue consisting of approximately 96% mineral that covers the anatomic crowns of the teeth.

Enamel cuticle: A thin coating of residual cellular and extracellular material on the enamel surface of newly erupted teeth that is quickly worn away.

Enamel lamella: A defect originating from the enamel surface, filled with organic material, that extends part way or all the way through the enamel.

Enamel rod (prism): The basic structural component of enamel, consisting of enamel crystals and residual enamel proteins, produced by ameloblasts and extending from the dentinoenamel junction to the tooth surface.

Enamel spindle: Extension of a dentinal tubule across the dentinoenamel junction into enamel, created when enamel matrix is deposited around an odontoblast process lying between adjacent ameloblasts.

Enamel tuft: A bush or tree-like structure containing residual enamel matrix, originating from the dentinoenamel junction and extending for a short distance into enamel.

Enamelin: An enamel matrix protein thought to be involved in initiation of mineral crystal formation and elongation; rapidly degraded and present mainly at the growing enamel surface.

Enamelysin (MMP-20): An enamel proteinase (matrix metalloproteinase-20) produced by secretory ameloblasts that degrades enamel matrix proteins during the secretory stage of amelogenesis.

Gnarled enamel: Enamel at sites of high tooth surface curvature that in ground sections exhibits apparent twisting paths of enamel rods due to the variation in direction of adjacent rods.

Ground sections: Because highly mineralized tissues such as enamel and adult bone are difficult to section using standard embedding and sectioning procedures, the mineral content typically is removed using acid or chelating agents. In order to study the mineral distribution, ground sections are prepared. The sample of enamel or bone is cut with a diamond saw blade to produce a section of 0.5 to 1 mm in thickness. The section is then thinned to a thickness of approximately 100 μm or less by polishing with fine abrasive paper or using a grinding plate. The section is placed on a glass microscope slide and a coverslip is mounted. Only the mineralized components are visible;

the surrounding or included soft tissues and cells are not preserved.

Hunter-Schreger bands: Bright and dark bands seen in ground sections of enamel viewed by reflected light, due to variations in the direction of groups of enamel rods.

Hydroxyapatite: The mineral form of calcium phosphate, $Ca_{10}(PO_4)_6(OH)_2$, found in skeletal tissues and teeth of vertebrates.

Incremental lines (striae of Retzius): Long-period growth lines in enamel occurring every 7 to 11 days, indicating the position of the enamel surface when the lines were formed during the secretory stage of amelogenesis.

Interrod enamel: Enamel secreted from the sides of Tomes' processes, surrounding the enamel rod, containing mineral crystals with a different orientation than those of the rod.

Junctional epithelium: The epithelium, originally derived from the reduced enamel epithelium on eruption of the tooth, that is attached to the tooth surface, either enamel or cementum, and seals the bottom of the gingival sulcus.

Kallikrein 4 (KLK4): An enamel proteinase produced by secretory ameloblasts that functions to degrade enamel matrix proteins during the maturation stage of amelogenesis.

Neonatal line: The prominent incremental line in enamel (and dentin) present in teeth that are forming at the time of birth.

Odontogenic ameloblast-associated protein (ODAM): A protein produced by ameloblasts that is present in the basal lamina formed at the end of the secretory stage of amelogenesis.

Papillary layer: A combination of the three outer layers of the enamel organ (outer enamel epithelium, stellate reticulum, stratum intermedium), which is deeply penetrated by blood vessels from the dental follicle, giving the appearance in sections of papillae.

Perikymata: Horizontal grooves that encircle the tooth at the intersections of striae of Retzius with the enamel surface.

Presecretory ameloblast: Cell of the inner enamel epithelium undergoing differentiation to a secretory ameloblast, including elongation of the cell and migration of the nucleus to a proximal location and the Golgi complex to a supranuclear position.

Plaque: The microbial layer (biofilm) adherent to the tooth surface through attachment to the acquired enamel pellicle.

Reduced (protective) ameloblasts: Ameloblasts of the final stage of amelogenesis that adhere to the enamel surface and contribute to the formation of the junctional epithelium on eruption of the tooth.

Reduced enamel epithelium: The cells of the enamel organ at the completion of maturation, including the reduced ameloblasts and the papillary layer, that forms the junctional epithelium upon eruption of the tooth.

Rod sheath: The space around the occlusal three-fourths of the enamel rod, created by the abrupt change in the direction of enamel crystals between the rod and interrod enamel, and containing a slightly greater amount of enamel proteins than the rod or interrod enamel.

Ruffle-ended ameloblast: A maturation stage ameloblast with an infolded or "ruffled" distal surface (adjacent to the enamel); responsible for the transport of mineral into the enamel.

Secretory ameloblast: Ameloblasts with distal Tomes' processes that secrete and partially mineralize the enamel matrix and create the rod structure of enamel.

Smooth-ended ameloblast: An ameloblast with a relatively smooth distal surface, that actively or passively participates in the removal of water and degraded enamel proteins during the maturation stage.

Substituted hydroxyapatite: Hydroxyapatite mineral in which some of the calcium, phosphate, or hydroxyl ions are replaced by other ions.

Tomes' process: The elongated distal process of an ameloblast from which enamel matrix is secreted to form the enamel rod and the interrod enamel.

Tuftelin: A putative enamel matrix protein associated with enamel tufts and thought to be important for early mineralization.

Chapter 5 Dentin, Pulp, and Tooth Pain[1]

Michel Goldberg

Biomédicale des Saints Pères, Université Paris Descartes, INSERM UMR-S 1124

Dentin forms the bulk of the tooth. It supports the enamel which covers the crown and the cementum that constitutes the superficial layer of the root of the tooth (Fig 5.1). Although dentin is a mineralized tissue, it contains less mineral and is more resilient than enamel, providing resistance to fractures and cracks. Dentin is a vital tissue, containing cytoplasmic processes of the cells that produce it, **odontoblasts,** and nerve endings (Figs. 5.2 and 5.3). Dentin encloses the pulp, which has an abundant blood and nerve supply, as well as immunologic and regenerative properties. The pulp maintains the vitality of the dentin and the odontoblasts. Dentin, as enamel, is susceptible to dental caries, may develop sensitivity when exposed, and is affected by several hereditary diseases.

Evolution of dental structures

From an evolutionary point of view, scales covering the whole body were gradually restricted to the oral cavity. A mineralized bony structure appeared in the so-called odontodes, the primitive teeth of early vertebrates. At later stages of evolution, the formative cells polarized and developed long processes within the mineralized part, which was gradually transformed into **osteodentin,** a bone-like structure that implies that cells similar to osteocytes are located within lacunae. The cell bodies moved out from the mineralized structure, polarized, and contributed to the formation of a continuous layer at the surface of the pulp. The next step of evolution was the formation of a true **orthodentin**, with the

cell bodies outside the mineralized dentin and long processes extending within dentinal tubules.

Dentin structure and composition

Different types of dentin are present in normal and pathologic teeth (Fig. 5.2 and Tables 5.1 and 5.2).

Outer layers

In the coronal part of the teeth, beneath the enamel and under the dentinoenamel junction (DEJ), the **mantle dentin**, 30 to 150 μm thick, displays resilient properties. This is the first layer of dentin deposited, and it is less mineralized than the circumpulpal dentin. Lower calcium phosphate content is found, and the phosphorylated non-collagenous proteins implicated in mineralization are reduced (Fig. 5.4a).

In the root, beneath the cementum and along the dentin-cementum junction, two different dentinal structures have been identified, with some variations related to species differences: the **hyaline Hopewell–Smith zone** appearing as a thin border (8–15 μm thick), and **Tomes' granular layer** (8–15 μm in width) (Fig. 5.4b). The two peripheral layers contain a few bent, minute dentinal tubules. Globular structures (**calcospherites**) are grouped in these outer layers, which possibly result from the increased size of matrix vesicles. Calcospherites merge more or less homogeneously, but between the mineralized globules, defective large **interglobular spaces** are not mineralized. This is reminiscent of what is seen in X-linked hypophosphatemia teeth (hypophosphatemic rickets) where globular structures are seen, isolated by large interglobular spaces containing non-collagenous proteins and proteoglycans (Table 5.2).

---

[1] With a contribution by Bradley K. Formaker, Ph.D., University of Connecticut School of Dental Medicine, Farmington, CT.

Fundamentals of Oral Histology and Physiology, First Edition. Arthur R. Hand and Marion E. Frank.
© 2014 John Wiley & Sons, Inc. Published 2014 by John Wiley & Sons, Inc.

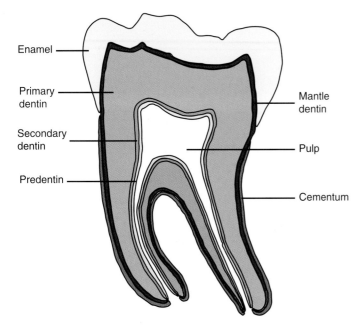

Figure 5.1   General organization of a tooth. Beneath the coronal enamel, the different layers of dentin are found. Mantle dentin is the first dentin deposited; circumpulpal or primary dentin constitutes the bulk of the tooth. Secondary dentin is deposited at a slow rate after primary dentin formation is complete. A layer of predentin separates the dentin from the pulp. The root is covered by cementum.

Circumpulpal dentin

The bulk of dentin is constituted of **circumpulpal dentin** exclusively produced by the odontoblasts (Fig. 5.5a). Odontoblasts initially form **predentin**, which undergoes mineralization and becomes dentin. The daily production of dentin decreases from 10 µm/day at the onset of dentin formation to 4 µm/day. This generates a rhythmic formation, and at each 4 µm a daily incremental (**von Ebner's**) line appears. This circadian rhythm is interacting with another longer-period rhythm forming **Owen's lines**, appearing each 16–20 µm, due to unknown mechanisms. The continual centripetal formation of **primary dentin** results in gradual reduction of the pulp volume (Figs. 5.2 and 5.3).

As each odontoblast deposits dentin matrix and retreats toward the central pulp, it extends an elongated process from the distal end of the cell body. Continual deposition and mineralization of dentin matrix around the odontoblast process creates a tubule within the dentin, from near the dentinoenamel junction to the pulpal surface of the dentin. Dentin contains about 20,000 **dentinal tubules** per mm², with variations between the outer and inner parts of the dentin layer. Due to space restriction, more tubules are present in the inner third than in the outer third (between 18,000 and 21,000/mm²). The tubules are curved, displaying a gradual S shape from the dentinoenamel junction to the pulp. The primary dentin of the crown and most of the root

Dentin location, types and structures

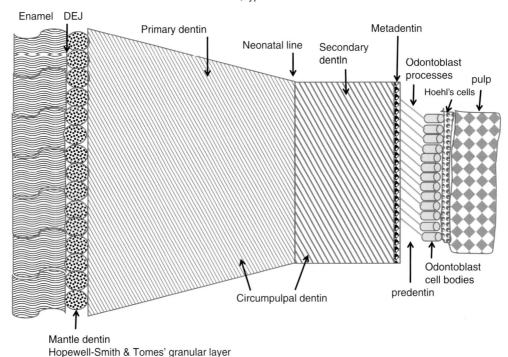

Figure 5.2   Schematic distribution of the different dentin layers located between the dentinoenamel junction (DEJ) and the dental pulp. Two atubular peripheral layers are located beneath the enamel or cementum: the mantle dentin in the crown and the peripheral layers in the root, including the atubular hyaline Hopewell-Smith layer and/or the Tomes' granular layer. Primary dentin includes the atubular peripheral layers and the tubular circumpulpal dentin of the crown and root. The neonatal line separates dentin formed before birth from dentin formed after birth. Secondary dentin is formed continuously after the completion of primary dentin formation. The mineralization front, or metadentin, is the border where dentin mineralization is initiated. Odontoblast processes cross the predentin (15-20 µm in width) and enter the dentinal tubules. Hoehl's cells may differentiate into odontoblasts, the dental pulp being located beneath.

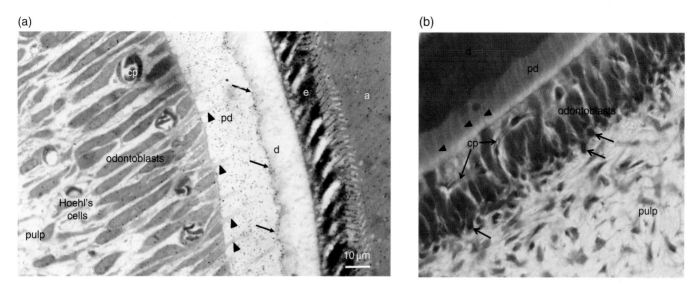

Figure 5.3   Light micrographs of odontoblasts and forming dentin. (a) One-μm-thick section of a rat incisor. On the right, enamel (e) is formed by secretory ameloblasts (a) The mineralization front (arrows) located at the edge of the dentin layer (d) is covered by silver grains (radioautography using (³H) serine as phosphoprotein precursor). Odontoblast processes (arrowheads) extend through the predentin (pd). Dentin extracellular matrix molecules are synthesized in odontoblast cell bodies. Hoehl's cells may differentiate into odontoblasts. The odontoblast and Hoehl's cell layers include endothelial cells forming capillaries (cp). The dental pulp is located more centrally. Bar = 10 μm. (b) Hematoxylin- and eosin-stained section of a human molar. Labels as in 5.3(a). Arrowheads indicate odontoblast processes, and arrows indicate Hoehl's cells.

Table 5.1   Schematic distribution of the successive layers and types of sound dentin in longitudinal section between the dentinoenamel (DEJ) and the pulp

Location	Dentin Type	Structure
Peripheral dentin	Crown: • Mantle dentin	Atubular dentin, 30–150 μm thick. Initial dentin formed in the crown. Non-phosphorylated proteins. Resilient border.
	Root: • Hopewell-Smith layer: 8–15 μm and/or • Tomes' Granular layer: 8–15 μm	Initial atubular dentin. Calcospherites or globular structures and interglobular spaces. A few bent minute tubules.
Circumpulpal dentin	Primary dentin	The dentin formed between the creation of initial peripheral dentin and early tooth functioning. The tubules display a longitudinal S-shaped curvature. The formation of primary dentin is limited by the outer DEJ and the initiation of secondary dentin deposition.
	Secondary dentin	Formed normally and continuously after completion of the crown and root. Results from the daily 4-μm dentin formation. The S-shape of the tubules is more accentuated, and the tubules are less numerous, due to space restriction.
Peripheral dentin	Atubular dentin	• Mantle dentin • Hopewell-Smith & Tomes' granular layers • Fibrodentin formation in the mesial and distal surfaces of the root canal
Circumpulpal dentin	Tubular dentin	Intertubular dentin: a collagen-rich dentin associated with non-collagenous proteins along and between the collagen fibrils. The hydroxyapatite crystallites are 3–5 nm thick and 60 nm long. Peritubular dentin: 25–30 nm crystallites, and an amorphous network without collagen fibrils lining the lumina of dental tubules.

Table 5.2   Pathologic dentin

Causative Event	Response	Structural Alteration
Genetic alterations: • dentinogenesis imperfecta • dentin dysplasia • X-linked hypophosphatemia	Gene deletion of collagen I, or phosphorylated proteins (SIBLINGs) (DSPP, DSP, DMP1)	Abnormal dentin properties and tooth structure
Environmental effects: • fluorosis • dioxin • other toxic agents	Odontoblast gene expression changes	Hyper/hypomineralization, structural alterations
Loss of tooth structure: • caries • abrasion • restorative dental material	Reactionary dentin	Ortho- or osteodentin formed beneath a calciotraumatic line
Pulp exposure	Reparative dentin	Dentinal bridge, partial or total pulp mineralization

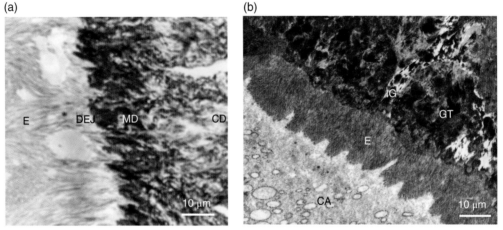

(a)   (b)

Figure 5.4   Electron micrographs of a rat molar. (a) Atubular mantle dentin (MD) in the coronal part of the forming molar. DEJ: dentinoenamel junction. E: enamel. CD: circumpulpal dentin. (b) Beneath the forming enamel (E) and cervical ameloblasts (CA), calcospherites contribute to the formation of the superficial Tomes' granular layer (GT). An interglobular space (IG) is located between the granules. Bar = 10 μm.

is formed before eruption. The curvature is more accentuated in tubules formed after the eruption of the tooth.

Secondary dentin formation begins after completion of primary dentin formation. The structure and composition of secondary dentin are similar to those of primary dentin. A slight change in the direction of the dentinal tubules occurs when secondary dentin formation begins. The formation of secondary dentin continues at a slow rate throughout life, but is gradually reduced in later years (Fig. 5.2 and Table 5.1).

Between the tubules, **intertubular dentin** is found (Figs. 5.5a, 5.6 and Table 5.1). This dentin specifically results from the continuous apposition of predentin components at the mineralization front (Fig. 5.3). It is a collagen-rich structure, containing fibrils about 80 to 100 nm in diameter (Fig. 5.6). Non-collagenous proteins are associated either with the surface of collagen fibrils and holes due to the quarter-stagger transversal bands of collagen fibrils, or they fill the spaces between collagen fibrils (Fig. 5.7). The dentin organic matrix plays a crucial role in promoting crystal nucleation and allowing limited growth to

hydroxyapatite crystallites. The needle-like crystallites are 3 nm in thickness and 60 nm in length. Each crystallite is formed by the association of two plates (each 1 nm thick) separated by a thin electron-lucent layer (Fig. 5.8a).

The lumen of the dentinal tubules contains non-mineralized collagen fibrils and some amorphous proteins forming a periodontoblastic structure around the odontoblast process. **Peritubular dentin** forms a highly mineralized ring around the tubules but never completely fills the lumen. Isodiametric crystals about 25 nm in width and 9 to 10 nm in length resist abrasive forces and occlusal pressures (Fig. 5.5b and Table 5.1). These crystallites have high magnesium and carbonate content. They display high solubility in acid and chelating solutions. Peritubular dentin formation begins within the tubules, a few micrometers from the predentin-dentin junction. Present mostly in the inner two-thirds of the dentin, it is reduced in the outer one-third and almost lacking in the mantle dentin. Peritubular dentin does not contain collagen fibrils, but is comprised of non-collagenous proteins, namely phospholipids or lipoproteins and proteoglycans (Fig. 5.5b).

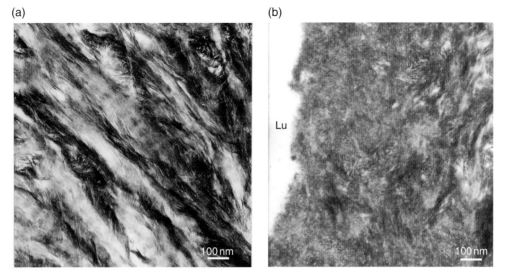

Figure 5.5   Electron micrographs of unstained ultrathin sections of human dentin. (a) Intertubular dentin. Crystallites are located along and between collagen fibrils. The periodic banding of collagen is apparent. Bar = 100 nm. (b) Peritubular dentin displays isodiametric crystallites about 35 nm in diameter. Lumen of dentinal tubule (Lu). Bar = 100 nm.

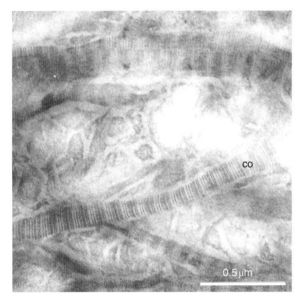

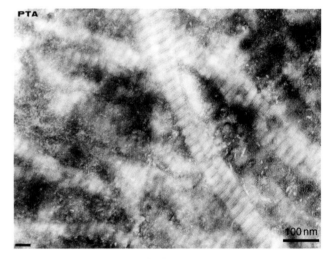

Figure 5.7   Electron micrograph of phosphorylated extracellular matrix proteins stained with phosphotungstic acid–chromic acid (PTA) in intertubular dentin. The electron-dense staining is located along and between the collagen fibrils. Bar = 100 nm.

Figure 5.6   Electron micrograph of type I collagen fibrils (co) in intertubular dentin. Demineralized section. Bar = 0.5 μm.

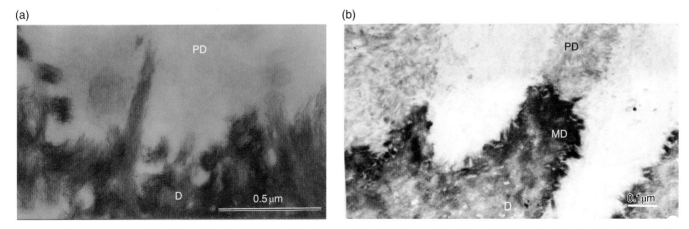

Figure 5.8   Electron micrographs of rat molar dentin. (a) Unstained section. Needle-like crystallites located at the mineralization front between the predentin (PD) and dentin (D) are seen along the collagen fibrils. Bar = 0.5 μm. (b) The distal border (metadentin: MD) located between the predentin (PD) and intertubular dentin (D) is densely stained by the phosphotungstic acid–chromic acid mixture. Bar = 0.1 μm.

In the sclerotic zone of carious decay, or after pathologic abrasion, or as a consequence of the aging process, the tubules may be filled by intratubular mineralization. Such heterogeneous mineralization results from the occurrence of pathologic processes that favor the precipitation of calcium and phosphate ions into non-apatitic forms within the lumen of the tubules.

The reparative process occurs in arrested carious lesions, or in response to the preparation of cavities. It also may be due to the effects of the release of resin monomers by restorative dental materials. These events lead to the formation of **tertiary dentin**, classified as either **reactionary dentin** or **reparative dentin**. **Hoehl's cells** (Fig. 5.3) and surviving secretory odontoblasts form reactionary dentin, which appears either as orthodentin or osteodentin (Table 5.2). If both the odontoblastic and Hoehl's cell layers are irreversibly altered, pulp progenitor cells contribute to the formation of reparative dentin.

> Dentin includes atubular peripheral dentin (the mantle dentin in the crown and Hopewell-Smith and/or Tomes' granular layers in the root) and tubular circumpulpal dentin. After the formation of primary dentin, secondary dentin is formed during the entire life of the functioning tooth. Between the tubules, there is a network of intertubular dentin, whereas around the lumen of the tubules peritubular dentin increases resistance to occlusal pressures. After a mild lesion (caries, abrasion, and/or restorative material), odontoblasts and Hoehl's cells contribute to the formation of reactionary dentin (also named tertiary dentin) beneath a calciotraumatic line. After irreversible alteration of these cells, or a pulp exposure, pulp cells contribute to the formation of reparative dentin.

Dentin composition

Dentin consists of an organic matrix composed largely of **Type I collagen**, within which hydroxyapatite mineral crystals are deposited. Mature dentin contains more organic substance than enamel, but less mineral (Table 5.3). In addition to Type I collagen, small amounts of Type III and Type V collagen are present. Non-collagenous components, including phosphorylated and non-phosphorylated proteins, proteoglycans, lipids, **growth factors**, and enzymes, account for about 10% of the organic matrix (Table 5.4). While many of the non-collagenous components also are present in bone and other tissue, products of the dentin sialophosphoprotein gene are specific to odontoblasts and dentin. These non-collagenous components have important functions in mineral nucleation and crystal growth.

Dentin formation

Pre-odontoblast differentiation and tooth morphogenesis

As described in Chapter 3, at early stages of tooth formation, neural crest-derived mesenchymal cells migrate toward the first branchial arch. Interaction between these cells (condensing mesenchyme) and epithelial cells located specifically at placode sites leads to the proliferation of the epithelial cells and formation of a dental lamina. The two tissues form the rudiment of the embryonic tooth, epithelial cells forming the enamel organ and mesenchymal cells forming the dental papilla, or embryonic pulp (Fig. 5.9).

Crown morphogenesis starts with the formation of dental buds, followed by the cap stage, and later by early and late bell stages. The lateral proliferation of epithelial cells occurring at the periphery contributes to increase the diameter of the enamel organ. Four epithelial layers form the enamel organ: the outer enamel epithelium, the stellate reticulum, the stratum intermedium, and the inner enamel epithelium, the latter eventually differentiating to ameloblasts (Figs. 5.9–5.12). The cells undergo a series of divisions, leading to the formation of folds, the onset of shaping grooves and cusps. In the mouse molar, cell division in the embryonic mesenchymal pulp stops before it does in the enamel organ, leading to a larger surface of inner enamel epithelium compared with pre-odontoblasts. Folds begin to form, leading to cusp formation. In the central area of the enamel organ, the enamel knot regulates the morphogenetic process, influencing the process through cell proliferation and apoptosis.

Epithelial-mesenchymal interactions are instrumental in the transition from mesenchymal embryonic pulp cells to a pre-odontoblastic stage. The cells at the periphery of the embryonic pulp undergo asymmetric division. After the last mitosis, the larger cells in contact with the **basement membrane** (BM) (**basal lamina**) become early **pre-polarized odontoblasts** (Figs. 5.10 and 5.11). These cells ultimately differentiate into **polarized secretory odontoblasts** (Figs. 5.13a and b). The cells some distance away from the BM are smaller and retain their potential as **stem cells**. They are grouped in the sub-odontoblastic cell layer of Hoehl (Figs. 5.2 and 5.3), which may differentiate ultimately toward the odontoblastic lineage. It is crucial to highlight that odontoblasts are post-mitotic cells. In case of carious decay or odontoblast injury, differentiation of Hoehl's cells is reactivated and polarized secretory odontoblasts are implicated in reactionary dentin formation (Figs. 5.14–5.16b and 5.16c). If both the odontoblastic and Hoehl's cell layers are irreversibly

Table 5.3   Summary of the global composition of dentin.

Component	By Weight	By Volume
Mineral content	68–70%	50%
Organic content	21%	30%
Water (free and bound)	11%	20%

Note: Substantial differences occur between the different types of dentin described in the text.

> Early tooth development involves reciprocal interactions between neural crest-derived mesenchymal cells and oral ectoderm-derived cells of the enamel organ. The peripheral mesenchymal cells of the dental papilla proliferate and become pre-polarized odontoblasts, subsequently differentiating into odontoblasts. Cells in the sub-odontoblastic layer retain their potential as stem cells.

Table 5.4   Components of the extracellular organic matrix

Component	Protein Family	Specific Proteins
Collagen (90%)	Collagens	Type I (~90%) and Type I trimer (~11%) Type III and V (1–3%): During dentin formation and detected in some pathology
Non-collagenous proteins (10%)	Phosphorylated SIBLINGs (Implicated in mineral nucleation and crystal growth, but also inhibitors in some cases)	Dentin sialophosphoprotein (DSPP): cleaved immediately after secretion into *Dentin SialoProtein (DSP), *Dentin Glycoprotein (DGP) and *Dentin Phosphoprotein (DPP) Dentin matrix protein1 (DMP1) Bone sialoprotein (BSP) Osteopontin (OPN) Matrix Extracellular Phosphorylated Glycoprotein (MEPE)
	Transient phosphorylated protein expressed by young odontoblasts	Amelogenin
	Other ECM proteins (non-phosphorylated)	Osteonectin Osteocalcin Serum-derived proteins (α_2HS glycoprotein, albumin)
	Proteoglycans	Decorin, biglycan, fibromodulin, osteoadherin
	Growth factors	Transforming growth factor β (TGFβ), fibroblast growth factors (FGFs), insulin-like growth factors 1 & 2 (IGF-1 & -2), vascular endothelial growth factor (VEGF), bone morphogenetic proteins (BMPs)
	Enzymes	Acid & alkaline phosphatases, matrix metalloproteinases (MMPs), tissue inhibitors of metalloproteinases (TIMPS), A disintegrin and metalloproteinase (ADAMs), A disintegrin and metalloproteinase with thrombospondin motifs (ADAMTS)
	Proteolipids/phospholipids	Intracellular (membrane) and extracellular

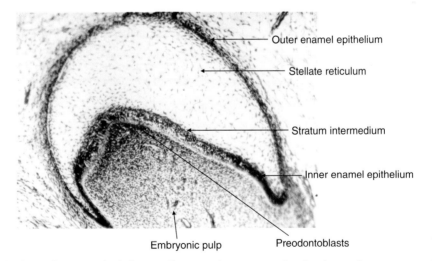

Figure 5.9   Light micrograph of a tooth germ at the bell stage. The enamel organ comprises four layers: the outer enamel epithelium, the stellate reticulum, the stratum intermedium, and the inner enamel epithelium. A basement membrane separates the inner enamel epithelium from the pre-odontoblasts at the tip of the pulp horn. These cells line the periphery of the embryonic pulp.

altered, pulp progenitors contribute to the formation of reparative dentin (Fig 5.16a). As odontoblasts become older they gradually are reduced in number. Hoehl's cells then may become activated and differentiate into new odontoblast-like cells.

Polarizing post-mitotic odontoblasts

Odontoblasts are grouped in a restricted layer at the periphery of the pulp. The odontoblast layer includes three to four rows of cell bodies. In the distal cell body, **polarizing post-mitotic**

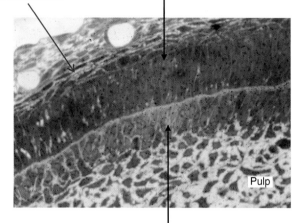

Figure 5.10   Light micrograph of developing rat incisor. The stratum intermedium and presecretory ameloblasts are facing pre-polarized odontoblasts. Between the two layers of cells, the formation of predentin has already been initiated. Numerous pulpoblasts (fibroblasts) are present within the dental pulp.

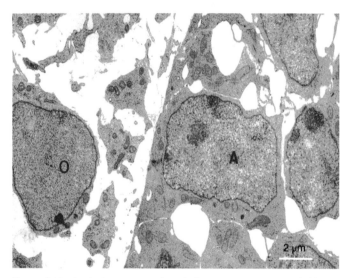

Figure 5.11   In the inner enamel epithelium, presecretory ameloblasts (A) establish a series of intercellular junctions. At the surface of the embryonic pulp polarizing presecretory odontoblasts (O) have not yet begun to produce dentin. Bar = 2 μm.

odontoblasts establish intercellular junctional complexes, including a series of gap and desmosome-like junctions. Initially, odontoblast processes are short, coated with carbohydrates/oligosaccharides, and adherent to the BM. As newly formed dentin is deposited, **odontoblast cell bodies** move backward toward the central part of the pulp, and the cell processes elongate. Secretory molecules are initially released all around the cell bodies. Thick interodontoblastic collagen fibers (**von Korff fibers**), consisting of Type III collagen, contribute to the anchorage of the cellular compartment to the initial forming dentin (Fig. 5.13b). During the terminal cell polarization, the secretion of collagen and

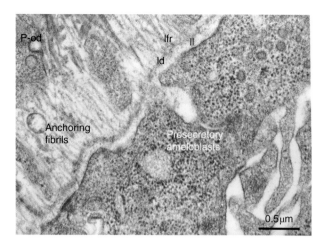

Figure 5.12   Ribosome-rich presecretory ameloblasts form a continuous cell layer. They produce the three parts of the basement membrane (lamina lucida, ll; lamina densa, ld; lamina fibroreticularis, lfr). Anchoring fibrils are the earliest components synthesized by the pre-odontoblasts (p-od). They are at right angles with the basement membrane. Bar = 0.5 μm.

non-collagenous proteins is gradually restricted to the distal part of the cell bodies. Secretion then occurs in the predentin and along the mineralization front.

Polarized secretory odontoblasts

Odontoblasts form dentin, a mineralized structure resulting exclusively from the biological activities of these cells. Schematically, intertubular dentin formation occurs within a three-layer system, consisting of the cell bodies, the predentin, and the dentin. Most extracellular matrix (ECM) molecules are synthesized and secreted by the odontoblasts (Figs. 5.2, 5.17–5.19). Very few molecules are synthesized elsewhere and take an interodontoblastic pathway, cross the terminal intercellular barrier, and diffuse in the predentin/dentin areas. Although this is the case for albumin and α_2HS glycoprotein (fetuin), serum-derived molecules are a very minor component of dentin ECM.

The cell body layer

At the periphery of the dental pulp, odontoblast cell bodies form a layer infiltrated by capillaries (Fig. 5.3). Odontoblast cell bodies 3 μm wide and 20 to 40 μm in length display three anatomically distinct parts, as follows.

1. The basal part, where mitochondria accumulate around the nucleus, whereas rough endoplasmic reticulum (rER) occupies the lateral borders.

2. The central part, with lateral stacks of rER cisternae, a few supranuclear Golgi complexes randomly oriented, immature secretory vesicles, and lysosomal multivesicular bodies. Some vesicles contain abacus-like structures showing periodicity. The repeated 1000-nm banding suggests accumulation of procollagen, larger than the periodic 640-nm banding pattern of collagen fibrils. Immunolabeling reveals a close link between the intracellular collagen and the abacus-like vesicles, also identified as acid-phosphatase-containing structures. Hence, it was first believed that

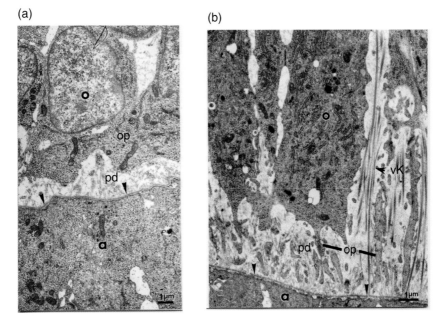

Figure 5.13   (a) Early dentinogenesis. A basement membrane (arrowheads) is present at the distal surface of the presecretory ameloblasts (a). Polarizing odontoblasts (o) display developing processes (op). A few fibrils are located in the initial predentin (pd). Bar = 1 μm. (b) At a later stage, polarizing odontoblasts (o) display an increase in rER cisternae. Between cell bodies, bundles of thick collagen fibrils are probably representative of the von Korff fibrils (vK). Bar = 1 μm.

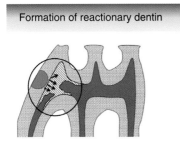

Figure 5.14   Schematic drawing showing the formation of reactionary dentin (brown-hatched area) after the preparation of a cavity (blue semicircle) in the mesial aspect of the first maxillary molar of a rat. Pulp (magenta). (Based on: Decup, F., Six, N., et al. (2000) Bone sialoprotein-induced reparative dentinogenesis in the pulp of rat's molar. *Clinical Oral Investigations*, 4(2), 110–119.)

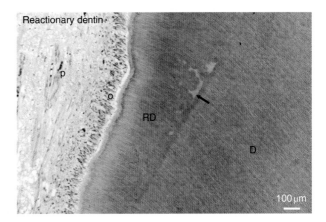

Figure 5.15   Formation of reactionary dentin (RD) in the dental pulp of a human premolar 90 days after the filling of a cavity. Dentin (D); pulp (P); odontoblasts (o); interglobular spaces (arrow). Bar = 100 μm.

these abacus-like vesicles were implicated in the collagen secretory pathway, but now it is clear that the nonsecreted collagen is stored and destroyed within these vesicles, actually recognized as lysosomes (Figs. 5.17 and 5.18). Cytoskeletal proteins are implicated in the cell body in the formation of cilia, but also shape the cells. These include tubulin in the form of microtubules and molecules implicated in secretion/re-internalization: actin microfilaments and vimentin intermediate filaments, all of them contributing to space information, exocytosis, and endocytotic events (Fig. 5.19).

3. The distal part contains clusters of mitochondria. They accumulate together with large lysosomes and small secretory vesicles containing procollagen microfibrils. Near the predentin, gap and desmosome-like intercellular junctions seal the lateral membranes (Fig. 5.19). In a few non-human species, some tight junctions are also identified.

A sub-plasmalemmal undercoat is formed by microfilaments. Inside the odontoblast processes, microtubules and intermediate filaments, such as nestin, constitute a developed network. Mitochondria are smaller compared to those present in the cell body. Internalization of clathrin-coated vesicles contributes to the uptake of degraded molecules or cleaved peptides, which are transferred to the large lysosomes located in the distal cell bodies. Secretion of extracellular matrix proteins occurs by exocytosis of secretory vesicles. Because exocytosis occurs within a few milliseconds, it is very difficult to detect under a microscope. Empty membrane ghosts or electron-lucent areas may characterize the secretory vesicles at the electron microscope level.

Extracellular matrix precursor molecules are delivered by blood vessels, diffuse through the fenestrations of endothelial

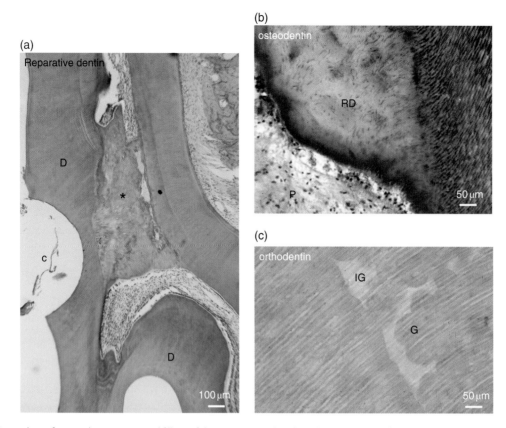

Figure 5.16   (a) Ninety days after a pulp exposure and filling of the cavity (c) with a dental cement, reparative dentin (*) partially occludes the exposure of the mesial root pulp. Dentin (D). Bar = 100 μm. (b) Human tooth: Reactionary osteodentin (RD), stains as a pink/violet structure, whereas orthodentin (right part of the figure) contains purple tubular dentin. Pulp, (P). "Stains all" method. (c) After the preparation of a cavity in a human premolar and glass ionomer filling, reactionary orthodentin is formed, characterized by globular structures (G) and interglobular spaces (IG). Bars in b and c = 50 μm.

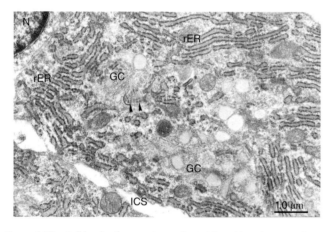

Figure 5.17   Cell body of a secretory odontoblast. Abundant rough endoplasmic reticulum (rER) fills the cytoplasm, and a prominent Golgi complex (GC) is present. Arrowheads indicate the collagen-like content of an abacus-like vesicle. Nucleus (N); intercellular space (ICS). Bar = 1 μm.

cells, and cross the semipermeable BM limiting the capillaries. Amino acids are incorporated into the forming protein in the rER of the odontoblasts. The addition of initial sugars such as mannose occurs within the rER, whereas the terminal sugars, e.g., fucose, are added in the Golgi complex. Sulfate and phosphate are incorporated into the proteins directly in the Golgi saccules. The newly synthesized ECM components are conveyed from the presecretory to secretory vesicles where they

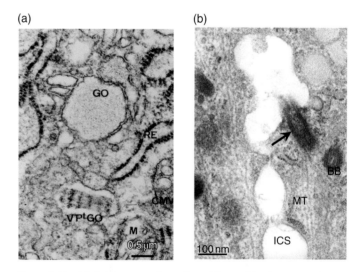

Figure 5.18   (a) Golgi region of an odontoblast cell body. Accumulation of procollagen abacus-like bundles in post-Golgi vesicles (VP'GO) is characteristic of collagen secreting cells. Rough endoplasmic reticulum (RE); Golgi vesicle (GO); mitochondrion (M). Bar = 0.5 μm. (b) Cytoskeletal proteins in the cell body. A cilium (arrow) and basal body (BB) are located near the intercellular space (ICS) between odontoblast cell bodies. Microtubules (MT). Bar = 100 nm.

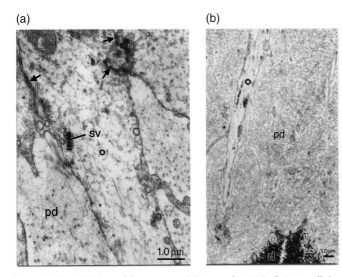

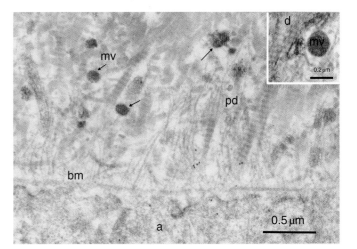

Figure 5.19   (a) Odontoblast process (o) in predentin (pd). Intercellular junctions (arrows) hold adjacent cells together. Secretory vesicle (sv). Bar = 1 μm. (b) Odontoblast process (o) extends through the predentin (pd) and reaches dentin (d). Bar = 1 μm.

Figure 5.20   Matrix vesicles (mv) (arrows) are present in the predentin (pd) at the onset of dentinogenesis. Electron microscopic immunogold labelling for MMP20 (small black particles) is discrete at that stage. Basement membrane (bm); presecretory ameloblasts (a). Bar = 0.5 μm. **Inset:** higher magnification of a matrix vesicle (mv) in the mineralizing dentin (d). Bar = 0.2 μm.

mature and are secreted after enzymatic processing. The C-terminal non-helical extensions of the procollagen are cleaved in the distal cell bodies by a procollagen peptidase, identical to a bone morphogenetic protein (BMP). After secretion, the N-terminal extensions are cleaved by a peptidase in the proximal predentin. The non-helical extensions are recaptured by the cells and transferred to the distal lysosomes. This recapture provides feedback information to the odontoblasts.

Odontoblast cell processes expand some distance away within the tubules. The actual length of the process is still a matter of discussion. Processes may extend from the pulp to the dentinoenamel junction, but most are probably limited to the inner one-third or one-half of the dentin.

The predentin compartment

Between the cell bodies and dentin, the predentin forms a layer with a constant thickness (15–20 μm in width). The collagen molecules in this non-mineralized compartment are secreted from the odontoblast processes. After secretion into the predentin, the native collagen fibrils increase in thickness (lateral aggregation) and elongate (end-to-end association due to telopeptide interactions, consequently contributing to the lengthening of the collagen fibrils). Initially, just after their assembly, collagen fibrils in the inner predentin display a 20-nm average diameter. At the end of the fibrillation process, in the distal predentin, collagen fibers show a 70- to 80-nm mean diameter. Proteoglycans such as decorin, biglycan, and fibromodulin are implicated in collagen fibrillation, and constitute a gradient of amorphous gel allowing the sliding and migration of the collagen fibrils toward the distal mineralization front. This orientation is under the control of forces resulting from secretion, distortion of the gel network, and pushing the fibrils toward the dentin edge. Dissipative forces contribute to the formation of calcospherites at the mineralization front (Figs. 5.2 and 5.19).

The dentin layer

The junction between predentin and dentin is not linear, but appears as a wavy profile produced by successive salient globular calcospherites. Most non-collagenous proteins (**SIBLINGs** and proteoglycans) are secreted in the 3- to 5-μm-thick **metadentin**, a thin border located at the mineralization front. Some of these non-collagenous proteins are added at the surface of fibrils and within the gaps between the quarter-staggered collagen molecules. Consequently, needle-like mineral crystallites contribute to the onset of intertubular dentin mineralization. Crystallite maturation occurs in the dentin located deep to the metadentin. The crystallites fill the interfibrillar spaces. The ECM limits growth of the mineral phase, which also provides some elastic properties to dentin.

As is the case in other calcified tissues such as cartilage and bone, **matrix vesicles** (MVs) are implicated at early stages of the crown and root formation in the mineralization of the peripheral dentin layers. MVs appear as membrane-bounded vesicles arising from budding processes from the plasma membrane of non-polarized young odontoblasts (Fig. 5.20). They act as nucleating centers, and the transition from amorphous calcium phosphate to crystalline phase takes place within MVs. The interaction of heparan sulfate proteoglycans, calpactin I and II, tissue non-specific alkaline phosphatase (TNAP), Ca^{2+}-ATPase, annexins II, V, and VI, metalloproteinases (MMP-1, -2, -3, and -9), BMPs and their receptors, and calcium-phosphate-lipoprotein complexes (CPLX) promotes the transformation of amorphous calcium phosphate into hydroxyapatite. After the initial formation of bundles of crystallites, MVs are no longer needed for dentin mineralization to proceed.

Formation of peritubular dentin

The three-layer compartment structure is well adapted to the formation of intertubular dentin. The mechanism of formation of peritubular dentin is less clear. This dentin does not form at the predentin border, but starts to be formed a few

(a)   (b)

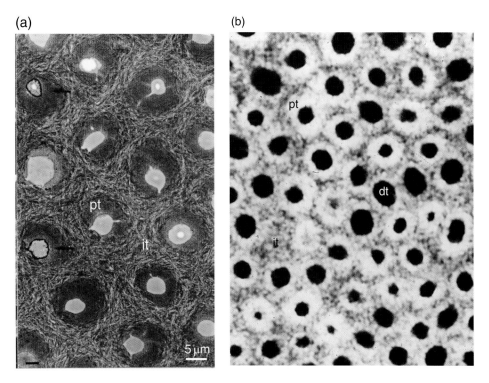

Figure 5.21   Dentinal tubules and peritubular dentin (a) Electron micrograph of human dentin. Intertubular dentin (it); peritubular dentin (pt). Bar = 5 μm. (b) Microradiograph of human dentin. Peritubular dentin has a greater mineral content and appears whiter than intertubular dentin. Dentinal tubule (dt).

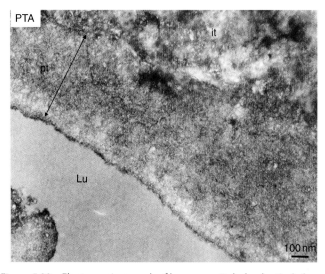

Figure 5.22   Electron micrograph of human peritubular dentin (pt). Intertubular dentin (it); lumen of dental tubule (Lu). The section was stained with phosphotungstic acid (PTA), revealing phosphorylated extracellular matrix proteins. Bar = 100 nm.

Pre-odontoblasts are mitotic cells. After the last division, post-mitotic presecretory polarizing odontoblasts synthesize and secrete collagen and non-collagenous proteins, including the phosphorylated SIBLINGs implicated in the mineralization process. Synthesis of extracellular matrix (ECM) proteins occurs in the cell body of secretory odontoblasts, whereas secretion of ECM molecules and re-internalization of fragmented molecules after enzymatic cleavage occur in the cell processes. The processes elongate as dentin is deposited and the odontoblast cell bodies move toward the pulp. Deposition and mineralization of dentin around the processes creates the dentinal tubules. The formation of intertubular dentin is a two-step process: collagen and some ECM are secreted in the predentin, whereas other ECM molecules are secreted more distally at the mineralization front (metadentin). The formation of peritubular dentin is less clear, occurring by secretion of some molecules or deposition of plasma-derived molecules along the walls of the tubules.

micrometers away from the mineralization front. Minute tubules perforate the peritubular dentin, indicating that branches of vital odontoblast processes are present during peritubular dentin formation. This suggest that either extracellular matrix molecules are secreted by the processes along the tubule walls, or that components originating from the blood plasma diffuse within the tubules and are subsequently deposited along the walls of the tubules (Figs. 5.21 and 5.22).

Type I collagen is lacking in the peritubular dentin, whereas phospholipids, proteoglycans, and a few SIBLINGs are detected. The organic matrix forms an amorphous thin network between isodiametric crystals differing from the collagen-associated crystallites of the intertubular dentin. Peritubular dentin is more mineralized than intertubular dentin, and consequently better resists abrasion or attrition. The distribution varies among species, forming between 2 to 10% of the dentin surface in humans, a gradient being detectable when moving from the outer to the inner dentin.

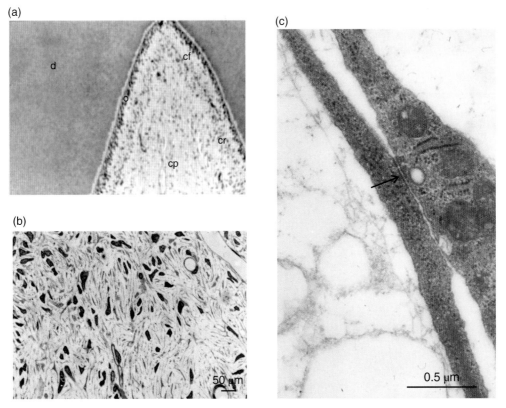

Figure 5.23   (a) Light micrograph of dental pulp. Beneath the odontoblast layer (o), cell-free (cf) and cell-rich zones (cr) are seen at the pulp periphery. The central pulp (cp) contains structural pulp cells of the fibroblast-type (pulpoblasts). (b) Heterogeneity of the pulp cells: pulpoblasts, endothelial cells and pericytes. Semi-thin section. Bar = 50 μm. (c) Intercellular junction (arrow) between two fibroblasts. Bar = 0.5 μm.

Pulp structure and function

Many publications refer to a dentin-pulp complex. However, this concept does not take into account the following facts.

- In contrast with dentin, the dental pulp is a soft connective tissue that normally is not mineralized.
- Dentin is formed by the odontoblasts and Hoehl's cells, which are neural crest-derived, post-mitotic cells, with a limited lifespan. In contrast, a variety of pulp cells are from different origins. They are continuously renewed with a rapid turnover.
- Odontoblasts are implicated in dentin formation, including primary, secondary, and reactionary dentin, whereas pulp cells stimulate reparative dentin formation, pulp stones, or diffuse mineralization.
- Dentin is not vascularized, whereas two structurally different vascular networks supply the pulp.

Therefore, from a biological point of view, pulp and dentin are very different (Figs. 5.2 and 5.23).

Coronal pulp development

At the bell stage, the epithelial enamel organ surrounds the mesenchymal embryonic pulp or dental papilla. The initial coronal pulp has a dual origin.

- The neural crest-derived pre-odontoblasts migrate toward the periphery of the dental papilla where they undergo a fixed number of cell divisions and finally become post-mitotic odontoblasts with a long lifespan, implicated in dentin formation.
- The structural pulp cells exhibit a short lifespan. They take origin from the mesenchyme of the first branchial arch and from the frontonasal process. The **fibroblast-like pulp cells (pulpoblasts)** appear in the central part of the pulp, and migrate toward the sub-odontoblastic region. They are continually renewed.

Three regions are identified in the pulp: (1) the acellular layer of Weil, called a **cell-free pulp area**, located beneath the odontoblast Hoehl's cell layer in the superficial pulp; (2) this peripheral pulp layer covers a **cell-rich pulp zone** wrapping the bulk of the pulp; and (3) this also is identified as **central pulp** (Fig. 5.23a).

Root pulp development

At the end of the bell stage, the edges of the inner and outer enamel epithelium merge and form the cervical loop. Upon completion of the crown, proliferation and apical extension of the cells of the cervical loop results in the development of Hertwig's epithelial root sheath. The root sheath cells induce the adjacent mesenchymal cells of the dental papilla to differentiate

Table 5.5 Composition of the extracellular matrix (ECM) of the dental pulp

Component	Protein Family	Specific Proteins
Collagen	Collagen	Type I (56%) Type III (41%) Type V (2%) Type VI (0.5%) (associated with microfibrillin)
Non-collagenous proteins	Phosphorylated ECM proteins	Bone sialoprotein (BSP) Osteopontin (OPN) (DSPP, DPP, DSP, DMP1, MEPE not detected, except in case of compensatory mechanisms or during the formation of reparative dentin)
	Non-phosphorylated ECM proteins	Fibronectin Osteonectin Osteocalcin (limited to odontoblast/Hoehl's cell layer)
	Proteoglycans Glycosaminoglycan	Versican Chondroitin sulfate-4 (CS-4) CS-6 (60%) Dermatan sulfate (DS) (34%), Keratan sulfate (KS) (2%) Hyaluronic acid
	Growth factors	BMPs Type IA & II receptors for TGFβ Activin
	Protein taking origin from the plasma	Fibronectin
	Enzymes	Metalloproteinases (MMPs: collagenases, gelatinases, stromelysin-1) Tissue inhibitors of metalloproteases (TIMPs) Alkaline and acid phosphatases Catalytic lysosomal and extracellular enzymes
	Phospholipids	Membrane and ECM phospholipids (proteolipids)

into odontoblasts and initiate root formation. Initially, the root elongates above a fixed position where the epithelial diaphragm is found. The short pre-eruptive phase is followed by the eruptive phase, closely associated with the formation of the root and radicular pulp. The vascular network of the pulp displays an increased complexity, appearing in the root as a fishnet-like structure. In the root, innervation appears to be located centrally, near the blood vessels.

Two different more or less independent innervation and vascularization pathways have been identified at those stages: the first is linked to crown formation whereas the second is associated with root formation.

The adult pulp: composition and cells

Similar to connective tissue in other locations, the extracellular matrix of the dental pulp consists of collagens, non-collagenous proteins, glycoproteins, proteoglycans, enzymes, growth factors, various phospholipids and proteolipids, and components derived from plasma (Table 5.5). Additionally, some components characteristic of bone are typically present, whereas several components characteristic of dentin are present only in certain situations, such as during the formation of reparative dentin.

Fibroblast-like pulp cells (or pulpoblasts), and pulp stem cells

The spindle-shaped fibroblast-like pulp cells synthesize and secrete collagenous and non-collagenous proteins (Fig. 5.23b). Collagen fibrils are thin and punctuated by proteoglycans. The pulpoblasts contain numerous free ribosomes and a few rough endoplasmic reticulum cisternae (Figs. 5.24 and 5.25). Secretion vesicles fill most of the cells, whereas others seem to contain mostly electron-dense lysosomes. The two structures are simultaneously present. Cytoskeletal proteins are present throughout the cell. Many cells appear to be ciliated. The pulpoblasts are firmly linked by intercellular junctions (Fig. 5.23c). This implies that pulpal cells bound to each other appear in the central part of the crown, migrate together toward the pulp periphery, and undergo apoptosis.

After tooth formation is completed, beneath the peripheral layer comprising odontoblasts and Hoehl's cells, the pulp includes a central part containing fibroblast-like cells, a few axons, and blood vessels lined by endothelial cells (Fig. 5.23a). Inflammatory and immune cells also contribute to the cellular heterogeneity of the pulp (Figs. 5.24 and 5.26). The life span of pulpal fibroblast has not been determined accurately, but *in vitro* studies suggest a mean lifetime of 24 ± 11 days. Thus, pulpoblasts

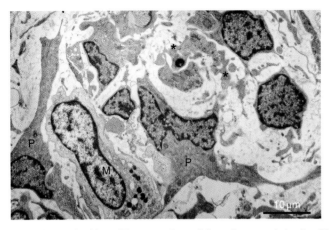

Figure 5.24   Pulpoblasts (P), macrophage (M), and apoptotic bodies (*) within the dental pulp. Bar = 10 μm.

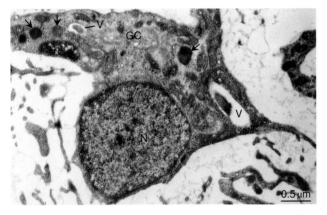

Figure 5.25   Numerous vacuoles (V) and lysosomes (arrows) implicate pulp fibroblast-like cells in phagocytosis and degradation of the ECM. Nucleus (N); Golgi complex (GC). Bar = 0.5 μm.

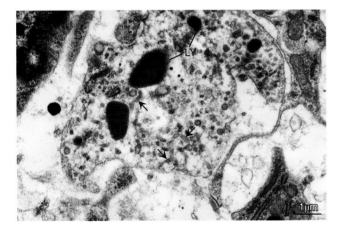

Figure 5.26   Macrophage in the pulp, displaying tubulovesicular structures (arrows) and lysosomes (LY). Bar = 1 μm.

are not immobilized cells, but display a dynamic outcome. Even if they are structural cells, they proliferate, migrate and end their life by apoptosis.

The fibroblast-like cells may be mesenchymal cells related to mononuclear phagocytes/histiocytes. They are elongated, with thin spinous processes. They are highly mobile and contain numerous lipid vesicles. Pulp cells are implicated in the turnover of the tissue, secreting new ECM proteins, and degrading old or damaged proteins through production and secretion of matrix metalloproteinases (Fig. 5.25).

In this heterogeneous population of cells, most pulpoblasts are structural. However, 1 to 2% of these cells are stem cells, progenitors of cells of osteoblast-like lineage. These cells display self-renewal capabilities, with a concomitance of multipotent and monopotent cells. They may differentiate into osteoblasts, odontoblasts, chondrocytes, adipocytes, neurons, and a few other phenotypes.

Little is known of the *in vivo* biology of **pulp stem cells**. It is unknown whether these cells, which are highly proliferative *in vitro*, proliferate and form *in vivo* a tissue with a defined phenotype; or if short intercellular contacts between the stem cell and structural pulpoblasts allow the release and diffusion of paracrine messages provoking their later transformation. All these cells may contribute to a bony/dentin tissue, implicated in reparative osteodentin formation.

Inflammatory cells

Immune defense cells have been identified in the dental pulp, forming a population including pulpal dendritic cells, histiocytes/macrophages, and T-lymphocytes. Other **pulp inflammatory cells** include polymorphonuclear neutrophilic leukocytes and mast cells, which are also implicated in the defense mechanisms.

Lymphocytes are classified as B-lymphocytes or T-lymphocytes. T-lymphocytes include peripheral T-cells, helper/inducer T-cells ($CD4^+$) and cytotoxic/suppressor T-cells ($CD8^+$). The B-lymphocytes are rare or lacking in the normal pulp and during an early inflammatory reaction of the pulp, whereas they are increased in advanced phases. In contrast, the T-lymphocytes are revealed by immunostaining both in normal and inflamed pulps.

Immune cells of the family of dendritic cells (DCs) take origin in the bone marrow, and migrate into the pulp. Dendritic cells are seen in the odontoblast layer and in the central part of the pulp. DCs and macrophages share several morphologic and phenotypic properties. Macrophages are scavenger cells with phagocytic capacities. The DCs eliminate the antigen immune complexes. They produce microbicidal enzymes and several cytokines and growth factors implicated in tissue repair, and they activate the T-lymphocytes. DCs are concentrated at the periphery of the coronal pulp. Their number increases with the formation and eruption of the teeth. Then an age-related decrease parallels an increased susceptibility to infection. All these cells express antigenic peptides at their membrane surface, and they are members of the **class I and class II major histocompatibility complex (MHC)** cells. Macrophages and MHC Class II-expressing dendritic cells constitute the majority of the pulp cells implicated in the immune reaction. The immune cells engulf (phagocytose) and eliminate the apoptotic bodies; they are also implicated in phagocytosis of bacteria.

Resident macrophages appear at perivascular locations. In addition to histiocytes, macrophages expressing lysosomal membrane-associated markers are present mostly in the sub-odontoblastic zone. Nonresident macrophages and monocytes expressing MHC class II molecules constitute minor macrophage populations (Figs. 5.24 and 5.26).

In uninflamed dental pulp, lymphocytes have been found as normal resident cells. T-lymphocytes are located near blood vessels in the inner portion of the pulp. The B-lymphocytes are rarely encountered in the normal pulp and therefore display a questionable potential role.

Mast cells containing histamine, leukotrienes, and platelet-activating factor, are implicated in immediate hypersensitivity reactions. They express serine proteases and the pro-inflammatory cytokine tumor necrosis factor α (TNFα). Histamine is released in response to neurogenic inflammation. Mast cells do not contribute to early vascular or specific immune responses in the initial pulp pathology, whereas cytolytic T-lymphocytes, memory T-cells, and helper T-lymphocytes contribute to the late (chronic) pulp response.

Polymorphonuclear leukocytes are mostly involved in the capture and degradation of caries-associated bacteria invading the dental pulp.

Pulp vascularization

Blood vascularization

During development of the crown, the penetration of vascular cells into the tooth germ at the late bell stage leads to the construction of a network forming the rudiment of vessels. **Pulp vascularization** starts from single CD34+ cells forming vascular cords inside the developing connective tissue. During root formation, a capillary network occupies the peripheral areas, whereas arterioles and venules are located in the central part of the pulp. In the adult the process of vasculogenesis persists and contributes to a continuous adjustment of vessels in response to functional needs.

In the adult, vessels enter the pulp via the apical and accessory foramina. The primary feeding arterioles (35–45 μm in diameter) divide into secondary arterioles (35–25 μm) and end as terminal arterioles (15–25 μm). Pre-capillaries (12–15 μm) are in continuity with capillaries (>8 μm), followed by post-capillary venules (12–23 μm). Collecting venules (24–50 μm) enlarge to form venules (>50 μm), which exit from the pulp via the apex of the tooth. Red cell velocity decreases and in capillaries attains values one-tenth of those of the feeding arteries. The maximum value for red cell velocity in the large collecting veins is only one-fifth of that of the large arterioles. This functional organization is linked to the diameter of the different parts of the microvasculature (Figs. 5.27 and 5.28).

Resin casts of the vascular network in the coronal part of molars reveal at the pulp periphery discontinuous round areas forming loops of terminal capillaries about 100 to 150 μm in diameter (Fig. 5.28a). Fenestrated capillaries infiltrate the odontoblast layer, allowing ECM precursor molecules to diffuse near the basal part of odontoblasts. In contrast, in the roots, capillaries are in continuity, displaying a fishnet-like arrangement (Fig. 5.28b).

The pulp microvasculature is composed of endothelial and periendothelial cells. Periendothelial cells include pericytes, embedded within the capillary basement membrane, transitional cells partially surrounded by the basement membrane, and fibroblasts. Endothelial cells contain Weibel-Palade bodies and

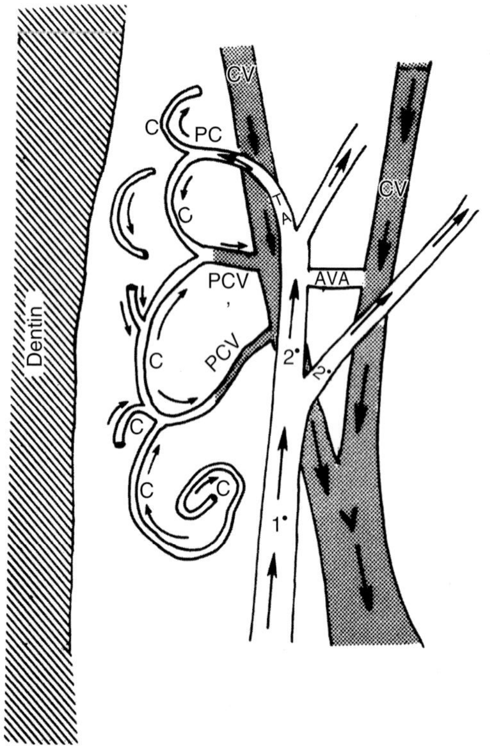

Vessel type	Diameter (μm)	Vm (mm/sec)	Q (10⁻⁴mm³/sec)	$\frac{Qa}{Q}$
1° Feeding Arteriole	35~45	1.46 ± 0.11	16.68 ± 1.79	1.0
2° Feeding Arteriole	24~34	1.08 ± 0.09	6.31 ± 0.71	2.6
Terminal Arteriole (TA)	16~23	0.58 ± 0.06	1.71 ± 0.21	9.8
Pre-Capillary (PC)	12~15	0.48 ± 0.13	0.82 ± 0.27	20.3
Capillary (C)	> 8	0.27 ± 0.03	0.16 ± 0.01	104.2
Post-Cap.Venule (PCV)	12~23	0.20 ± 0.02	0.57 ± 0.06	29.2
Collecting Venule (CV)	24~50	0.37 ± 0.03	3.56 ± 0.54	4.7
Venule (V)	> 50	0.57 ± 0.05	16.83 ± 1.75	1.0

$Vm = \dfrac{VCL}{1.6}$ (Mean velocity)

$Q = Vm \cdot \dfrac{\pi D^2}{4}$ (Volumetric flow rate)

Mean ± Sem

Figure 5.27   Schematic representation of the vascular bed in the coronal part of the pulp. The vessel diameter and speed of blood flow in the successive vessel types are indicated. (From Kim, S., Lipowsky, H.H., Usami, S. & Chien, S. (1984) Arteriovenous distribution of hemodynamic parameters in the rat dental pulp. *Microvascular Research*, 27(1), 28–38. Reproduced by permission from Elsevier Science Publishers.)

(a)

(b)

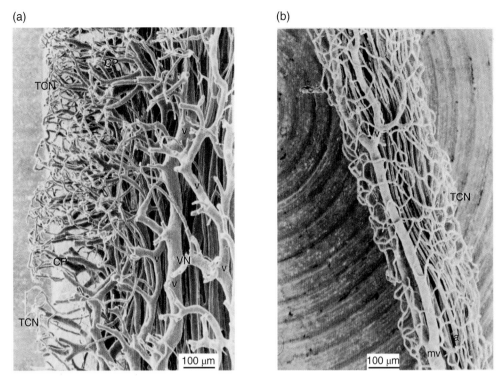

Figure 5.28   (a) Coronal pulp. Resin replica of the blood vessels and capillaries. Vessels of the terminal capillary network (TCN) penetrate the odontoblast layer. (b) Root pulp. Resin replica showing the fish net-like vascularization. Capillary plexus (CP); arteriole (a); main venule (mv); venular network (VN); venules (v). Scale bars = 100 μm. (From Takahashi, K. (1985) Vascular architecture of dog pulp using corrosion resin cast examined under a scanning electron microscope. *Journal of Dental Research*, 64 (Special Issue), 579–584. Reproduced by permission from SAGE Publications.)

express the platelet α-granule membrane protein, GMP-140. Gap and desmosome-like junctions seal the hollowed tubular-like endothelial cells. The basement membrane lining the capillaries is continuous and acts as a semipermeable membrane. Inflammatory cells pass through the space located between endothelial cells and pericytes. The release of neuromediators by autonomic axon terminal endings regulates the pulpal circulation (vasoconstriction or vasodilatation). Compared to arterioles, the nerve terminals are denser around venules.

Lymph vascularization

Lymph angiogenesis occurs in the dental papilla at the bell stage. Formation of lymphatic vessels from mesenchymal cells is regulated by vascular endothelial growth factors (VEGF-C, VEGF-D) and their receptor (VEGFR-3). The number of lymph capillaries increases and lumen expansion is noted early after birth. In the adult pulp, lymphatic vessels are always present in the apical region but are sometimes missing in the coronal and middle regions. None are found in the pulp horn regions. Lymph capillaries begin in the sub-odontoblastic cell-free zone of Weil, in the coronal pulp. Lymph collected in interstitial tissues is captured and drained toward the apex via lymph capillaries. This anatomical distribution suggests that lymph captured by unsealed lymph endothelial cells flows in the apical direction and moves toward the neck lymph node chains.

Lymphatic endothelial cells are thinner, and more irregular than capillary endothelial cells. Intercellular junctions are of the gap type, with large intercellular clefts and irregular discontinuities of the basement membrane. No pericytes are seen. The route of exit of lymphatic capillaries has functional importance. Collected in the apical part of the pulp, calculations suggest that the lymph flows faster in the apical root canal, due to increasing lymph pressure.

Beneath the sub-odontoblastic Hoehl's cell layer the pulp comprises a cell-free and a cell-rich area. The central pulp occupies the rest of the pulp. Spindle-shaped fibroblast-like cells (pulpoblasts) are structural, but also feeder cells, providing nutriments to a few stem cells (1–2%) that possibly differentiate into osteoblast-like cells implicated in pulp mineralization. Inflammatory cells such as T-lymphocytes express antigenic molecules of the class I and II major histocompatibility complex. This is also the case for dendritic cells, resident macrophages and histiocytes, mast cells, and polymorphonuclear leukocytes. In the adult pulp, primary feeding arterioles precede pre-capillaries, capillaries, and post-capillary venules. Collecting venules exit from the pulp, in the direction of larger veins. Arterioles and veins are located centrally. At the periphery of the pulp, in the crown, terminal capillaries form round loops about 100–150 μm in diameter. In the root, capillaries form a fishnet-like arrangement. Lymph capillaries originating in the sub-odontoblastic region collect the lymph in the apical direction, moving it toward the neck lymph chains.

Innervation of the dentin and pulp

The dental pulp is innervated by afferent sensory fibers that are branches of the fifth cranial (trigeminal) nerve, and sympathetic and parasympathetic fibers that travel with the trigeminal nerve. After the trigeminal (Gasserian or semilunar) ganglion, the nerve divides into three branches: ophthalmic, maxillary, and mandibular. The pulps of maxillary teeth are innervated by the maxillary branch of the trigeminal nerve, and the pulps of mandibular teeth are innervated by the mandibular branch. After the entrance of the inferior alveolar nerve into the mandibular canal, the nerve subdivides into a mental nerve and an inferior dental nerve. The inferior dental nerve branch sends nerves to the different mandibular teeth. Axons enter the pulp via the apical foramina. They initially are located in the central part of the pulp, near the blood vessels. The branching terminals of ascending axons are especially dense near the pulp horn tips, forming the **plexus of Raschkow** in the sub-odontoblastic area (Fig. 5.29a).

Nerves are implicated in tooth sensitivity. Axon endings establish gap junctions with odontoblast cell bodies and Hoehl's cells. Some nerve termini penetrate the odontoblast layer (Fig. 5.29a) and enter the dentin, displaying brush-like or fan-like shapes (Fig. 5.29b). Ultrastructural studies have revealed the presence of nerve fibers and their endings closely associated with odontoblast processes within the lumina of dentinal tubules. They terminate exclusively as free endings and never develop junctional complexes. The concomitance of odontoblast cell bodies and axon endings is related to dentin sensitivity and to the mechanisms implicated in pain (see below).

In the pulp, axons are partially or totally embedded in Schwann cells and grouped into bundles wrapped by a perineurium (Figs. 5.30a, 5.30b). In the root, the nerve density decreases, and axons are mostly associated with the blood vessels ascending in the center of the pulp. Approximately 70 to 80% of pulpal axons are unmyelinated, whereas 20 to 30% of nerves are myelinated.

The cell bodies of axons are located in the trigeminal ganglion. Six distinct types of nerves have been identified in the dental pulp.

- Sensory nerve fibers responsible for the sensitivity of dentin are implicated in events associated with early aspects of pain and sharp pain (**A-β, A-δ fast nerves**).

- **A-δ slow, intradental C fiber polymodal** and **silent**, and **C fiber nerves** are concerned with ache.

- In addition, postganglionic intradental **sympathetic C fiber nerves** act as inflammatory mediators.

Unmyelinated and myelinated axons are considered to be sensory afferents, activated by the hydrodynamic mechanism (see "Mechanisms of Tooth Pain" below). They are responsible for immediate dentin sensitivity and respond to application of bradykinin and histamine.

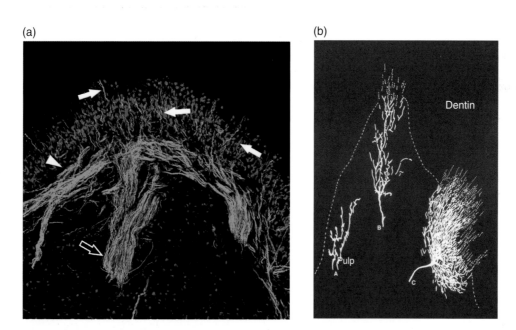

(a) (b)

Figure 5.29   The distribution of nerves in the pulp and dentin. (a) Immunofluorescent labeling of neurofilament 200 kD and GAP-43 in nerve fibers (green) in the coronal pulp of a human molar. Nerve bundles in the pulp (black arrow) enter the subodontoblastic plexus (arrowhead); some of these fibers (white arrows) enter and traverse the layer of odontoblasts (large blue nuclei). (b) Schematic drawing showing the types of nerve endings at the pulp-dentin junction. Endings present in odontoblast layer or below it in pulp (A); endings branching in pulp and extending into dentin in a narrow pattern (B); fan-shaped endings with numerous branches in pulp and extensions into dentin (C). (a) Courtesy of Dr. Michael A. Henry. In Byers, M.R., Henry, M.A, & Närhi, M.V.O. (2012) Dental innervation and its responses to tooth injury. In: *Seltzer and Bender's Dental Pulp* (eds. K.M. Hargreaves et al.) 2nd edn. pp. 133–157. Quintessence, Chicago. Reproduced with permission from Quintessence Publishing Co., Inc. (b) From Byers, M.R. (1985) Terminal arborization of individual sensory axons in dentin and pulp of rat molars. *Brain Research*, 345(1), 181–185. Reproduced by permission from Elsevier Science Publishers.)

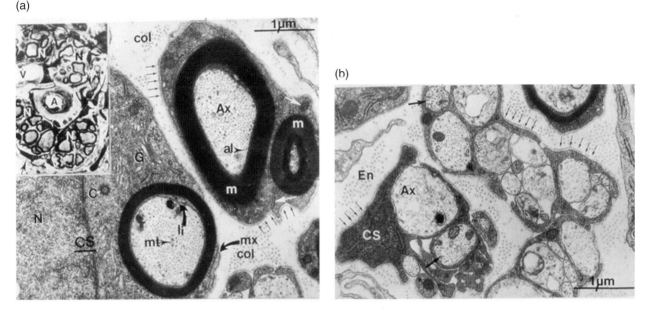

Figure 5.30   Electron micrographs of pulpal nerves. (a) Myelinated nerves. Inset: light micrograph of a nerve bundle. Nerves (N); arteriole (A); venule (V). (b) Unmyelinated nerves. Axons (ax); collagen (col); Schwann cell (CS); myelin sheath (m); endoneurium (En). Bar = 1 μm. (From Goldberg, M., Héritier, M., Farge, P., & Magloire, H. (1989) La pulpe. In: *Manuel d'Histologie et de Biologie Buccale* (ed. M. Goldberg) p. 82. Masson, Paris.)

Innervation of the developing tooth

Trigeminal axons are present in the maxillary and mandibular processes before any structural evidence of tooth formation and mineralization. In the condensing mesenchyme, axons sprout and grow toward the mesenchyme. At the cap stage, axons form a plexus at the base of the dental papilla. Sensory axons enter the dental papilla at the late bell stage, at the onset of enamel formation. They develop rapidly and a network is formed in the sub-odontoblastic- odontoblastic-predentin region during the last few weeks of dentinogenesis. In the coronal dentin the development of pulp innervation starts at the tips of cusps, extending up to 160 μm into the dentin. After initial occlusion, sensory axons located in the central pulp are associated with blood vessels.

Innervation of the erupted mature tooth

In the adult molar, the fibers arborize extensively in the coronal pulp. Many nerve terminals penetrate into the predentin, for about 10 to 20 μm. Others penetrate directly into the dentinal tubules for a distance of about 100 μm. Still other nerve fibers take transverse and complicated courses across dentin. Some simply penetrate within the predentin and end at the predentin-dentin border, or thick nerve fibers penetrate the predentin and undergo dendritic ramification. Tree-like structures expand at the predentin-dentin junction and appear to have no relationship with the dentinal tubules. Innervation is extensive in the crown and scarce or lacking in the root. Neurotransmitters, including nerve growth factor (NGF), calcitonin gene-related peptide (CGRP), enkephalin, C-terminal flanking peptide of neuropeptide tyrosine, neuropeptide Y (NPY), vasoactive intestinal polypeptide (VIP), substance P, somatostatin, serotonin, acetylcholine, and norepinephrine and glial-derived neurotrophic factor (GDNF) are associated with nerves present in the dental pulp.

Mechanisms of tooth pain

Although the dentin/pulp complex is innervated, the mechanisms of tooth sensitivity and pain are not fully elucidated. Tooth sensitivity occurs when dentin is exposed to the oral environment due to loss of the covering enamel or cementum. The nociceptor nerves enter the dental pulp through the apex and fan out in the sub-odontoblastic region. Gap junction contacts should provide a clear-cut explanation for the transmission between axons and retrograde information carried by the fifth cranial nerve. A few nerves penetrate the inner 100- to 120-μm dentin border. Nerve endings are located within the lumina of the dentinal tubules, but apparently they do not develop intercellular junctions with odontoblast processes.

The number of nerve terminals ending within dentin has not been determined accurately. One hundred to two hundred intratubular nerves were recorded per 2000 to 2500 tubules, but this was probably an overestimation. The remaining open question, therefore, is why and how dentin sensitivity appears in the outer dentin, especially at the dentinoenamel junction (DEJ), a non-innervated region of the crown. The same question arises concerning the cervical zone. Again, although they are very sensitive regions, no innervation has been found in these areas. Direct and indirect mechanisms have been proposed.

Direct mechanisms

Odontoblasts as sensor cells

Odontoblasts are neural crest-derived cells. It was therefore hypothesized that these cells may retain some traits as neurons. Indeed it has been shown that isolated rat and human odontoblasts display cholinesterase and choline acetylase activity, characteristic of the cholinergic system. Monoamine oxidase A and B were identified in samples obtained from young patients and rats. Hence, odontoblasts have characteristics of both sympathetic and parasympathetic neurons, and may release neurotransmitters instrumental in the onset of pain.

Odontoblasts play a role in tooth pain transmission as mediators of mechanotransduction, identified on the basis of mechanosensitive ion channels associated with a primary cilium and movements of dentinal fluid within tubules.

Neuromediators released by nerve ending

Many neuromediators are released inside the pulp and the molecules trigger both sensitivity and pain. However, differences between the specific roles that nerves play suggest that the following.

1. A-fibers are responsible for the sensitivity of dentin and for the mediation of sharp pain induced by dentinal stimulation.

2. Pre-pain (non-painful sensations) results with the activation of the lowest threshold A-fibers, some of which are classified as Aβ-fibers. Aβ- and Aδ-fibers belong to the same functional group.

3. Intradental C fibers are activated only when the external stimuli reach the pulp itself. They induce a dull pain by intense thermal stimulation associated with pulpal inflammation.

Activation of transient receptor potential (TRP) channels is involved in tooth pain. The melastatin (TRPM8) receptor is found on Aδ fibers in dentin and on C fibers in the pulp; this fiber segregation suggests a physiological substrate for the sensation that

occurs from cooling a tooth (Fig. 5.31). First, Aδ fibers mediate a sharp shooting pain, followed by C fibers mediating a dull persistent pain. Myelinated Aδ fibers transmit information faster (5–30 m/sec, or 70 mph) than unmyelinated C fibers (<2 m/sec, or < 4.5mph) and it takes longer for physical cooling to reach the pulp. Thus, the time lag between sharp and dull pain sensations is due to the transmission speed and segregation of the detecting nerve fibers within the tooth.

Indirect mechanisms

When the dentin surface of a tooth is exposed, small droplets may be seen. This dentinal fluid or "dentinal lymph" originates from the interstitial fluid in the pulp. Brännström (1968) has shown that the preparation of cavities or dentin surface exposure leads to the displacement of the dentinal fluid (Figs. 5.32 and 5.33). The movement of the dentinal fluid stimulates an odontoblast-nerve mechanosensory complex, resulting in pain sensation. Movements of the odontoblasts toward the pulp or into the dentinal tubules were visualized experimentally after drilling, cooling or heating, and desiccation with dental air spray. The high number of dentin tubules per mm² provides some explanation to movements of odontoblast cytoplasm and/or nuclei. Gap junctions allow crosstalk between the odontoblasts/sub-odontoblastic cell bodies and nerve endings located in Raschkow's plexus. The set of experiments elaborated by Brännström has established a clear link between the clinical and neurobiological considerations (Figs. 5.32 and 5.33).

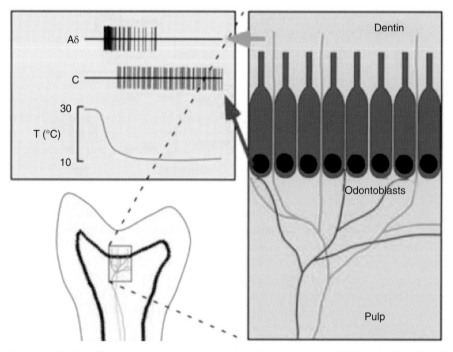

Figure 5.31   TRP channels in teeth. *Blue box*: Diagram of mouse molar showing the segregation of C fibers (red) and Aδ fibers (green). The odontoblast layer, separating pulp from dentin, is shown as blue cells. The transient receptor potential channel melastatin 8 (TRPM8) is found on both fiber types, but C fibers are restricted to the pulp and do not penetrate the odontoblast layer. In contrast, Aδ fibers pass through odontoblast layer and terminate in the dentin. *Green box*: Responses of C fibers to tooth cooling lagging behind responses of Aδ fibers. The responses of Aδ fibers mediate the initial sharp pain felt upon cooling of the tooth while the responses of C fibers mediate the dull pain that follows. (From Takashima, Y., Daniels, R.L., Knowlton, W., Teng, J., Liman, E.R., & McKemy, D.D. (2007) Diversity in the neural circuitry of cold sensing revealed by genetic axonal labeling of transient receptor potential melastatin 8 neurons. *Journal of Neuroscience*, 27(51), 14147–14157. Reproduced by permission of the Society for Neuroscience, Washington DC.)

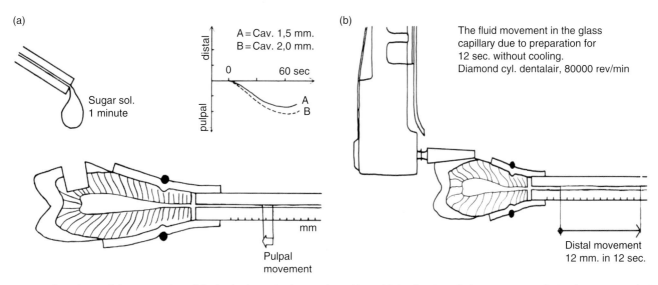

(a)

Sugar sol.
1 minute

A = Cav. 1,5 mm.
B = Cav. 2,0 mm.

0   60 sec

distal

pulpal

A
B

mm

Pulpal
movement

(b)

The fluid movement in the glass
capillary due to preparation for
12 sec. without cooling.
Diamond cyl. dentalair, 80000 rev/min

Distal movement
12 mm. in 12 sec.

Figure 5.32   Experimental demonstration of the hydrodynamic theory of sensitivity. (a) Application of a hyperosmotic solution (e.g., sugar solution) to exposed dentin draws fluid from the pulp into the dentinal tubules. Evaporation of dentinal fluid from the surface of exposed dentin by an air blast causes even more extensive fluid movement from the pulp into the dentinal tubules, also forcing odontoblast cell bodies into the tubules. (b) Heat generated from cavity preparation without cooling forces dentinal fluid toward the pulp (and away from the tooth in the capillary tube). (a) From Brännström, M. (1986) The hydrodynamic theory of dentinal pain: sensation in preparations, caries, and the dentinal crack. *Journal of Endodontics*, 12(10), 453–457. Reproduced by permission from Elsevier Science Publishers. (b) From Brännström, M. et al. (1968) Movement of dentinal and pulpal fluid caused by clinical procedures. *Journal of Dental Research*, 47(5), 679–682. Reproduced by permission from SAGE Publications.)

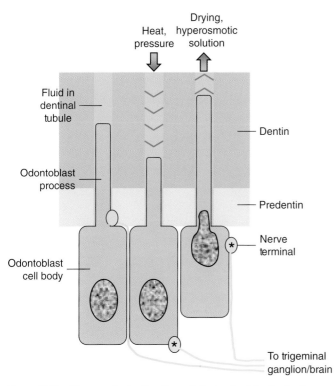

Drying,
Heat,   hyperosmotic
pressure   solution

Fluid in
dentinal
tubule

Odontoblast
process

Odontoblast
cell body

Dentin

Predentin

Nerve
terminal

To trigeminal
ganglion/brain

Figure 5.33   Diagram illustrating the cellular basis of the hydrodynamic theory of tooth pain. The odontoblast and its process form a mechanoreceptor complex with nerves innervating the tooth and contacting the odontoblast cell body or its process in predentin or in dentin. Movement of fluid in the dentinal tubules (dentinal lymph) results in displacement of the processes and cell bodies, which activates the nerves, resulting in pain sensation.

Many Aδ- and C fiber nociceptors dominate intrinsic pulp innervation and consequently the rapid switch to sharp pulp pain. Among the few Aβ fibers present in dental tissues, some might be nociceptive, but most are low-threshold mechanoreceptors, providing pre-pain information. The concept of mechanoreceptors behaving as algoneurons (neurons implicated in algia, or pain) is consistent with the **hydrodynamic theory**.

Distinct types of nerves have been identified in the dental pulp: the A-*β* A-*δ* fast fibers implicated in pain; A-*δ* slow fibers, intradental C-fiber polymodal and silent, and C-fibers are concerned with ache; postganglionic intradental sympathetic C-fibers are implicated in the release of inflammatory mediators. Neurotransmitters are associated with nerves in the dental pulp. Activation of TRP channels is involved in tooth pain.

Odontoblasts may act as sensor cells, being involved in pulp mechanotransduction. Neuromediators may be released by nerve endings. The hydrodynamic hypothesis provides a possible explanation, together with the concept of algoneurons.

Clinical correlations

Caries

Initially, the carious lesion starts to develop in enamel. Acid produced by dental plaque bacteria disrupts specifically some rod enamel structures, membrane, and extracellular matrix protein remnants. Microchannels form across the whole thickness of dental enamel. The carious lesion reaches the dentinoenamel junction (DEJ) and spreads between the inner enamel surface and the outer mantle dentin. The two structures separate, the DEJ enlarges, and bacterial colonies initiate the destruction of the dentin outer surface (Fig. 5.34).

Two different colonization factors contribute to the progress of the lesion. Firstly, the mantle dentin is destroyed by bacterial exoenzymes. The collagen fibrils are cleaved by bacterial collagenase into three-quarter and one-quarter segments. The resulting peptides are further degraded by gelatinases A and B. In the enlarged DEJ, bacteria increase in number, taking their nutriments from food, liquid and solid residues, saliva, and from the demineralized mantle dentin acting as substrate (Figs. 5.34a, 5.34b). Secondly, dentinal tubules allow for bacterial penetration into the circumpulpal dentin (Figs. 5.34c, 5.34d).

The production of acids leads to the demineralization and disappearance of the peritubular dentin. Enlarged tubules favor bacterial diffusion within the tubules, producing an acidic adhesive polysaccharide gel within the lumen of the tubules. This second front is not linear, but structured as a glove, with degradation "digits" penetrating deep inside dentin. Beneath the **soft carious dentin** easily removed by hand curettes, the dentin layer displays a gradient of demineralization. The peritubular dentin, destroyed near the surface of the lesion, reappears gradually in deeper regions as a thin ring that finally displays its whole thickness and appears to be less affected (Figs. 5.35 and 5.36). The residual needle-like crystallites of the intertubular dentin are more numerous in the depth of the carious lesion, and appear to be less destroyed in this intermediate zone. In the deepest part of the slowly progressing or arrested carious dentin, dentin tubules are filled by

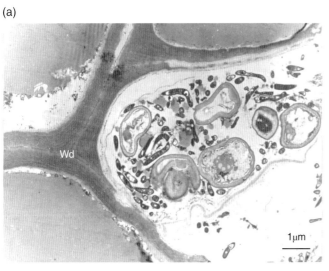

(a)

(b)

(c)

(d)

Figure 5.34   (a) Cell wall debris (Wd) originating from food intake present in the carious cavity. (b) Accumulation of bacteria and the lytic front. Tubules are enlarged and filled with bacteria. (c) Some tubules are filled with bacteria while others are empty. (d) Bacteria in the enlarged lumen of a tubule. Demineralized intertubular dentin (dID) is the bulk of the soft carious dentin. Peritubular dentin (PD) has mostly disappeared, and only remnants are seen. (a–c) bars = 1 μm; (d) bar = 0.5 μm.

mineral re-precipitations occluding the lumen of the tubules (Figs. 5.35 and 5.36a, 5.36b). The intraluminal mineral is whitlockite, a non-apatitic crystalline form of calcium phosphate, or amorphous calcium phosphate. Only a few of the intraluminal mineral deposits are hydroxyapatite. The resulting **sclerotic dentin layer** limits the deeper part of the lesion and slows the progression of the lesion (Figs. 5.36a, 5.36b). However, in the lesion that is still active, bacteria might find their way laterally, bypass the occluding precipitate, and pursue the tissue destruction.

Beneath the sclerotic zone, dentin is apparently normal. Some distance away, beneath what has been named a calciotraumatic line (a spatiotemporal interruption of dentinogenesis, leading to the formation of a line similar to an incremental–or a reversal–line in bone) (Figs. 5.14–5.16), the tubular reactionary dentin is formed by odontoblasts that

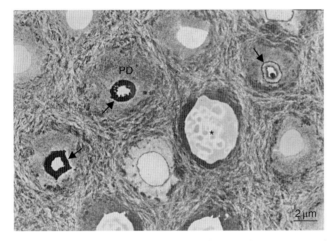

Figure 5.35   Transition between the zone of bacterial invasion (*) and the sclerotic zone of the carious decay. Some dentinal tubules contain re-precipitations of mineral (arrows). Peritubular dentin (PD). Bar = 2 μm.

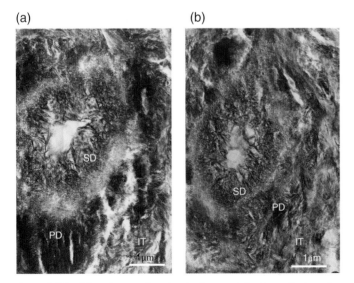

Figure 5.36   Sclerotic zone. Intraluminal re-precipitations of mineral (SD) occlude partially or totally the lumina of the tubules. Peritubular dentin (PD) and intertubular dentin (IT) were not demineralized by the carious process. Bar = 1 μm.

recover their biologic properties, or by sub-odontoblastic Hoehl's cells. This type of reactionary dentin is similar to orthodentin. The dentin may also appear heterogeneous, formed by calcospherites with large defective interglobular spaces. Osteocyte-like cells located within lacunae are embedded in a bony structure, which consequently appears as osteodentin.

For many years the clinical concept was that the preparation of cavities should follow mechanical rules after careful removal of the infected dentin. With the development of adhesives and resin-containing materials, the principles directing therapy have changed. Instead of drilling geometrical cavities, it is now mandatory to keep the sclerotic dentin after careful elimination of the bacteria-contaminated soft carious dentin. Sclerotic dentin limits the effects on the pulp of the free monomers released by dental resins. The permeability of the tissue is decreased in the sclerotic zone, and the adhesive properties of this zone are high enough to ensure stability to the restorative procedures even after minimal preparation.

> Successive layers have been identified in carious dentin. Food debris is located in the cavity. Dissolution of the mantle dentin is concomitant with the enlargement of dentinal tubules filled with bacteria. In the soft carious dentin peritubular dentin is totally dissolved. Deeper in the tubules, peritubular dentin gradually reappears. Finally sclerotic dentin occludes the lumina of the tubules, slowing the carious process. In the subjacent dental pulp, reactionary dentin appears beneath a calciotraumatic line.

Preparation of dental surfaces: effects of etching

Acidic solutions or gels improve the adhesion of resin components to enamel structures. Instead of a flat surface, alternate projecting or depressed rods and interrod spaces (rods 3–5 μm in width and/or interrod spaces 0.5–1 μm thick) contribute to create a scalloped profile. The restorative resin fills the depressions, approximately 5 to 10 μm in depth. In addition, enlarged intercrystal spaces enhance deeper penetration of minute resin tags into intercrystallite porosities (Type I and II etched enamel).

The same etching concept applies to the preparation of dentin surfaces. The crystallographic differences between the inter- and peritubular mineral phases accounts for the greater acid solubility of crystals in the peritubular dentin. Consequently, acid or chelating solutions enlarge the diameter of the tubules, with a diameter increasing from 4 μm to 6–8 μm (Fig. 5.37). This allows deeper penetration of resin tags within the lumen of dentinal tubules (Fig. 5.38). The rough surface of the tags reflects the lateral penetration within the intercollagenic spaces. This contributes to the formation of a **hybrid layer**, composed of the collagen network, remnants of non-collagenous components, and resin tags at different stages of polymerization. This situation is observed exclusively when flat dentin surfaces are sliced experimentally with a diamond disk or when flat surfaces of

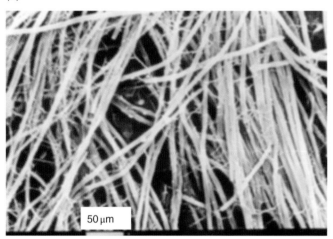

Figure 5.37 Scanning electron microscopy of human dentin after acid etching. The tubules are enlarged. Intertubular dentin forms a continuous network. Bar = 20 μm.

(a)

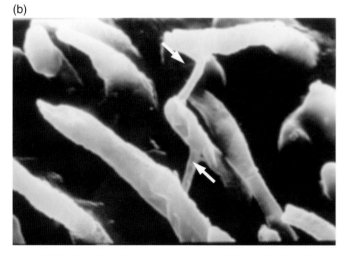

(b)

Figure 5.38 Scanning electron micrographs of the penetration of restorative resin into tubules of etched dentin. (a) Removal of the dentin matrix reveals long resin tags in the dentinal tubules. Bar = 50 μm. (b) Higher magnification showing resin in small lateral branches (arrows) connecting the major dentinal tubules.

cavities are drilled with diamond or tungsten burs. In reality, once the demineralized dentin has been removed manually or chemically (collagenase, pronase, or sodium hypochlorite), cleaned dentin surfaces are subjected to acid or chelating solutions. The formation of resin tags and a variable hybrid layer contribute to increase the adhesion of resin-containing materials to the dentin surfaces.

However, this advantage is counterbalanced by the diffusion of free polymers released by the resin restorative material, which are cytotoxic and therefore noxious for the pulp cells. Odontoblasts are injured and degenerate, and/or the cell-rich border of the pulp displays severe alterations. In addition to inflammatory cells, numerous apoptotic cells are detectable in areas of the pulp affected by the diffusion of resin components through the enlarged dentinal tubules. With time, either a layer of reparative dentin is formed, or the pulp degenerates. Large vacuolar areas appear, and finally the whole dental pulp disappears.

Cervical sensitivity

Cervical erosions or **abfractions** (**mylosis**) gradually develop after gingival recession. At the enamel-dentin-cementum junction, four interrelations between dentin and enamel have been reported. In most cases, a thin border of cementum covers the cervical enamel (60%). An end-to-end situation is also observed, with continuity between enamel and cementum (30%). The reverse situation is far less frequent, with the enamel edge covering the cervical cementum (2–5%). In about 10% there is a gap between the enamel and cementum, and the peripheral dentin is exposed. This latter distribution favors cervical sensitivity.

The cervical region displays specific lesions named erosion or mylolysis. The cervical destruction shows two surfaces: the upper surface forming a wide angle with the long axis of the tooth, starting in enamel, and forming a half-moon structure. The lower surface is at a right angle with the long axis of the tooth. The surfaces are smooth, generally not covered by dental plaque. The coronal acellular cementum and the cervical dentin are implicated in the destroyed areas. The depth of the lesion increases with time.

Pulp sensitivity seems to be related with the opening or closure of dentinal tubules. Intratubular mineralization reduces the sensitivity, whereas open tubules contribute to increased tooth sensitivity. Mylolysis occurs (1) with dentin exposure at the dentinoenamel junction, (2) with the tissue softening due to acid beverages or solutions displaying chelating properties, and (3) finally the slow loss of tooth structure is due to the combined action of horizontal brushing and the abrasive particle content of toothpastes.

Initially, fingernail or instrument contact with the junction gives rise to sensitivity. In the naked cervical region, or after mylolysis formation, thermal variations induce pain. There is no terminal innervation at that location, and the hydrodynamic theory readily explains the symptoms.

Varnishes or chemically induced mineral precipitation inside the tubules contribute to reduce the symptoms. Fluoride or strontium induced re-precipitations are limited to a thin outer layer. Temporary improvements may be observed, and repeated treatments are necessary for acceptable results.

Reparative dentin formation and pulp mineralization

The response of odontoblasts and Hoehl's cells to a mild carious lesion is the formation of reactionary dentin. Two to three days after the preparation of a cavity, the pulp cells express **osteocalcin** and some pulp cells are differentiating toward the odontoblast-like phenotype. Extracellular matrix proteins produced during reactionary dentin formation include Type I collagen, DSP and DMP1; DSPP does not appear to be present.

These results emphasize the difference between the odontoblast/Hoehl's cell layer and the pulp. If the odontoblasts/Hoehl's cells are irreversibly injured, some pulp stem cells are committed. Pulp progenitor cells produce either reparative osteodentin or contribute to the formation of a mineralized tissue filling the pulp cavity.

Reactionary dentin recapitulates the early formation of the peripheral mantle dentin, including globular structures and interglobular spaces. This dentin is formed by polarizing or polarized odontoblasts, and therefore it is a tubular dentin. In contrast, reparative dentin is reminiscent of the ancestral development of osteodentin. Non-polarized cells are located in lacunae, communicating by minute lateral processes, allowing response to mechanical stresses.

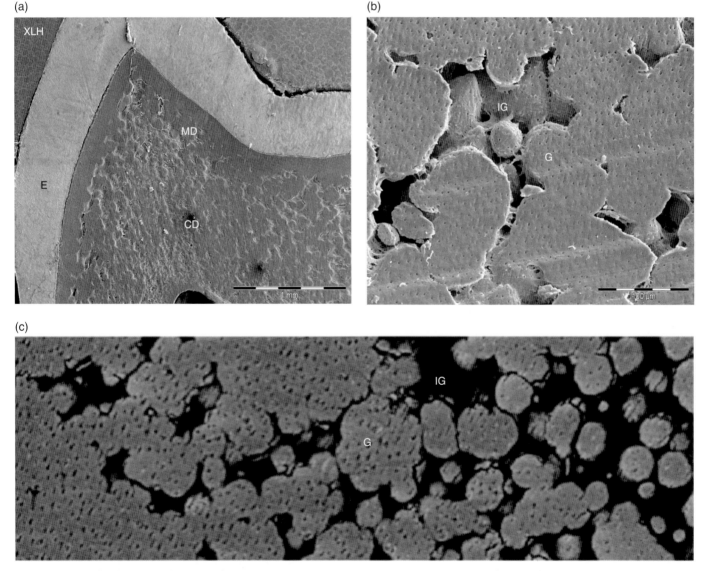

Figure 5.39   X-linked hypophosphatemic rickets (XLH). Human tooth, scanning electron microscopy. (a–b) Secondary electron imaging. Beneath the enamel layer (E), the mantle dentin (MD) looks normal, but globular structures (G) and interglobular (IG) spaces are detected in the circumpulpal dentin (CD). (c) Backscattered electron imaging. The globular structures (with dark dentinal tubules) appear gray due to their higher mineral content, whereas the hypomineralized interglobular spaces are black.

Part of the embryonic pulpal cell population expresses markers characteristic of stem cells, such as Oct-4, Nanog, SSEA-3, SSEA-4, TRA-1-60 and TRA-1-81. Embryonic and adult stem cells, and induced pluripotent stem cells (iPSC) provide alternative strategies to obtain cells that have high potential for pulp healing and regeneration. Successful experimental approaches include the following pulp stem cell populations:

- postnatal dental pulp stem cells (DPSCs): display differentiation potential to become odontoblasts/osteoblasts, chondrocytes, adipocytes, and neurons
- stem cells from human exfoliated deciduous teeth (SHEDs): cells are similar to, but more immature than, DPSCs
- stem cells from the apical papilla (SCAP).

In addition, some positive results were also obtained with stem cells from the periodontal ligament (PDLSCs) and dental follicle progenitor cells (DFPCs). Pulp regeneration also may be derived from mesenchymal stem cells (MSCs) or from bone marrow stem cells (BMSCs). To this list should be added the circulating endothelial/skeletal progenitor cells.

Dentin pathology: dentinogenesis imperfecta, dentin dysplasia, hypophosphatemic rickets

Gene alterations are at the origin of structural pathologies of dentin. **Dentinogenesis imperfecta** (DGI) and **dentin dysplasia** (DD) implicate mostly gene deletions of human chromosome 4q21. This is the location where genes coding for the SIBLING family proteins are grouped. When the molecules are deleted or abnormal, three forms of DGI are recognized. Short roots and early pulp closure are one of the most frequent DGI pathologies. Yellow-brown to blue-gray color of the crown has been observed, with few dentinal tubules and hypomineralization of the tissue. Type I collagen gene mutation is implicated in type 1 DGI, whereas DSPP gene mutations characterize type II and type III DGI.

X-linked hypophosphatemic rickets, due to mutation of PHEX (phosphate regulating gene with endopeptidase activity on the X chromosome), is characterized by the presence of globular structures (calcospherites) isolated by large interglobular spaces (Fig. 5.39). Inside the calcospherites, dentinal tubules are normally present, whereas in the interglobular spaces, DSP, DMP1, BSP, MEPE, and osteocalcin accumulate, showing in addition alterations of post-translational processing. The major alteration identified is due to DMP1 mutation and its interaction with FGF23. Deep fissures are detected between structural parts of teeth. Unmineralized pulp horns facilitate the penetration of bacteria and subsequently pulp necrosis.

Experimentally it was also shown that deletion of the gene encoding sphingomyelin phosphodiesterase 3 causes both osteogenesis imperfecta and dentinogenesis imperfecta in mice.

DGI and DD are seldom seen as a single genetic disease. They are usually associated with other defects (osteogenesis imperfecta, deafness, blue sclera, etc.). The mutation being identified, these defects are targets for gene therapies.

Dentin pathologies are due to genetic mutations (including a series of 4q21 deletions), environmental pathologies (fluorosis, dioxin, and other toxic agents), or resulting from bacterial carious lesions, abrasions, or pulp calcification inducing local (pulp stones) or diffuse mineralization. Dentinogenesis imperfecta, dentin dysplasia, and X-linked hypophosphatemic rickets are the most frequently observed pathologies due to genetic mutations.

References

1. Baume, L.J. (1980) The biology of pulp and dentine: a historic, terminologic-taxonomic, histologic-biochemical, embryonic and clinical survey. *Monographs in oral science*, 8, 1–220. Basel, Karger.
2. Brännström, M. (1968) Physio-pathological aspects of dentinal and pulpal response to irritants. In: *Dentin and pulp* (ed. N.B.B. Symons) pp. 231–246. Thomson, Dundee, Scotland.
3. Byers, M., Suzuki, H., Maeda, T. (2003) Dental neuroplasticity, neuro-pulpal interactions, and nerve regeneration. *Microscopy Research and Technique*, 60, 503–515.
4. Goldberg, M., & Smith, A.J. (2004) Cell and extracellular matrices of dentin and pulp: a biological basis for repair and tissue engineering. *Critical Reviews in Oral Biology and Medicine*, 15, 13–27.
5. Goldberg, M., Kulkarni, A.B., Young, M., & Boskey, A. (2011) Dentin: structure, composition and mineralization,– the role of dentin ECM in dentin formation and mineralization. *Frontiers in BioSciences*, 3, 711–735.
6. Huang, G.T.-J., Gronthos, S., & Shi, S. (2009) Mesenchymal stem cells derived from dental tissues vs. those from other sources: their biology and role in regenerative medicine. *Critical Reviews in Oral Biology and Medicine/ Journal of Dental Research*, 88, 792–806.
7. Jontell, M., Okiji, T., Dahlgren, U., et al. (1998) Immune defense mechanisms of the dental pulp. *Critical Reviews in Oral Biology and Medicine*, 9, 179–200.
8. Mackenzie, A., Ferguson, M.W.J., & Sharpe, P.T. (1992) Expression patterns of the homeobox gene, Hox-8, in the mouse embryo suggest a role in specifying tooth initiation and shape. *Development*, 115, 403–420.
9. Maeda, T., Iwanaga, T., Fujita, T., et al. (1986) Immunohistochemical demonstration of nerves in the predentin and dentin of human third molars with the use of an antiserum against neurofilament protein (NFP). *Cell and Tissue Research*, 243, 469–475.
10. Magloire, H., Maurin, J.C., Couble, M.L., et al. (2010) Topical review: dental pain and odontoblasts, facts and hypotheses. *Journal of Orofacial Pain*, 24, 335–349.
11. Ruch, J.V., Lesot, H., Karcher-Djuricic, V., et al. (1982) Facts and hypotheses concerning the control of odontoblast differentiation. *Differentiation*, 21, 7–12.
12. Silverstone, L.M., Saxton, C.A., Dogon, I.L., & Fejerskov, O. (1975) Variation in the pattern of acid etching of human dental enamel examined with the scanning electron microscope. *Caries Research*, 9, 373–387.
13. Takahashi, K. (1985) Vascular architecture of dog pulp using corrosion resin cast examined under a scanning electron microscope. *Journal of Dental Research*, 64, 579–584.

Glossary

Basement membrane/basal lamina: A three-dimensional molecular structure produced by epithelial cells, consisting of collagen IV, laminin, nidogen/entactin and perlecan. The basement membrane serves to attach the epithelium to the underlying mesenchyme/connective tissue and allows diffusion of molecules between epithelium and connective tissue.

Calcospherite: A globular or spherical accumulation of mineral in dentin.

Cell-free pulp area: A thin border located between the Hoehl's cell layer and the central pulp, where pulp cells are reduced in number.

Cell-rich pulp zone: A region just beneath the cell free area with increased numbers of cells.

Central pulp: The bulk of the pulp, internal to the odontoblasts, Hoehl's cell layer, and cell-free pulp border.

Cervical erosions or abfractions, or mylolysis: The loss of dental substance at the cervical region, increasing risk of tooth sensitivity.

Circumpulpal dentin: The bulk of tooth dentin, lying between the peripheral mantle dentin and secondary dentin at the pulpal surface.

Class I and class II major histocompatibility complex (MHC): Proteins expressed at the surface of cells, including pulp cells, that bind antigenic peptides for recognition by the immune system.

Dentinal tubules: Tubular spaces extending through the dentin, created as dentin matrix is deposited around the odontoblast processes.

Dentinogenesis imperfecta, dentin dysplasia, X-linked hypophosphatemic rickets: Three forms of genetic alterations leading to dentin pathologies.

Fibroblast-like pulp cells (pulpoblasts): Structural pulp cells; may provide nutriments for stem cells.

Growth factors: Proteins or hormones capable of stimulating cell proliferation and differentiation; growth factors association with dentin include TGFβ, FGFs, IGF I & II, VEGF, and BMPs.

Hoehl's cells: Cells resulting from the last division of preodontoblasts. They may remain dormant, or may differentiate if odontoblasts are injured or unable to secrete new layers of dentin.

Hyaline Hopewell-Smith zone: A superficial border of atubular dentin beneath cementum in the root.

Hybrid layer: A superficial zone where the restorative resin penetrates between the collagen fibrils of the softened dentin surface, and resin tags anchors the restorative resin within the enlarged tubules.

Hydrodynamic theory: An explanation for the mechanism by which tooth pain is perceived. Stimulation of dentin causes displacement of fluid within the dentinal tubules, activating the odontoblast-nerve mechanoreceptor complex.

Hydroxyapatite: The calcium phosphate mineral phase found in normal dentin, organized as needle-like crystallites.

Interglobular spaces: Poorly mineralized regions of dentin between normally mineralized regions resulting from the failure of adjacent calcospherites to merge.

Intertubular dentin: The dentin resulting from predentin mincralization. Intertubular dentin constitutes the bulk of the dentin layer.

Mantle dentin: The most superficial atubular dentin layer in the crown.

Matrix vesicles: Cell-derived membrane vesicles, serving as nucleating centers associating a series of molecules and producing bundles of mineral crystallites; present in the early outer dentin.

Metadentin: The 3–5 µm wide mineralization front between predentin and dentin, where non-collagenous proteins associate with the collagen fibrils and initiate dentin mineralization.

Nerves: Present in the central pulp and at the pulp periphery. Implicated in pain: A-β, A-δ fast, A-δ slow, intradental C fiber polymodal and silent, C fiber, and sympathetic C fiber.

Odontoblasts: The cells responsible for the synthesis, secretion, and reuptake of the dentin extracellular matrix proteins. As sensor cells, they synthesize mediators characteristic of cholinergic and parasympathetic nerves and released by nerve endings.

Odontoblast cell bodies: The cell areas where precursors are incorporated into nascent extracellular matrix proteins.

Odontoblast cell process: Distal extension of the odontoblast, traversing predentin and present in dentinal tubules. Secretion and re-internalization of fragmented extracellular matrix proteins by the odontoblast process occurs in predentin (collagen and proteoglycans) or in dentin (molecules implicated in mineralization).

Orthodentin: Tubular dentin formed by the odontoblasts.

Osteocalcin: An ECM molecule that may be a mineralization inhibitor.

Osteodentin: A bone-like dentin structure that includes osteocytes within lacunae.

Osteonectin: A non-phosphorylated ECM molecule.

Owen's lines: Accentuated contour lines in dentin resulting from disturbances in mineralization.

Peritubular dentin: The layer of dentin deposited in the presence of odontoblasts along the luminal wall of the tubules.

Plexus of Raschkow: A network of sub-odontoblastic nerves.

Polarized secretory odontoblasts: After organization of the cytoskeleton, odontoblasts start to synthesize and secrete the dentin ECM.

Polarizing post-mitotic odontoblasts: At the end of the ultimate cell division, polarization of the odontoblasts is initiated. At the end of this process, the polarized cells are able to synthesize and secrete the dentin ECM.

Predentin: The initial unmineralized matrix deposited by odontoblasts.

Pre-polarized odontoblasts: These cells arise from the last division. They are not yet polarized and the terminal junctions need to be firmly established.

Primary dentin: The external tubular dentin layer formed between the beginning of dentin formation near the dentino-enamel junction and after eruption, when the tooth becomes functional.

Pulp inflammatory cells: These cells include dendritic cells, histiocytes/macrophages, T-lymphocytes, polymorphonuclear neutrophilic leukocytes, and mast cells.

Pulp stem cells: No more than 1–2% of the pulp cell population. Pluripotent or monopotent cells that display the capacity to differentiate into osteoblasts, chondrocytes, adipocytes, and odontoblasts. Five groups of stem cells have been identified in the tooth. They may contribute to pulp regeneration and also to tissue engineering.

Pulp vascularization: Central ascending arterioles and collecting venules. Small independent capillaries loops are seen in the crown periphery, whereas a continuous fishnet-like arrangement is present in the root.

Reactionary dentin: Produced by the odontoblasts and/or Hoehl's cells in response to carious decay or abrasion or in reaction to the cytotoxic molecules of a restorative biomaterial.

Reparative dentin: Dentin formed in response to a pulp exposure. Pulp capping activates pulp cells, which form a dentinal bridge. Reparative dentin formation may not be restricted to the surface of the pulp, but may form a limited reparative dentin structure within the pulp (pulp stone or pulpolith), or a diffuse mineralization of the pulp.

Sclerotic dentin layer: Intraluminal re-precipitations in dentinal tubules slow the progression of the carious lesion.

Secondary dentin: The tubular dentin formed between the completion of tooth formation and the remaining life of the tooth.

Soft carious dentin: Demineralized dentin found in the upper layers of the carious lesion.

SIBLINGs: Small Integrin-Binding LIgand, N-linked Glycoproteins, a family of phosphorylated proteins that includes dentin sialophosphoprotein (cleaved after secretion mainly into dentin sialoprotein and dentin phosphoprotein), dentin matrix protein 1, bone sialoprotein, osteopontin, and matrix extracellular phosphorylated glycoprotein (MEPE).

Tertiary dentin: Reactionary or reparative dentin.

Tomes' granular layer: Superficial layer of atubular dentin formed by calcospherites and interglobular dentin.

Type I collagen: and type I trimer: The major collagen found in dentin ECM.

von Ebner's lines: Incremental lines occurring at five-day intervals during dentin formation; believed to be due to changes in collagen fiber orientation.

von Korff fibers: Thick fibers of type III collagen running between adjacent odontoblasts and inserting into mantle dentin.

PART III
TOOTH AND JAW SUPPORT

Chapter 6 Structure and Physiology of the Periodontium[1]

Arthur R. Hand

Department of Craniofacial Sciences and Cell Biology, School of Dental Medicine, University of Connecticut

The **periodontium**, literally "around the tooth," comprises the tissues that invest and support the teeth in the maxilla and mandible. The relationship between the teeth and their supporting tissues is complex, involving multiple systems: vascular, neurological, and immunological, to nourish, control, and protect this "joint." The focus of this chapter is on cementum, the mineralized tissue that covers the root dentin, the **periodontal ligament (PDL)**, the structure that attaches to and holds the tooth in its socket (**alveolus**), and the **alveolar bone**, the portion of the jaws that forms the alveolus. The **gingivae**, the portion of the oral mucosa adjacent to the teeth, also is part of the periodontium; its structure and function are presented in Chapter 9.

Cementum structure, composition and formation

Structure of cementum

Cementum is a collagen-based, mineralized tissue, with similarities to bone. Cementum may be **acellular**, consisting only of extracellular matrix components and mineral, or it may be **cellular**, with its forming cells, **cementoblasts**, trapped within the matrix as **cementocytes** (Figs. 6.1 and 6.2). Acellular cementum, also called **acellular extrinsic fiber cementum**, is the first cementum deposited on the dentin of the forming root, and is the predominant form found on the coronal

portion of the root. Cellular cementum, also called **cellular intrinsic fiber cementum**, is most abundant on the apical one-third to one-half of the root and in the **furcation** areas of multirooted teeth. Cellular cementum may be deposited on top of acellular cementum, especially in response to functional demands and post-eruptive tooth movements. Alternating layers of cellular and acellular cementum may occur (Figs. 6.2 and 6.3); this type of cementum is called **cellular mixed stratified cementum**. A fourth cementum variety, **acellular afibrillar cementum**, may be found near the cervical margin, covering small areas of enamel and dentin. Acellular afibrillar cementum has a mineralized matrix that lacks collagen fibrils.

Cementum, unlike bone, is avascular, lacks innervation and undergoes little remodeling. Its nutrition comes by diffusion from nearby blood vessels in the periodontal ligament. In regions where the cementum is very thick, such as the root apices or furcation areas, cementocytes in the deeper layers may not receive sufficient nutrition to survive. The cementocytes, like osteocytes of bone, are located within **lacunae** and have long cellular processes present in **canaliculi** that extend toward the periodontal ligament (Fig. 6.4).

> Cementum is a collagen-based mineralized tissue produced by cementoblasts. Acellular cementum covers the dentin of the coronal portion of the root; cellular cementum, containing cementocytes located in lacunae, is present on the apical portion of the root and in the furcation areas of multirooted teeth.

[1] With a contribution by Bradley K. Formaker, Department of Oral Health and Diagnostic Sciences, University of Connecticut, School of Dental Medicine

Fundamentals of Oral Histology and Physiology, First Edition. Arthur R. Hand and Marion E. Frank.
© 2014 John Wiley & Sons, Inc. Published 2014 by John Wiley & Sons, Inc.

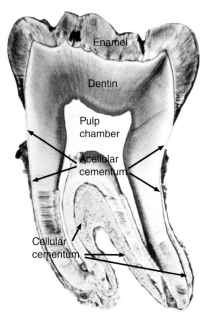

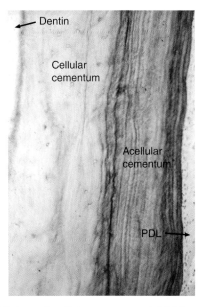

Figure 6.1   Cementum location. Low magnification image of a ground section of a mandibular molar tooth. Cementum covers the surface of the root dentin. Acellular cementum is located on the coronal one-half to two-thirds of the root; cellular cementum is located on the apical one-third to one-half of the root and in the furcation area between the two roots. Note that cellular cementum is considerably thicker than acellular cementum. (From Moss-Salentijn, L. (1972) *Orofacial Histology and Embryology: A Visual Integration.* Reproduced with permission from F.A. Davis Company, Philadelphia, PA.)

Figure 6.3   Cellular and acellular cementum. A thick layer of cellular cementum is covered by acellular cementum with many incremental lines. Periodontal ligament (PDL).

collagen accounts for about 90% of the organic matrix of cementum. Other constituents include several proteins also found in bone and/or dentin, growth factors, and cementum-specific proteins.

Formation of the tooth root

Initial cementum formation occurs concomitantly with root formation. Upon completion of the crown, the cervical loop of the enamel organ, consisting of the inner and outer enamel epithelia, exhibits significant cell proliferation and grows in an apical direction, forming **Hertwig's epithelial root sheath** and the **epithelial diaphragm** (Figs. 6.5a and 6.5b). At the advancing apical extent of the developing root, the cells of the epithelial root sheath lie adjacent to the ectomesenchymal cells of the dental papilla, separated only by a basal lamina. The root sheath cells induce the adjacent dental papilla cells to differentiate into odontoblasts. Following secretion of the initial root predentin, the epithelial root sheath becomes discontinuous and the epithelial cells migrate away from the root surface (Fig. 6.6a). Components of their basal lamina, such as the glycoprotein laminin and possibly small amounts of enamel matrix proteins, are thought to serve as chemoattractants for dental follicle cells, which migrate in to contact the surface of the root predentin. As described below, these cells from the dental follicle initiate the formation of acellular cementum.

The two-cell-layer thick epithelial diaphragm extends inward beneath the dental papilla (Fig. 6.5b), separating the dental papilla from the dental follicle. The epithelial diaphragm serves to delineate the morphology of the developing root. In multi-rooted teeth, the diaphragm grows together at specific points to create the **furcation**, or branch point, between the roots (Fig. 6.6b).

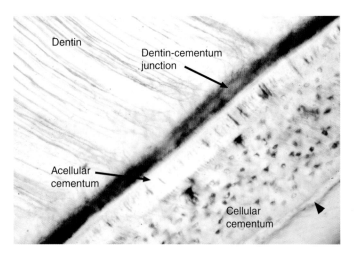

Figure 6.2   Cellular and acellular cementum. Ground section from the apical portion of a root. A layer of acellular cementum adjacent to the dentin is covered by a thicker layer of cellular cementum containing cementocyte lacunae. A thin layer of acellular cementum (arrowhead) is present on the surface of the cellular cementum.

Composition of cementum

The composition of cementum is shown in Table 6.1. Cementum consists of about 45 to 50% mineral (hydroxyapatite) and about 45 to 50% organic material and water. Type I

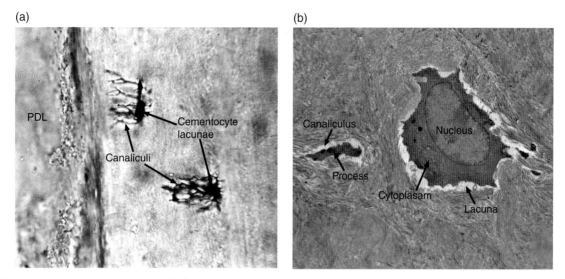

Figure 6.4   Cementocytes. (a) Ground section of cellular cementum showing cementocyte lacunae with canaliculi extending toward the cementum surface and the site of the periodontal ligament. (b) Electron micrograph of demineralized cellular cementum of a mouse molar tooth showing a cementocyte in a lacuna surrounded by the collagenous cementum matrix. One of the cementocyte processes within a canaliculus is indicated. (a) From Moss-Salentijn, L. 1972. *Orofacial Histology and Embryology: A Visual Integration.* Reproduced with permission from F.A. Davis Company, Philadelphia, PA.)

Table 6.1   Composition of cementum

Constituent	Properties and function
Hydroxyapatite	Hardness
Collagen I	Tensile strength; substrate for mineralization
Other collagens (III, V, VI, XII, XIV)	Associated with collagen I
Non-collagenous proteins	
Tissue nonspecific alkaline phosphatase	Hydrolysis of pyrophosphate and dephosphorylation of osteopontin, both inhibitors of mineralization
Bone sialoprotein	Recruitment and adhesion of cells to root surface; mineralization initiator
Dentin matrix protein 1 (DMP-1)	Regulation of mineralization
Dentin sialoprotein	Regulation (inhibition?) of mineralization
Fibronectin	Cell adhesion
Osteocalcin	Regulation of mineralization
SPARC/Osteonectin	Collagen binding; regulation of collagen content and fibril size; modulation of growth factor signaling
Osteopontin	Recruitment and adhesion of cells to root surface; mineralization inhibitor
Proteoglycans	Regulation of cell-cell and cell-matrix interactions; regulation of mineralization; binding of growth factors
Proteolipids	Cell membrane constituents
Tenascin	Cell adhesion
Cementum attachment protein	Cementoblast proliferation and differentiation
Cementum protein 1	Proliferation and differentiation of PDL cells toward cementoblast, osteoblast, and chondroblast lineages
Growth factors (insulin-like growth factor-1, fibroblast growth factors -1, -2, platelet-derived growth factor, transforming growth factor-ß, bone morphogenetic proteins -2, -3, -4, epidermal growth factor)	Promotion of cell proliferation; growth and differentiation; matrix synthesis

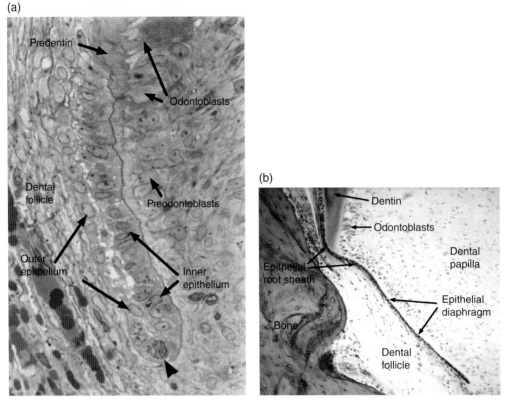

Figure 6.5 Epithelial root sheath and epithelial diaphragm. (a) The epithelial root sheath consists of two cell layers derived from fusion of the inner and outer enamel epithelia. The root sheath induces differentiation of root odontoblasts from the dental papilla cells. A mitotic cell (arrowhead) indicates the growth of the root sheath at its apical tip. (From Bosshardt, D.D. & Selvig, K.A. (1997) Dental cementum: the dynamic tissue covering of the root. *Periodontology 2000*, 13, 41–75. Reproduced by permission of John Wiley and Sons.) (b) The epithelial diaphragm is a continuation of the root sheath beneath the dental papilla. The diaphragm determines the formation of single versus multiple roots.

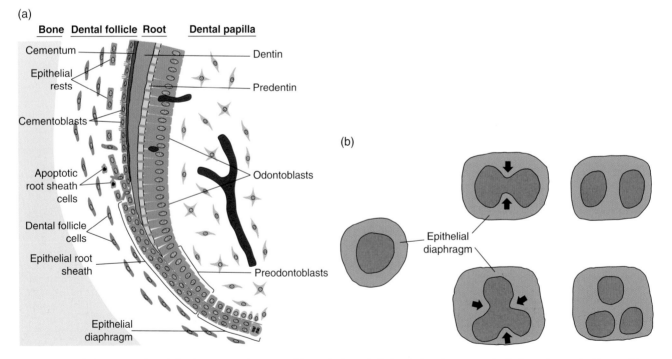

Figure 6.6 Epithelial root sheath and diaphragm. (a) The two-cell layer thick epithelial root sheath grows apically from the cervical loop of the former enamel organ and induces mesenchymal cells of the dental papilla to differentiate into pre-odontoblasts and odontoblasts. After odonto-blasts secrete the predentin matrix, the root sheath fragments and the cells migrate away from the root surface. Some root sheath cells undergo apoptosis, whereas others remain in the dental follicle (and subsequently the periodontal ligament) as a network of epithelial cell rests. As the root sheath fragments, dental follicle cells migrate to the root surface, differentiate into cementoblasts, and begin deposition of cementum and formation of a fringe of collagen fibrils (orange fibers in diagram). Some root sheath cells may transform into mesenchymal cells, which differentiate to cementoblasts (not shown). (b) The epithelial diaphragm seen in an apical view of developing teeth with a single root (left) and two or three roots (center and right). In multirooted teeth, the epithelial diaphragm grows inward (arrows) at two or three sites and fuses to delineate the roots.

After the initiation of root dentin formation and migration away from the root surface, the epithelial root sheath cells have three possible fates.

1. Some cells undergo apoptosis.

2. Some cells remain viable and may exist within the periodontal ligament for as long as the tooth remains in the alveolus. These cells, called the **epithelial rests of Malassez**, typically are seen in small clusters or short strands extending along and close to the root surface (Fig. 6.7a). In sections parallel to the root surface, the epithelial rest cells are seen to form a network of branching and anastomosing strands (Fig. 6.7b), probably a result of the apoptotic death of some cells. Although the number of epithelial rest cells is reduced with age, mitotic activity has been observed in these cells. It is not known if the epithelial rest cells have a specific function in the periodontal ligament.

3. Some root sheath cells may undergo transformation to mesenchymal cells, which then differentiate to cementoblasts. Such epithelial-mesenchymal transformations occur during development of other craniofacial structures, such as the transformation of ectodermal neural crest cells to craniofacial mesenchymal cells. These transformed epithelial root sheath cells may deposit acellular or cellular cementum, and may be incorporated as cementocytes in cellular cementum.

> Apically directed growth of the cervical loop forms the epithelial root sheath, which induces differentiation of odontoblasts to form the dentin of the root. The root sheath extends beneath the dental papilla as the epithelial diaphragm and creates the furcation of multirooted teeth. After deposition of the first root predentin, the root sheath cells migrate away from the root surface; some undergo apoptosis, leaving others to form a network of epithelial rests lying parallel to the root surface. Other root sheath cells may transform into mesenchymal cells and produce cementum.

Cementum formation

The formation of cementum occurs over an extended period of time. Depending upon the tooth, the prefunctional phase, before the tooth reaches the occlusal level, occurs over a period of about 3-1/2 years to almost 8 years. The deposition of acellular cementum occurs at a slow but constant rate of about 3 μm per year on single-rooted teeth; the rate varies, however, with tooth type and root surface area. The postfunctional phase, when the tooth becomes attached to bone via the periodontal ligament, lasts for the life of the tooth.

As the epithelial root sheath begins to break up and move away from the predentin surface, cells with the appearance of fibroblasts, originating from the dental follicle, migrate in between the epithelial cells and differentiate to cementoblasts. The expression of bone morphogenetic protein 3 (BMP-3) by dental follicle cells, and later by cells lining the root surface, has been linked to the differentiation of cementoblasts. These newly differentiated cementoblasts begin to deposit collagen fibrils oriented perpendicular to the root surface (Figs. 6.8 and 6.9). This fringe of collagen fibers intermingles with the collagen fibrils of the predentin, forming a firm attachment at the **dentin-cementum junction**. Mineralization of the mantle predentin begins internally and proceeds in a peripheral direction, encompassing the dentin-cementum junction and spreading into the cementum. The cementoblasts on the root surface continue to

> Fibroblasts from the dental follicle migrate to the developing root surface and differentiate into cementoblasts. These cells produce the initial acellular cementum, secreting collagen and inserting the fibrils into the peripheral dentin matrix. The developing periodontal ligament fiber bundles connect with this fiber fringe as the tooth emerges into the oral cavity; the fibers inserting into cementum are called Sharpey's fibers.

(a)

(b)

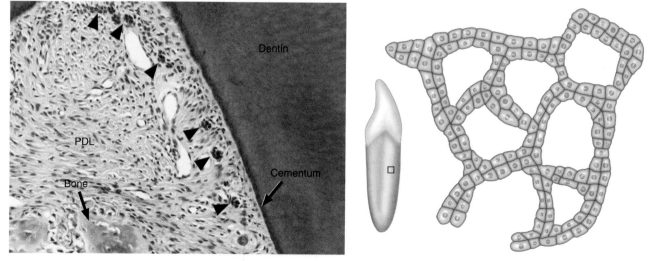

Figure 6.7   Epithelial rests of Malassez. (a) Light micrograph of the furcation region of the first permanent molar of a young child. Several clusters of epithelial rest cells (arrowheads), remnants of the epithelial root sheath, are present along the root surface. The crest of the interradicular bony septum is indicated. Periodontal ligament (PDL). (b) Drawing of the distribution of epithelial rest cells on the root surface. The rests form a network in the periodontal ligament that parallels the root surface. The box on the root of the tooth shows the approximate location of the main drawing.

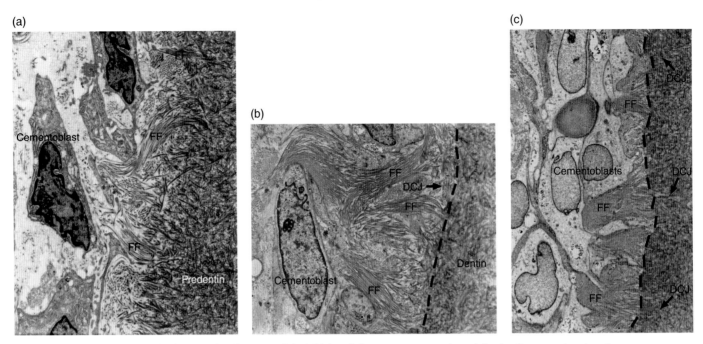

Figure 6.8   Electron micrographs showing development of the initial acellular cementum matrix and the dentin-cementum junction.
(a) Cementoblasts on the root surface produce and implant collagen fibrils into the predentin, forming a fiber fringe (FF) oriented roughly perpendicular to the developing root. (b) Cementum matrix almost completely covers the predentin matrix, and the external mineralizing front (dashed line) of the dentin has almost reached the dentin-cementum junction (DCJ). (c) The fiber fringe extends into the space of the immature periodontal ligament. The mineralization front (dashed line) of the dentin has passed the dentin-cementum junction. ((a), (b), and (c) From Bosshardt, D.D. & Selvig, K.A. (1997) Dental cementum: the dynamic tissue covering of the root. *Periodontology 2000*, 13, 41–75. Reproduced by permission of John Wiley and Sons.)

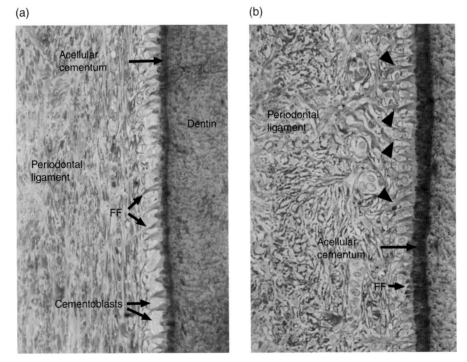

Figure 6.9   Light micrographs of developing cementum and periodontal ligament of unerupted human premolar teeth.
(a) A fiber fringe (FF) protrudes from a thin layer of mineralized acellular cementum. At this stage the periodontal ligament consists of a fibrocellular meshwork oriented parallel to the root surface. (b) A 15-μm-thick layer of mineralized cementum covers the root surface. The orientation of the periodontal ligament fibers has changed; many are now roughly perpendicular to the root. Some of the periodontal ligament fibers are continuous with the fiber fringe (arrowheads). ((a) and (b) From Bosshardt, D.D. & Selvig, K.A. (1997) Dental cementum: the dynamic tissue covering of the root. *Periodontology 2000*, 13, 41–75. Reproduced by permission of John Wiley and Sons.)

(a)

(b)

(c)

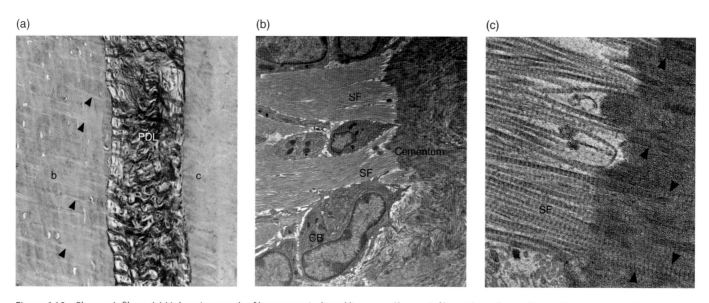

Figure 6.10 Sharpey's fibers. (a) Light micrograph of human periodontal ligament Sharpey's fibers. The collagen fibers of the periodontal ligament (PDL) are stained blue. Sharpey's fibers (arrowheads) are embedded in the alveolar bone (b). Sharpey's fibers also are present in cementum (c) but are less distinct. Azan stain. (From: Beertsen, W., McCulloch, C.A.G., & Sodek, J. (1997) The periodontal ligament: a unique, multifunctional connective tissue. *Periodontology, 2000*, 13, 20-40. Reprinted with permission from John Wiley and Sons.) (b) and (c) Electron micrographs of periodontal ligament fibers inserting into cementum (Sharpey's fibers, SF) of a mouse molar tooth. (a) The Sharpey's fibers pass between cementoblasts (CB) to enter the cementum. (b) At high magnification the individual banded collagen fibrils of the Sharpey's fibers can be seen in the cementum (arrowheads).

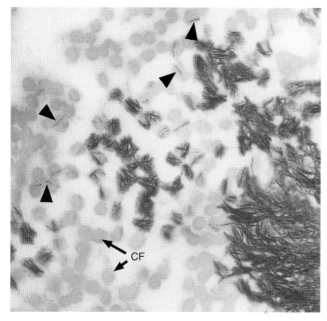

Figure 6.11 Electron micrograph of a section parallel to the root surface at the mineralization front of cementum. Cross-sectioned collagen fibrils (CF) appear as gray circles. Individual mineral crystals (fine dark lines) form within the collagen fibrils (arrowheads); additional mineral crystals are deposited within the fibrils (center), and finally between the fibrils to form the completely mineralized cementum (lower right). (From Bosshardt, D.D. & Selvig, K.A. (1997) Dental cementum: the dynamic tissue covering of the root. *Periodontology 2000*, 13, 41–75. Reproduced by permission of John Wiley and Sons.)

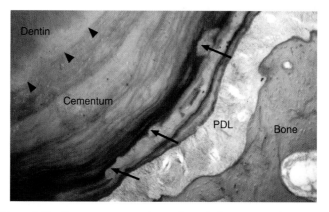

Figure 6.12 Cementum resorption and repair. Resorption of cementum by odontoclasts (similar to osteoclasts) may occur in a variety of conditions, including during orthodontic tooth movement. Resorbed areas (arrows) may be filled in later with newly deposited cementum. Arrowheads indicate the dentin-cementum junction.

deposit collagen, lengthening the fiber fringe, and also secrete non-collagenous proteins around the fibrils. When this initial layer of cementum achieves a thickness of 15 to 20 μm, at about the time that the cusp tip penetrates the oral mucosa, the fiber fringe connects with the principal fiber bundles of the developing periodontal ligament (Fig. 6.9). Acellular cementum thus serves as the main site of attachment of periodontal ligament collagen fibers. These fibers, inserting roughly perpendicularly into the cementum, are visible in histologic sections and are called **Sharpey's fibers** (Fig. 6.10).

Cellular cementum forms rapidly, up to 30 times faster than acellular cementum. Newly differentiated cementoblasts cover the root predentin in the apical and furcation regions and begin to deposit the initial matrix of cementum, with collagen fibrils intermingling with those of the predentin. Mineralization of the predentin extends across the dentin-cementum junction into the newly formed cementum. An irregular layer of unmineralized cementum, **precementum** or **cementoid**, is present between the cementoblasts and the mineralization front. Cementoblasts secrete matrix components completely around themselves, resulting in their entrapment in lacunae. The collagen fibrils of cellular cementum are mainly oriented parallel to the root surface, running in a circular direction around the tooth. Cellular cementum is deposited mainly as an adaptive tissue, in response to functional demands and to repair resorptive defects. Sharpey's fibers are fewer in number and more irregularly spaced in cellular cementum than in acellular cementum.

Cementum mineralization shares similarities with, but also differs from, the mineralization process in bone. For example, there is no evidence for a role of matrix vesicles in acellular cementum mineralization; mineral crystals are first deposited within the collagen fibrils, then between the fibrils (Fig. 6.11). Cementoblasts regulate the extracellular levels of the mineralization inhibitor inorganic pyrophosphate (PP_i) in order to control the amount of cementum deposition. Regulation of inorganic pyrophosphate levels is critical for proper acellular cementum formation, but less so for cellular cementum. Cementum mineralization is a very slow process; the width of the unmineralized precementum layer is 3 to 5 μm, roughly equivalent to the yearly deposition of cementum, and mineral crystals achieve their mature size between 1 and 4 μm deep to the mineralization front.

Tension transmitted through the periodontal ligament appears to stimulate cementum deposition. During orthodontic treatment, new cementum formation is greater on the tension side of the root than on the pressure side (the side toward which the tooth is being moved). Also, as a result of the normal **mesial drift** of teeth in the arch, cementum is thicker on the distal surface of the root than on the mesial surface. Cementum deposition, primarily cellular cementum, also occurs during repair of resorption defects (Fig. 6.12).

> Cellular cementum is mainly an adaptive and reparative tissue that is formed rapidly, trapping the cementoblasts as cementocytes in lacunae.

Periodontal ligament structure and function

The periodontal ligament attaches the tooth root to alveolar bone (Fig. 6.13), and it serves to absorb and resist the forces of occlusion on the tooth. It consists of collagenous fiber bundles containing hundreds or thousands of individual collagen fibrils (Fig. 6.14). The collagen fibrils and other extracellular matrix components are synthesized and maintained by periodontal ligament fibroblasts. Type I collagen is the major constituent of the fibers, but types III and XII collagen also are present. Type III collagen synthesis increases during periodontal ligament remodeling, whereas type XII collagen is thought to be important in maintaining the organization of the collagen fiber bundles. The fibroblasts are aligned along and between the fiber bundles and extend cytoplasmic processes that surround and organize the bundles. The periodontal ligament fiber bundles are embedded, as Sharpey's fibers, in cementum on the root and in the alveolar bone facing the tooth (Fig. 6.15). The embedded portions of Sharpey's fibers are fully mineralized in acellular cementum and partially mineralized in cellular cementum and bone. **Interstitial areas** containing loose connective tissue, blood vessels, and nerves are present between the fiber bundles in the periodontal ligament. These interstitial areas are continuous with openings through the alveolar bone (**Volkmann's canals**) to the marrow spaces of the alveolar process (Fig. 6.13).

Periodontal ligament fibers

Several distinct groups of fiber bundles are found in specific locations of the periodontal ligament (Fig. 6.16). These fiber bundles are known as the **principal fibers** of the periodontal ligament.

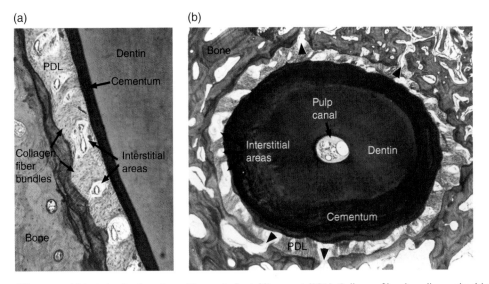

Figure 6.13 Periodontal ligament. (a) Longitudinal section of the periodontal ligament (PDL). Collagen fiber bundles embedded in alveolar bone extend across the space between the bone and the tooth and are embedded in cementum. Interstitial areas between the bundles consist of loose connective tissue and contain blood vessels and nerves. (b) Cross-section of the apical portion of a root and the surrounding alveolar bone. Interstitial areas are present between the fiber bundles of the periodontal ligament. Blood vessels from the bone enter and leave the periodontal ligament via Volkmann's canals (arrowheads). ((a) and (b) From Moss-Salentijn, L. (1972) *Orofacial Histology and Embryology: A Visual Integration.* Reproduced with permission from F.A. Davis Company, Philadelphia, PA.)

(a)

(b)

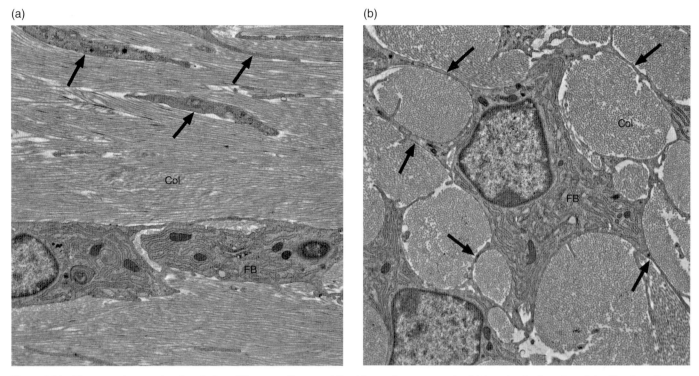

Figure 6.14   Electron micrographs of periodontal ligament fibers and fibroblasts of a mouse molar. (a) Longitudinal section of the fiber bundles shows the individual collagen fibrils (Col), with portions of two fibroblasts (FB) and several fibroblast processes (arrows). Fibroblast nucleus (N). (b) A cross-section reveals that each fiber bundle, with its individual collagen fibrils (Col), is surrounded by fibroblast processes (arrows).

(a)

(b)

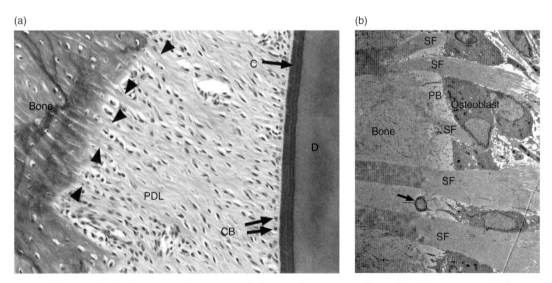

Figure 6.15   Sharpey's fibers in alveolar bone. (a) Light micrograph showing the insertion of periodontal ligament (PDL) fibers (arrowheads) into alveolar bone. Fibroblast nuclei are aligned along the fiber bundles of the PDL. Nuclei of cementoblasts (CB) are aligned along the surface of the cementum (C). Dentin (D). Hematoxylin and eosin stain. (b) Electron micrograph of the surface of alveolar bone surrounding a mouse molar. Several osteoblasts are seen on the surface of the bone. Unmineralized pre-bone (PB) (osteoid) is present between the osteoblasts and the (previously) mineralized bone to the left (this sample was demineralized prior to sectioning). Five Sharpey's fibers (SF) consisting of numerous collagen fibrils pass between the osteoblasts and are anchored in the bone. A small osteocyte (arrow) is embedded in the bone.

- *Alveolar crest fibers* extend from the crest of the alveolar bone obliquely, attaching to the cementum at a position more coronal than their attachment to the bone. These fibers resist occlusal or incisal displacement of the tooth.

- *Horizontal fibers* are located just below the alveolar crest fibers and extend in a more or less horizontal direction from the alveolar bone to the cementum. These fibers resist lateral displacement of the tooth.

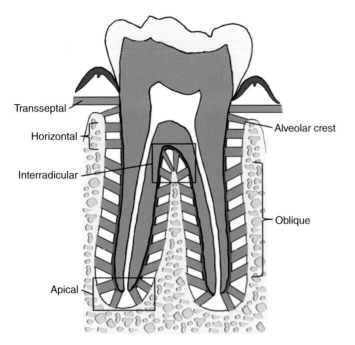

Figure 6.16   Principal fiber bundles of the periodontal ligament. The alveolar crest, horizontal, oblique, apical, and interradicular fiber bundles insert into the alveolar bone and the cementum. Transseptal fibers extend across the alveolar septum from the cementum on the mesial and distal surfaces to the cementum on the adjacent teeth in the arch.

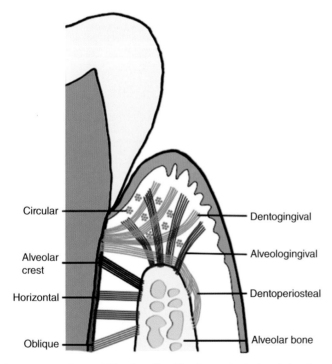

Figure 6.17   Gingival fiber bundles. The dentogingival and alveolo-gingival fibers, extending into the gingivae from the cementum and alveolar crest, respectively, bind the gingivae to the tooth and bone. Circular fibers, seen in cross-section, encircle the tooth, also holding the gingivae in place. The dentoperiosteal fibers extend from the cementum to the facial and lingual/palatal periosteum of the alveolar bone.

- *Oblique fibers* are the largest group of principal fibers. They extend obliquely from the bone to the cementum, attaching more apically to the cementum than to the bone. These fibers act like a sling or hammock, resisting intrusive forces during mastication.
- *Apical fibers* are arranged radially around the apical ends of the roots and resist displacement of the tooth in an occlusal or incisal direction.
- *Interradicular fibers* extend radially from the crest of the alveolar bone between the roots of multirooted teeth to the cementum in the furcation area of the tooth. These fibers also resist occlusal displacement of the tooth.

> The periodontal ligament attaches the tooth to the alveolar bone and absorbs forces applied to the tooth. The ligament consists of distinct principal fiber bundles consisting of type I collagen fibrils, separated by interstitial areas containing loose connective tissue, blood vessels, and nerves.

Although not strictly part of the periodontal ligament, there are other distinct groups of fibers that help to maintain the integrity of the periodontium (Figs. 6.16 and 6.17).

- *Transseptal fibers* extend across the crest of the alveolar bone from the cementum of one tooth to the cementum of the adjacent tooth. These fibers help to maintain the proximal surfaces of the teeth in contact.
- *Dentogingival fibers* extend from the cementum into the lamina propria of the free and attached gingivae, keeping these tissues in place around the cervical region of the tooth.
- *Alveologingival fibers* extend from the crest of the alveolar bone into the lamina propria of the free and attached gingivae, and also serve to hold these tissues in place.
- *Dentoperiosteal fibers* extend apically from the cementum over the alveolar crest and insert into the periosteum and bone of the outer cortical plate of the alveolar process.
- *Circular fibers* encircle the neck of the tooth, intermingling with the other fibers in this region and helping to hold the free gingivae against the tooth.

A second fiber system consisting of **oxytalan fibers** is present in the periodontal ligament (Fig. 6.18). Oxytalan fibers are similar to the microfibrils of elastic fibers and consist predominantly of the protein **fibrillin**. Oxytalan fibers are oriented in an apico-occlusal direction, but often insert perpendicularly into the cementum. These fibers frequently are associated with blood vessels in the periodontal ligament. Although their function has not been clearly established, they may serve to stabilize blood vessels or act as a mechanoreceptive system to regulate blood flow.

Blood supply

The periodontal ligament receives its blood supply from three different sources: branches of the alveolar arteries supplying the pulps of the teeth that enter the periodontal ligament at its

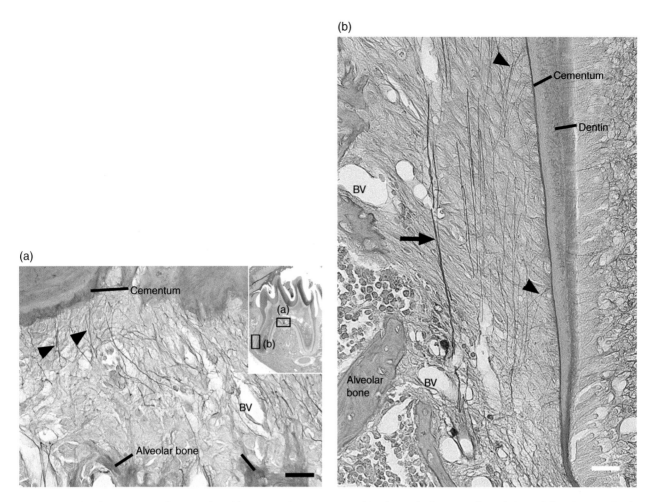

Figure 6.18   Oxytalan fibers in rat molar periodontal ligament. The inset in panel (a) shows the location of panels (a) and (b). (a) Interradicular region. Purple oxytalan fibers (arrowheads) connect forming cementum with alveolar bone. Blood vessel (BV). (b) Near the root apex many oxytalan fibers have an apico-occlusal orientation, with thick fibers (arrow) running along vessels near the alveolar bone. Other finer fibers (arrowheads) branch from the thicker fibers to insert into the cementum. ((a) and (b) From Inoue, K., Hara, Y., & Sato, T. (2012) Development of the oxytalan fiber system in the rat molar periodontal ligament evaluated by light- and electron-microscopic analyses. *Annals of Anatomy* 194(5), 482–488. Reprinted with permission from Elsevier.)

apical extent; branches of the arteries supplying the adjacent alveolar bone that perforate the wall of the alveolus and enter the periodontal ligament via Volkmann's canals; and via anastomoses between gingival vessels and periodontal ligament vessels (Fig. 6.19). The vessels run in an apico-occlusal direction, and tend to be clustered in the interstitial areas between collagen fiber bundles. The vessels branch and form an interconnected network consisting of arterioles, capillaries, and post-capillary venules.

The width of the periodontal ligament averages about 0.2 mm. It is slightly wider in the apical and gingival regions,

and somewhat narrower in the mid-root region. Changing functional demands can alter the width and structure of the periodontal ligament. Loss of an opposing tooth and the resultant lack of normal occlusal forces during mastication causes atrophy of the periodontal ligament. The width of the periodontal ligament decreases, the fiber bundles become thinner, and their orientation is altered. In some cases the fiber bundles may be oriented nearly parallel to the root surface (Fig. 6.20).

The periodontal ligament undergoes continual turnover and renewal. The rate of collagen turnover in the periodontal ligament is as much as eight times greater than other soft connective tissues. Several factors contribute to this rapid turnover: the periodontal ligament is subjected to continual tensile and compressive stresses from the forces of mastication; the slow wearing away of enamel on the occlusal surfaces of opposing teeth results in a slow but continual post-functional eruption; and the attrition of enamel on the proximal surfaces of adjacent teeth results in a continual mesial drift of the teeth (Fig. 6.21). The application of orthodontic forces to the teeth results in both

> Additional groups of collagen fiber bundles serve to maintain tooth alignment and hold the gingival tissues in place. Within the periodontal ligament, a second fiber system consisting of microfibrils, the oxytalan fibers, is oriented in an apico-occlusal direction. The periodontal ligament has a rich blood supply derived from branches of pulpal vessels, the adjacent alveolar bone, and the gingivae.

(a)

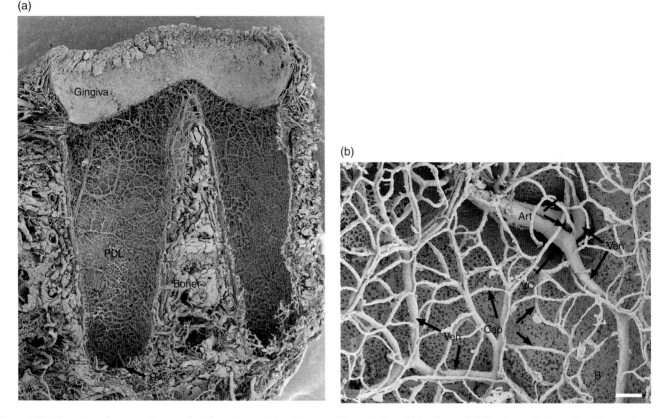

Figure 6.19   Scanning electron micrographs of a resin cast of canine premolar periodontal blood vessels following soft tissue digestion and removal of the tooth. (a) Low magnification image showing the vascular network of the periodontal ligament (PDL) surrounding the roots. The periodontal ligament vessels are supplied through connections with branches of the alveolar arteries in the bone that enter the ligament via Volkmann's canals, anastomoses with gingival vessels in the cervical region, and branches from alveolar arteries prior to their entry into the pulp at the root apex (RA). (b) High magnification image showing an arteriole (Art) entering the ligament from the alveolar bone via a Volkmann's canal (VC). Branches of the arteriole form a capillary network (Cap) adjacent to the cementum. Post-capillary vessels form a venular network adjacent to the bone of the alveolar wall (B). ((a) and (b) From Matsuo, M. & Takahashi, K. (2002) Scanning electron microscopic observation of microvasculature in periodontium. *Microscopy Research and Technique* 56(1), 3–14. Reprinted by permission of John Wiley and Sons.)

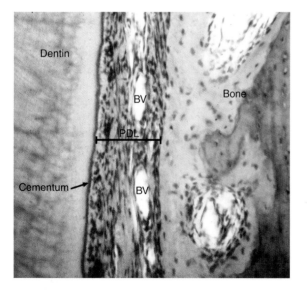

Figure 6.20   Atrophic periodontal ligament. Loss of function of the tooth has resulted in a thinning of the periodontal ligament (PDL) and a change in the orientation of the fiber bundles, which now nearly parallel the root surface. Blood vessels (BV).

tensile and compressive stresses in the periodontal ligament. Remodeling of the attachments of the periodontal ligament to cementum and bone are required in order to adapt to these stresses and movements.

> The width of the periodontal ligament is about 0.2 mm, and is dependent upon functional demands. The stresses of mastication and the slow postfunctional eruption and mesial drift of the teeth result in a high rate of periodontal ligament collagen turnover.

Cells of the periodontal ligament

The principal cell type of the periodontal ligament is the fibroblast. Other cells that are present in the periodontal ligament include cementoblasts along the root surface, **osteoblasts** along the bone surface, and **osteoclasts** or odontoclasts involved in bone or root resorption. Macrophages, undifferentiated mesenchymal cells, and epithelial cells that are remnants of the

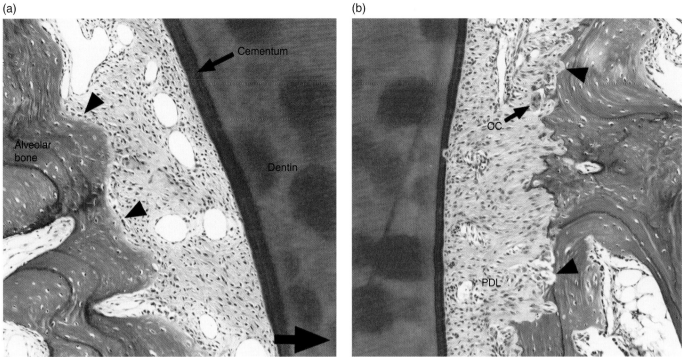

Figure 6.21 Mesial drift. (a) The continual mesial drift (direction of large arrow at bottom) of the teeth results in bone deposition by osteoblasts (arrowheads), a smooth bone surface, and cement lines in the alveolar bone on the distal side of the root. (b) Bone resorption and an irregular bone surface (arrowheads) are found adjacent to the mesial root. Osteoclast (OC).

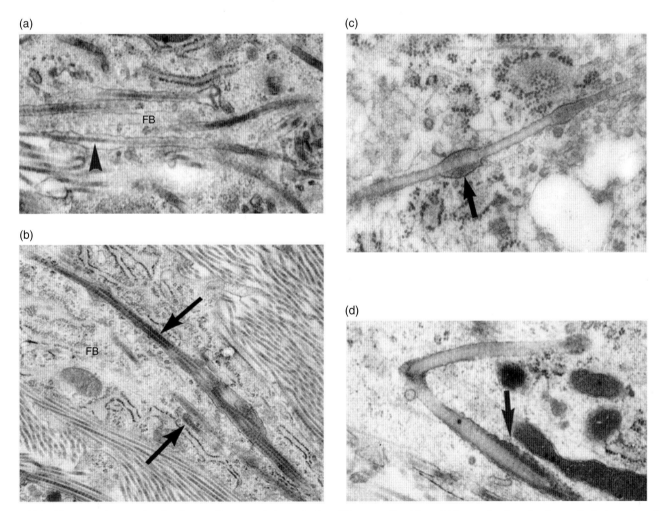

Figure 6.22 Electron micrographs of collagen phagocytosis by periodontal ligament fibroblasts. (a) Internalization of collagen fibrils (arrowhead). Fibroblast (FB). (b) Collagen fibrils within intracellular vacuoles (arrows). (c) and (d) Collagen containing vacuoles that have fused with lysosomes (arrows). (Courtesy of Dr. Wouter Beertsen.)

epithelial root sheath, the epithelial rests of Malassez, also are found in the periodontal ligament.

Fibroblasts synthesize and organize new collagen fibrils in the periodontal ligament, and are responsible for extracellular as well as intracellular degradation of collagen fibrils undergoing turnover. Fibroblasts produce and secrete members of the **matrix metalloproteinase** enzyme family that sequentially degrade collagen and other matrix molecules. Additionally, fibroblasts internalize matrix components, including collagen fibrils, and degrade them within their lysosomal system (Fig. 6.22).

An important but poorly understood function of the periodontal ligament, being situated between mineralized bone and cementum, is maintenance of its unmineralized state. Undifferentiated cells of the periodontal ligament and the adjacent marrow spaces of the alveolar bone can differentiate to form osteoblasts and cementoblasts (see below), but the activities of these cells remain localized to their respective tissue surfaces. It is believed that the periodontal ligament fibroblasts secrete factors that inhibit mineralization of the extracellular matrix.

Stem cells in the periodontal ligament

Experimental studies have shown that a population of progenitor cells with the potential to differentiate into several distinct mesenchymal cell types can be isolated from the periodontal ligament. In cell culture, periodontal ligament stem cells can differentiate into cells that form bone, cementum, cartilage, fat, muscle, and neuron- and glial-like cells. Recent work indicates that perivascular cells (pericytes) associated with the microvasculature of alveolar bone and periodontal ligament of mice can differentiate into osteoblasts, cementoblasts, cementocytes, and periodontal ligament fibroblasts in untreated animals, as well as after injury of the periodontium. Periodontal ligament stem cells on hydroxyapatite/tricalcium phosphate scaffolds implanted into periodontal defects in experimental animals or the alveolus after tooth extraction form cementum and periodontal ligament. Thus, there is considerable interest in the therapeutic potential of these stem cells for treatment of periodontal defects.

> Fibroblasts are the main cell type of the periodontal ligament. Other cells include cementoblasts, osteoblasts, osteoclasts, macrophages, epithelial rest cells, and stem cells.

Sensory functions of the periodontal ligament

In addition to its role in attaching the teeth to alveolar bone, the periodontal ligament has important sensory functions. It is well supplied with nerves that respond to touch, pressure, and tooth position. Stimuli sensed by periodontal nerves result in oral reflexes that facilitate chewing, biting, and other oral functions, including saliva secretion. Two types of sensory receptors are found in the periodontal ligament: free nerve endings, which presumably function as nociceptors; and specialized nerve terminals that are mechanoreceptors. Periodontal mechanoreceptors are activated by tooth

movement and are composed of **Ruffini endings** intertwined among periodontal ligament fibers (Figs. 6.23, 6.24). Periodontal Ruffini endings have an extensive axonal arborization, with thick axons, but lack a fibrous capsule. They are most often found in areas of dense collagenous fiber bundles, especially around the root apex, and also in the middle region of the periodontal ligament.

Periodontal mechanoreceptors respond to physical stretch and are directionally sensitive and slowly adapting. When a tooth moves in its alveolus it causes tension in the ligaments, which in turn activate the periodontal receptors. Most receptors are maximally sensitive in one direction, but some are bidirectional due to the arrangement of the ligaments (Fig. 6.24). For example, inferior alveolar and lingual nerve receptors are directionally sensitive in two, three, or four horizontal directions as well as up and down. In addition, more than half of all periodontal nerve fibers are spontaneously active and some respond to more than one tooth, most likely because of close coupling between teeth rather than a branching of axons. The neuronal cell bodies of the Ruffini endings are located in the trigeminal ganglion and the mesencephalic nucleus. Central branches of afferent mesencephalic units, whose receptors are concentrated near the apex of the root, contact motor cells in the trigeminal motor nucleus and provide feedback information about bite pressure to the muscles of mastication (see Chapter 12).

In addition to the sensory nerves described above, sympathetic nerve fibers are associated with periodontal ligament blood vessels.

> Nerve fibers innervating the periodontal ligament provide mechanosensory, proprioceptive, and pain information.

Structure and function of alveolar bone

The alveolar processes of the mandible and maxilla develop as the teeth erupt, and their maintenance is dependent upon the presence of the teeth. If a tooth is lost, the alveolar bone that formerly supported the tooth is resorbed, and the height of the alveolar process is reduced in that area. The alveolar processes consist of cortical plates of compact bone, central regions of trabecular, or cancellous, bone, and marrow spaces, and the alveolar bone proper that lines the alveoli, or tooth sockets (Fig. 6.25). Around the anterior teeth, trabecular bone is absent and the cortical bone and alveolar bone are joined. The cortical bone contains typical **Haversian systems (osteons)**, and lamellar bone can be found in the trabeculae and the alveolar bone. The alveolar bone is called **bundle bone** because of the insertions of Sharpey's fibers from the periodontal ligament.

The cells involved in the formation, maintenance, and resorption of alveolar bone, osteoblasts, **osteocytes**, and osteoclasts, are identical to those found in other bones throughout the body. Osteoblasts are found on the surfaces of bone where bone formation is occurring (Fig. 6.26). Active osteoblasts are cuboidal in shape, and have abundant rough endoplasmic reticulum. A layer of **pre-bone** or **osteoid**, the initial unmineralized matrix deposited by the osteoblasts, is present between the cells and the mineralized bone. The thickness of the pre-bone layer varies, being thicker during rapid bone formation and thinner during inactive periods. Inactive or resting osteoblasts, also called

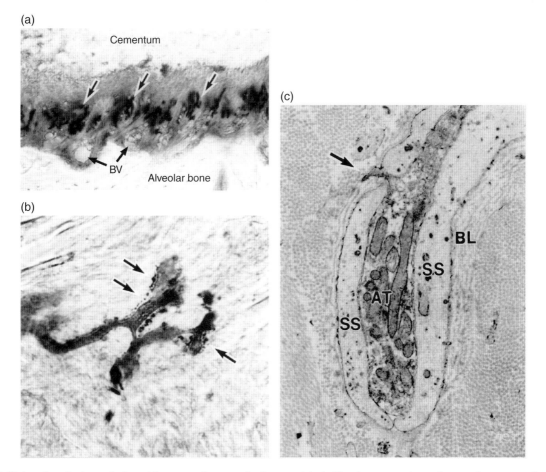

Figure 6.23 Ruffini endings in the periodontal ligament of a rat molar, immunolabeled for the neuronal protein, protein gene product 9.5 (PGP 9.5). (a) Light microscopic image of a cross-section through the periodontal ligament showing labeled nerve elements (arrows). Blood vessels (BV) are located adjacent to the alveolar bone. (b) High magnification image of a Ruffini ending. Microprojections of the axon terminal are indicated by the arrows. (c) Transmission electron micrograph of a Ruffini ending. The axon terminal (AT) is filled with mitochondria. Schwann cell sheaths (SS) enclose the terminal, and several layers of basal lamina (BL) separate the ending from the collagen fibrils of the periodontal ligament. An axonal microvillus (arrow) of the axon terminal extends through the Schwann cell sheath. ((a), (b) and (c) From Muramoto, T., Takano, Y., & Soma, K. (2000) Time-related changes in periodontal mechanoreceptors in rat molars after the loss of occlusal stimuli. *Archives of Histology and Cytology*, 63(4), 369–380. Reprinted by permission of *Archives of Histology and Cytology*/International Society of Histology and Cytology.)

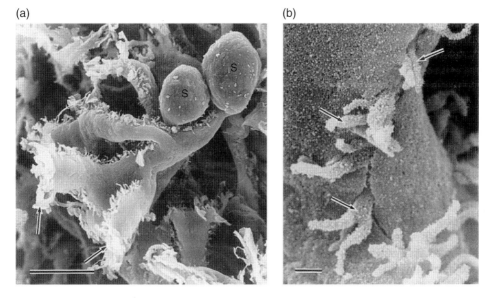

Figure 6.24 Scanning electron micrographs of periodontal Ruffini nerve endings of the rat incisor following removal of collagen fibers. (a) Arrows indicate Schwann cell processes extending from distal branches of Ruffini endings. The tongue-like segments of these "Venus fly trap" endings cradle periodontal ligament fibers and are considered the movement receptors. Schwann cell bodies (S). (b) Numerous axonal microvilli (arrows) projecting through a slit in the Schwann cell sheath. These microvilli come in contact with numerous periodontal ligament collagen fibrils and respond to motion as the fibrils scrape against them. Scale bars: a = 10 μm; b = 0.5 μm. (From Takahashi-Iwanaga, H., Maeda, T., & Abe, K. (1997) Scanning and transmission electron microscopy of Ruffini endings in the periodontal ligament of rat incisors. *Journal of Comparative Neurology*, 389(1), 177–184. Reprinted by permission of John Wiley and Sons.)

(a)   (b)

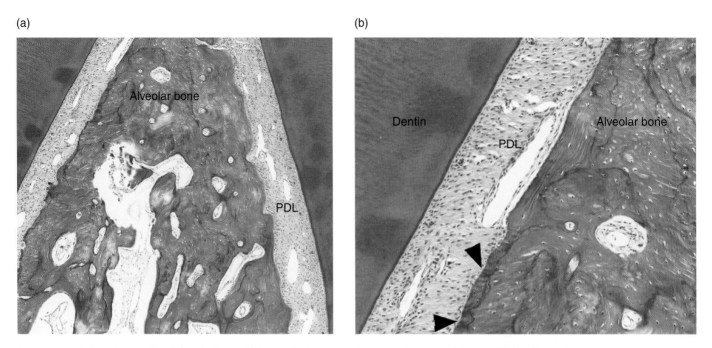

Figure 6.25   Light micrographs of alveolar bone. (a) Interradicular septum between the roots of the mandibular first molar. Marrow spaces are present between the bone trabeculae, and a few primary osteons appear to be forming. (b) Alveolar bone adjacent to the mesial surface of the distal root of the mandibular first molar. Osteocytes are present in lacunae, and bone lamellae are visible in some areas. Sharpey's fibers are visible between the arrowheads. The irregular basophilic lines in the bone are cement lines or reversal lines, formed when bone resorption ceases and bone deposition begins.

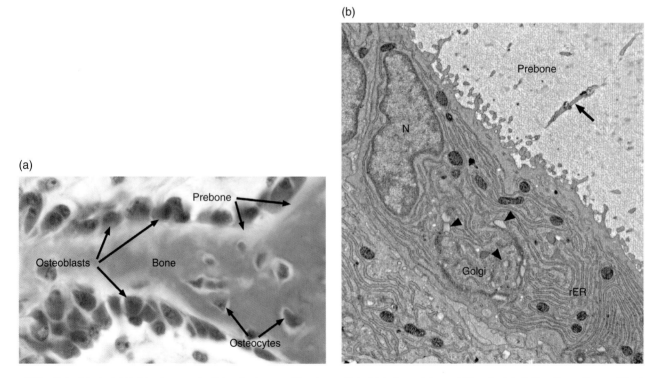

Figure 6.26   Osteoblasts. (a) Light micrograph of developing maxillary bone. Cuboidal-shaped, basophilic osteoblasts line the surfaces of the bone spicule. A layer of pale-staining pre-bone (osteoid) is present between the osteoblasts and the mineralized bone. Several osteocytes are located in lacunae within the bone. (b) Electron micrograph of an osteoblast on the surface of alveolar bone. The cytoplasm is filled with rough endoplasmic reticulum (rER) cisternae, and secretory vesicles (arrowheads) are forming in the Golgi complex. Pre-bone, at the upper right, contains abundant collagen fibrils and some cell processes (arrow).

endosteal or **bone lining cells**, form a thin layer on the surface of the bone. These cells can be activated and resume bone formation as the need arises.

Osteocytes are osteoblasts that have been surrounded by bone matrix and become embedded in the bone (Fig. 6.27). During the transition from osteoblast to osteocyte, the cells decrease the expression of type I collagen and alkaline phosphatase, and increase the expression of genes regulating mineralization (dentin matrix protein 1 [DMP1] and sclerostin [SOST]) and phosphate homeostasis (fibroblast growth factor 23 [FGF23], matrix extracellular phosphoglycoprotein [MEPE] and phosphate-regulating gene with homologies to endopeptidases on the X chromosome [PHEX]). Similar to cementocytes, osteocytes reside in spaces in the bone called lacunae, and cellular processes of osteocytes are enclosed in canaliculi. Osteocyte processes create a network throughout the bone, making contact with processes of adjacent osteocytes, with osteoblasts at the bone surface, and with blood vessels. Osteocytes maintain the lacunae and canaliculi in an unmineralized state, which is critical for diffusion of waste products and nutrients to and from the blood vessels in the periodontal ligament and Haversian canals. Although osteocytes do not have the synthetic capabilities of osteoblasts, they are essential for bone vitality and have an important signaling role. They regulate osteoblast and osteoclast function, act as mechanosensors to sense and respond to mechanical loading applied to the bone, and may be targets for parathyroid hormone.

Osteoclasts are large multinucleated cells (Fig. 6.28) that arise from fusion of bone marrow-derived precursors of the monocyte-macrophage lineage, under the control of specific cell surface ligands found on other cell types (e.g., osteoblasts, bone marrow stromal cells, certain immune cells) and receptors found on osteoclast precursors. The fusion of osteoclast precursors and their development into active osteoclasts requires interaction of the **receptor activator of nuclear factor kappa B ligand (RANKL)** on osteoblasts or bone marrow stromal cells with the **receptor activator of nuclear factor kappa B (RANK)** on the osteoclast precursors, and **macrophage colony stimulating factor (M-CSF)** on osteoblasts with **colony stimulating factor 1 receptor** on osteoclast precursors. Osteoblasts and bone marrow stromal cells also secrete **osteoprotegerin**, which binds to RANKL and prevents its interaction with RANK. The ratio of osteoprotegerin to RANKL is an important determinant of bone mass and skeletal integrity.

Osteoclasts adhere to extracellular matrix proteins at the bone surface via transmembrane **integrin receptors** at the **sealing zone**, an actin-filled ring-shaped cellular process that encloses the **ruffled border** where acid (protons) and proteolytic enzymes (matrix metalloproteinases and cathepsin K) are secreted, creating a degradative microenvironment. Their resorptive activity creates a depression or groove in the bone surface, a **Howship's lacuna**, within which the osteoclast sits.

> Alveolar bone supports the teeth, and is dependent upon the presence of the teeth. Osteoblasts produce the collagenous matrix of alveolar bone and mineralize it. Osteocytes and their processes, present in lacunae and canaliculi within the bone, form a network that has mechanosensory functions and regulates the activities of osteoblasts and osteoclasts. Osteoclasts are large multinucleated cells that arise by fusion of bone marrow-derived precursors and function to resorb bone.

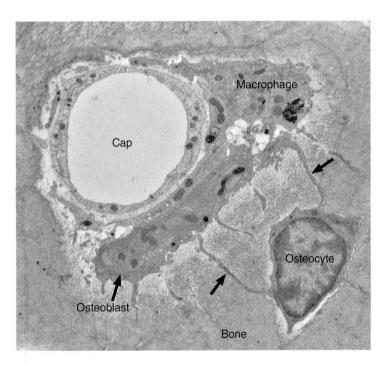

Figure 6.27   Electron micrograph of a small Haversian canal in alveolar bone. A capillary (Cap) and portions of an osteoblast and a macrophage are seen in the canal. An osteocyte is embedded in the bone. Osteocyte processes in canaliculi extend in several directions, and two processes contact similar processes of the osteoblast (arrows).

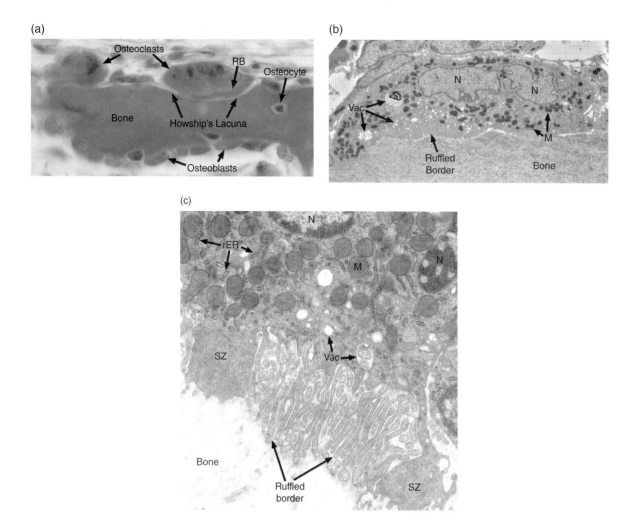

Figure 6.28   Osteoclasts. (a) Light micrograph of developing bone, showing two osteoclasts with multiple nuclei, osteoblasts, and osteocytes. The resorptive activity of the osteoclast on the right has created a Howship's lacuna. Ruffled border (RB). (b) Low magnification electron micrograph of an osteoclast on the surface of alveolar bone. Two nuclei (N) are present in this section; numerous mitochondria (M) and several small vacuoles (Vac) are seen in the cytoplasm. (c) Higher magnification of the ruffled border region of a similar osteoclast. The ruffled border is encircled by the sealing zone (SZ), seen as two broad cell processes filled with actin filaments. The cytoplasm contains numerous mitochondria (M), several small rough endoplasmic reticulum (rER) cisternae, and many small vacuoles (Vac) and vesicles.

Clinical correlations

Periodontal disease

The periodontal diseases, **gingivitis** and **periodontitis**, afflict a majority of adults. Recent epidemiological studies indicate that over 47% of adults in the United States have periodontitis, and 64% of adults aged 65 years and older have moderate or severe periodontitis. Many factors influence the development and course of these diseases, including a complex subgingival microbial biofilm, social and behavioral patterns, genetic and epigenetic host factors, and the host's immune and inflammatory responses. The presence and accumulation of pathogenic periodontal microorganisms in subgingival plaque induces an inflammatory response in the gingival and periodontal tissues (Fig. 6.29). Loss of the integrity of the junctional epithelium allows the microorganisms, their products, and antigens to spread into the lamina propria. The binding and recognition of bacterial products by cells of the periodontium, including cells of the innate immune system (polymorphonuclear neutrophilic leukocytes, macrophages, dendritic cells), results in the release of proinflammatory chemokines, cytokines, and other molecules, leading to an inflammatory response. Polymorphonuclear neutrophilic leukocytes accumulate in the gingival connective tissue, and vascular leakage results in an increased flow of gingival crevicular fluid. The release of additional proinflammatory factors and proteolytic enzymes by the cells of the periodontium, the inflammatory cells, and the invading microorganisms results in damage to the periodontal connective tissues. If the infection is not eliminated, macrophages and dendritic cells engage the adaptive immune system, and a chronic inflammatory state develops. The macrophages and lymphocytes of the chronic inflammatory infiltrate produce factors that result in differentiation of osteoclasts and subsequent resorption of alveolar bone. The junctional epithelium proliferates, elongates, and migrates apically along the root surface, disrupting periodontal ligament attachment to the root. The free surface of the epithelium also is displaced apically, increasing the depth of the gingival sulcus, and increasing

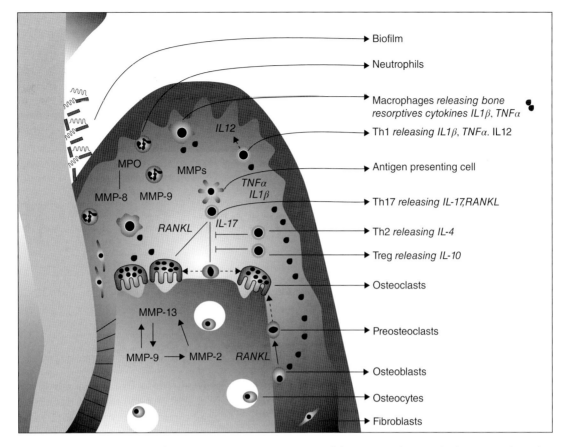

Figure 6.29   Diagram illustrating the cells and factors involved in the progression of chronic periodontitis. The formation of an infective bacterial biofilm on the tooth surface induces an inflammatory response in the periodontal tissues. Macrophages and T-lymphocytes (Th1 and Th17 cells) release pro-inflammatory cytokines (IL-1β, IL-12, IL-17, TNFα), and polymorphonuclear leukocytes (neutrophils) release matrix metalloproteinases (MMP-8, MMP-9), which degrade collagen and collagen fragments, and myeloperoxidase (MPO), which produces reactive oxygen species and inactivates the tissue inhibitor of MMPs (TIMP-1). The differentiation of Treg cells, which suppress inflammatory responses, is inhibited by the infection and immune activation. Expression of RANKL by Th17 cells and osteoblasts induces the formation and activation of osteoclasts, which resorb alveolar bone. Several cell types in the periodontium release MMP-13, which also has collagenolytic activity and promotes activation of other MMPs as well as osteoclasts. (From Hernández, M., et al. (2011) Host-pathogen interactions in progressive chronic periodontitis. *Journal of Dental Research*, 90(10), 1164–1170. © 2011 by International & American Associations for Dental Research. Reprinted by permission of SAGE Publications.)

the area of exposed tooth surface upon which plaque can form. The loss of bone and ligament attachment significantly reduces the support of the tooth, and is a major cause of tooth loss.

In addition to the local effects of periodontal disease, i.e., tissue destruction and tooth loss, several research studies have shown that periodontal disease is associated with increased risk for, or exacerbation of, several significant systemic diseases or conditions. These include cardiovascular disease, diabetes mellitus, adverse pregnancy outcomes, and respiratory diseases. However, at present, the statistical association between periodontal disease and systemic disease is weak, and it is unclear whether a major public health relevance exists.

Periodontal cysts

The remnants of the epithelial tissues associated with tooth development, e.g., the epithelial rests of Malassez and the dental lamina, can give rise to various types of cysts in the periodontal area. Periapical or radicular cysts develop from epithelial rest cells that are stimulated to proliferate by inflammatory mediators released during the response to degradation products from a necrotic tooth pulp. Lateral periodontal cysts and gingival cysts are believed to develop from remnants of the dental lamina. These cysts are most common in the mandibular premolar area; although rare, pressure from expansion of the cyst may lead to divergence of the roots of the adjacent teeth.

Genetic disease

The genetic disease hypophosphatasia, caused by mutations in the *ALPL* gene encoding tissue-nonspecific alkaline phosphatase, results in increased levels of the mineralization inhibitor inorganic pyrophosphate (PP_i). The reduced mineralization of bones leads to rickets and osteomalacia. Hypophosphatasia also causes premature tooth loss due to aplasia or hypoplasia of acellular cementum with resulting poor periodontal ligament attachment. Additionally, these teeth may show defects suggestive of poor dentin formation and mineralization, such as widened pulp chambers, increased interglobular spaces, and thin root dentin.

The most common diseases affecting the periodontium are the infectious diseases gingivitis and periodontitis. The inflammatory response to a microbial biofilm on the tooth surfaces results in destruction of the connective tissue and alveolar bone, with eventual loss of tooth support. Periodontal cysts may develop from remnants of the epithelial tissues associated with tooth development. The genetic disease hypophosphatasia causes reduced mineralization of bones and teeth and premature tooth loss.

References

1. Beertsen W., McCulloch C.A.G., & Sodek, S. (1997) The periodontal ligament: a unique, multifunctional connective tissue. *Periodontology 2000*, 13, 20–40.
2. Bosshardt, D.D. & Selvig, K.A. (1997) Dental cementum: the dynamic tissue covering of the root. *Periodontology 2000*, 13, 41–75.
3. Boyce, B.F. (2013) Advances in the regulation of osteoclasts and osteoclast function. *Journal of Dental Research*, DOI: 10.1177/0022034513500306.
4. Chen, F.-M., Sun, H-H., Lu, H., & Yu, Q. (2012) Stem cell-delivery therapeutics for periodontal tissue regeneration. *Biomaterials*, 33(27), 6320–6344.
5. Cho, M.-I. & Garant, P.R. (2000) Development and general structure of the periodontium. *Periodontology 2000*, 24, 9–27.
6. Dallas, S.L., Prideaux, M., & Bonewald, L.F. (2013) The osteocyte: an endocrine cell and more. *Endocrine Reviews*, DOI: 10.1210/er.2012-1026.
7. Dentino, A., Lee, S., Mailhot, J., & Hefti, A.F. (2013) Principles of periodontology. *Periodontology 2000*, 61(1), 16–53.
8. Diekwisch, T.G.H. (2001) Developmental biology of cementum. *International Journal of Developmental Biology*, 45, 695–706.
9. Foster, B.L., Nagamoto, K.J., Nociti, F.H.Jr., Fong, H., Dunn, D., Tran, A.B., Wang, W., Narisawa, S., Millan, J.L., & Somerman, M.J. (2012) Central role of pyrophosphate in acellular cementum formation. *PLoS One*, 7(6), e38393.
10. Foster, B.L., Popowics, T.E., Fong, H.K., & Somerman, M.J. (2007) Advances in defining regulators of cementum development and periodontal regeneration. *Current Topics in Developmental Biology*, 78, 47–126.
11. Grzesik, W.J. & Narayanan, A.S. (2002) Cementum and periodontal wound healing and regeneration. *Critical Reviews in Oral Biology & Medicine*, 13(6), 474–484.
12. Hernández, M., Dutzan, N., García-Sesnich, J., Abusleme, L., Dezerega, A., Silva, N., González, F.E., Vernal, R., Sorsa, T,. & Gamonal, J. (2011) Host-pathogen interactions in progressive chronic periodontitis. *Journal of Dental Research*, 90(10), 1164–1170.
13. Huang, X., Bringas, P. Jr., Slavkin, H.C., & Chai, Y. (2009) Fate of HERS during tooth root development. *Developmental Biology*, 334, 22–30.
14. Lekic, P. & McCulloch, C.A.G. (1996) Periodontal ligament cell populations: the central role of fibroblasts in creating a unique tissue. *Anatomical Record*, 245, 327–341.
15. Luan, X., Ito, Y. & Diekwisch, T.G.H. (2006) Evolution and development of Hertwig's epithelial root sheath. *Developmental Dynamics*, 235, 1167–1180.
16. Nanci, A. & Bosshardt, D.D. (2006) Structure of periodontal tissues in health and disease. *Periodontology 2000*, 40, 11–28.
17. Saygin, N.E., Giannobile, W.V., & Somerman, M.J. (2000) Molecular and cell biology of cementum. *Periodontology 2000*, 24, 73–98.
18. van den Bos, T., Handoko, G., Niehof, A., Ryan, L.M., Coburn, S.P., Whyte, M.P., & Beertsen, W. (2005) Cementum and dentin in hypophosphatasia. *Journal of Dental Research*, 84(11), 1021–1025.

Glossary

Alveolar bone: The portions of the maxilla and mandible that support the teeth, and into which the periodontal ligament fibers insert.

Alveolus: The tooth socket; formed by alveolar bone, to which periodontal ligament fibers attach.

Acellular cementum (acellular extrinsic fiber cementum): Cementum lacking cells, with collagen fibrils that originate in the periodontal ligament and insert into the cementum; found on the coronal one-half to two-thirds of the root.

Acellular afibrillar cementum: Cementum lacking embedded cells and collagen fibrils; restricted to the cervical region of the tooth, overlapping enamel.

Bundle bone: Bone with inserted collagen fibers (Sharpey's fibers) of tendons and ligaments, such as alveolar bone supporting the teeth.

Canaliculi: Unmineralized spaces in cementum (or bone) housing cytoplasmic processes of cementocytes (or osteocytes).

Cellular cementum (cellular intrinsic fiber cementum): Cementum containing cementocytes, with matrix collagen fibrils produced and secreted by cementoblasts.

Cellular mixed stratified cementum: Cementum consisting of alternating layers of acellular and cellular cementum.

Cementoblasts: Cells differentiated from fibroblasts of the dental follicle, or possibly from epithelial root sheath cells by epithelial-mesenchymal transformation, that produce and mineralize cementum.

Cementocytes: Cells located in lacunae in cellular cementum, originating from cementoblasts trapped in the matrix they produced.

Colony stimulating factor-1 receptor: A transmembrane protein that serves as the receptor for colony stimulating factor 1; regulates the differentiation and function of macrophages and osteoclasts.

Dentin-cementum junction: The interface between dentin and cementum, characterized by intermingling of collagen fibrils of cementum and dentin.

Endosteal (bone lining) cells: Inactive or resting osteoblasts lining the endosteal surfaces (marrow spaces, Haversian canals) of bone.

Epithelial diaphragm: Extension of the epithelial root sheath beneath the dental papilla; creates the furcation and determines the shape of the roots of multirooted teeth.

Epithelial rests (of Malassez): Remnants of the epithelial root sheath forming a network of cells in the periodontal ligament adjacent to the root surface.

Fibrillin: Glycoprotein component of elastin microfibrils; a major component of oxytalan fibers of the periodontal ligament.

Furcation: The region at the apical side of the tooth crown where the roots of multirooted teeth diverge.

Gingivae: The portion of the oral mucosa adjacent to the teeth, consisting of attached and free gingivae, and covered by stratified squamous keratinized epithelium.

Gingivitis: An inflammatory disease of the gingivae caused by a microbial biofilm adherent to the tooth surface, and characterized by edema, redness, tenderness, and easily induced bleeding of the tissues. Untreated gingivitis may progress to periodontitis.

Haversian system (osteon): The basic structural unit of compact bone, consisting of concentric lamellae of bone surrounding a central canal containing osteogenic cells, blood vessels, and nerves.

Hertwig's Epithelial root sheath: After completion of crown formation, the extension of the cervical loop of the enamel organ, consisting of the inner and outer enamel epithelial layers, that induces odontoblast differentiation and guides root formation.

Howship's lacuna: The depression or groove on a bone surface created by the resorptive activity of an osteoclast.

Integrin receptors: A family of cation-dependent (calcium- or magnesium-dependent) transmembrane cell proteins occurring as dimers of an alpha and beta subunit that mediate attachment of cells to the extracellular matrix via arginine-glycine-aspartic acid (RGD) sequences in extracellular matrix proteins. Some cells use integrin receptors to bind to other cells, and integrin receptors have important signaling functions in relation to cell growth, division, differentiation, and death.

Interstitial areas: Regions between principal fiber bundles of the periodontal ligament containing blood vessels and nerves.

Lacunae: Unmineralized spaces within bone or cementum occupied by osteocytes or cementocytes.

Macrophage colony stimulating factor (M-CSF): A growth factor produced by bone marrow stromal cells, osteoblasts, endothelial cells, fibroblasts, and some epithelial cells. M-CSF is required for the differentiation of progenitor cells into osteoclasts, regulation of osteoclast function, and osteoclast survival. Also called colony stimulating factor-1 (macrophage) (CSF1).

Matrix metalloproteinase: A member of a family of zinc-dependent proteolytic enzymes capable of degrading extracellular matrix components and other molecules.

Mesial drift: The slow movement of posterior teeth anteriorly and anterior teeth toward the midline, due to attrition of enamel on the proximal surfaces and pressure from the tongue and facial musculature.

Osteoblast: A cell derived from mesenchymal precursors that synthesizes and secretes the molecular components of bone matrix, and subsequently mineralizes the matrix.

Osteoclast: A large multinucleated cell, formed by fusion of bone marrow-derived precursor cells, whose function is to resorb bone and other mineralized tissues through the production and secretion of acid and proteolytic enzymes. Odontoclasts, cells that resorb the mineralized tissues of teeth, have the same structure as osteoclasts and also form from bone marrow precursors. However, some studies suggest that osteoclasts and odontoclasts differ in certain properties and responses to physiological and pathological conditions.

Osteocyte: The resident cell of bone, residing in a space (lacuna) within the bone, derived from an osteoblast that encloses itself in bone matrix; maintains the vitality of bone and has mechanosensory functions.

Osteoprotegerin: A soluble "decoy" receptor for RANKL produced by osteoblasts and other cells; binding of osteoprotegerin to RANKL blocks its interaction with RANK, inhibiting osteoclast formation and function.

Oxytalan fibers: Periodontal ligament fibers consisting mainly of fibrillin containing microfibrils, oriented longitudinally, parallel to the root surface; associated with blood vessels and occasionally inserting into cementum.

Periodontal ligament: The collagenous ligament attaching the cementum of the tooth root to the alveolar bone.

Periodontitis: An inflammatory disease of the periodontal tissues resulting from the response to a microbial biofilm adherent to tooth surfaces. Cytokines, chemokines, and proteolytic enzymes released by local tissue cells and by the invading inflammatory cells cause destruction of the connective tissue, formation and activation of osteoclasts, and alveolar bone resorption.

Periodontium: Supporting tissues of the teeth, including cementum, periodontal ligament, alveolar bone, and gingivae.

Pre-bone (osteoid): The initial unmineralized matrix deposited by osteoblasts during bone formation.

Precementum (cementoid): The unmineralized cementum matrix produced by cementoblasts during formation of cellular cementum.

Principal fibers: The main collagen fiber bundles of the periodontal ligament, including oblique, horizontal, alveolar crest, apical, and interradicular groups.

RANK (Receptor activator of nuclear factor kappa B): present on osteoclast precursor cells; binding of RANKL to RANK promotes fusion of the precursors and activation of the osteoclast.

RANKL (Receptor activator of nuclear factor kappa B ligand): RANKL is expressed by bone marrow stromal cells, osteoblasts, osteocytes, and some immune system cells and interacts with RANK on osteoclast precursor cells.

Ruffled border: The region of the osteoclast consisting of infolded cell membrane from which acid and proteolytic enzymes are secreted during active bone resorption.

Ruffini endings: Slowly adapting mechanoreceptors found in skin, joints, and the periodontal ligament; respond to stretch, sustained pressure, and mechanical deformation.

Sealing zone: An actin-filled, ring-shaped cellular process of osteoclasts forming an enclosure for the ruffled border. Osteoclasts attach to the bone surface via integrin receptors on the sealing zone.

Sharpey's fibers: Collagen fibers of the periodontal ligament (or other ligaments) inserting into alveolar bone (or other bones) and cementum.

Volkmann's canals: Channels containing blood vessels and nerves that enter bone from the surface or periosteum and make perpendicular connections with Haversian canals; Volkmann's canals also connect adjacent Haversian canals.

Chapter 7 Tooth Eruption and Shedding

Arthur R. Hand

Department of Craniofacial Sciences and Cell Biology, School of Dental Medicine, University of Connecticut

Tooth eruption is the movement of a tooth from its site of development in the maxilla or mandible to its functional position in the oral cavity. The eruption of a tooth requires a complex spatial and temporal coordination of molecular and cellular events among several tissues. This is made even more complicated when one considers that during much of our childhood, we have two sets of teeth in various stages of development, eruption, and shedding (Figs. 7.1, 7.2, and 7.3). That humans have two sets of teeth, twenty primary and thirty-two permanent teeth, is necessitated by the small size of the jaws in children compared to their substantially larger size in adults. The smaller size and fewer number of primary teeth can be accommodated in a child's jaws, whereas the larger size and number of permanent teeth provide optimum masticatory efficiency in an adult. However, throughout the vertebrate subphylum, the number, formation, and eruption of teeth is highly variable. Not all vertebrates have two sets of teeth. Most fish, amphibian, and reptilian species have multiple sets of teeth, continually replacing them throughout life. Alligators, for example, have as many as 80 teeth in their jaws at one time, and may grow more than 2,000 teeth over their lifetime. Some rodents (e.g., rats, mice, hamsters) have only one set of molars, and have continuously growing incisors; the tips of the incisors chip away as the animal gnaws and bites its food. Other rodents (e.g., guinea pigs, chinchillas) have a single set of teeth, but all of their teeth grow continuously to accommodate for the wear caused by their gritty diets. Similarly, all the teeth of rabbits grow continuously, however, they have a primary and a permanent dentition.

The location and timing of tooth development and eruption must be highly coordinated in order to achieve a functional and esthetic adult dentition. Eruption begins only after crown formation is complete, progresses at various speeds during different stages, and continues after occlusal contact to increase and maintain facial height throughout life and to compensate for wear of the enamel.

Normal eruption sequence

Tooth eruption occurs in a well-defined, although not invariant, temporal sequence (Tables 7.1 and 7.2). The mandibular primary central incisors are the first teeth to erupt, at about 6 months of age, followed by the lateral incisors at 7 months. The maxillary primary central and lateral incisors erupt at about 7.5 and 9 months, respectively. The mandibular and maxillary first primary molars emerge at 12 and 14 months, then the canines at 16 and 18 months, and the second primary molars at 20 and 24 months.

The permanent teeth erupt in a slightly different sequence than the primary teeth. Except for the third permanent molars, the same tooth erupts a few months to more than a year earlier in females than in males. The mandibular central incisors are the first teeth to emerge, at about 6-1/2 years (in females), followed by the mandibular and maxillary first molars at about 7 years. The mandibular lateral and maxillary central incisors emerge shortly after that, then the maxillary lateral incisors at about 8 years of age. Mandibular and maxillary canines are next, at a little after 9 years, then the maxillary and mandibular first premolars between 9-1/2 to 10 years. Both second premolars emerge at about 10-1/2 years. Thus, between approximately age 6-1/2 to 11 years, a **mixed dentition** of both primary and permanent teeth exists. The second molars emerge at about 12 years. Eruption of the third molars is quite variable, but on average, occurs at about 17-1/2 to 18 years of age.

Fundamentals of Oral Histology and Physiology, First Edition. Arthur R. Hand and Marion E. Frank.
© 2014 John Wiley & Sons, Inc. Published 2014 by John Wiley & Sons, Inc.

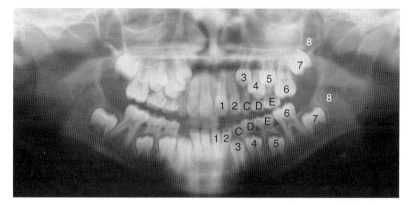

Figure 7.1 Panoramic X-ray of the mixed dentition of an 8- year-old child. The permanent teeth are indicated by the numbers (1, central incisor; 2, lateral incisor; 3, canine; 4, 1st premolar; 5, 2nd premolar; 6, 1st molar; 7, 2nd molar; 8, 3rd molar), and the remaining primary teeth by the letters (C, canine; D, 1st molar; E, 2nd molar). The four permanent incisors and the first permanent molars in each arch have erupted. The right mandibular primary canine has exfoliated, but the permanent canine has not yet erupted. The roots of the remaining primary canines and molars are undergoing resorption during the process of eruption of their permanent successors. The permanent premolars are developing between the roots of the primary molars. The roots of the second permanent molars are forming, and the earliest mineral deposition can be seen in the crowns of the developing third molars. (Courtesy of Section of Oral and Maxillofacial Radiology, University of Connecticut School of Dental Medicine.)

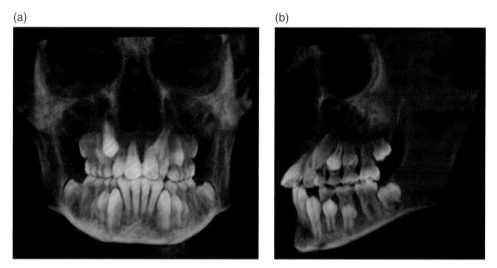

Figure 7.2 Cone beam computed tomographic (CBCT) images of the mixed dentition of an 8 year-old. (a) Frontal view. (b) Lateral view. (Courtesy of Section of Oral and Maxillofacial Radiology, University of Connecticut School of Dental Medicine.)

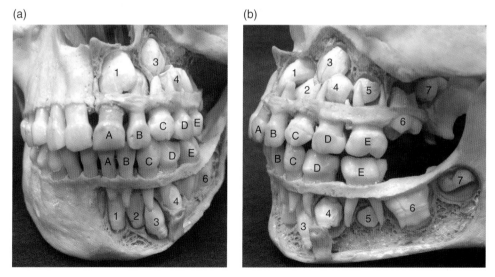

Figure 7.3 Photographs of the maxilla and mandible of a 5- to 5-1/2-year-old child with the facial cortical bone removed to reveal the developing permanent dentition. A, primary central incisor; B, primary lateral incisor; other teeth numbered as in Figure 7.1. (a) Frontal view. (b) Lateral view.

Eruption of the primary dentition begins with the mandibular incisors at about 6 months of age, and is completed at about 24 months with eruption of the maxillary second molars. Eruption of the permanent dentition begins with the mandibular central incisors at about 6 to 7 years, followed soon after by the first molars. Except for the third molars, eruption of the remaining teeth is completed when the second molars erupt at about 12 years. A mixed dentition of both primary and permanent teeth exists between 6-1/2 and 11 years of age.

Histology of tooth eruption

Pre-eruptive tooth movement

The teeth develop within bony crypts of the mandible and maxilla, surrounded by the dental follicles, and initially connected to the oral epithelium via the dental lamina. The permanent successors to the primary teeth initially are located in the same bony crypt as the primary tooth, lingual (palatal) to the primary tooth (Fig. 7.4). During eruption of the primary tooth, the permanent tooth becomes enclosed in its own bony crypt. While the crown is forming the tooth undergoes small, pre-eruptive, gyratory

Table 7.1   Chronology of primary tooth formation and eruption

Tooth*		Mineralization Begins (weeks in utero)	Enamel Complete (months postnatal)	Emergence (months postnatal)	Eruption Sequence	Root Complete (years)
Maxillary	C. Incisor	14	1.5	7.5	3	1.5
	L. Incisor	16	2.5	9	4	2
	Canine	17	9	18	8	3.25
	1st Molar	12.5–15.5	6	14	6	2.5
	2nd Molar	12.5–19	11	24	10	3
Mandibular	C. Incisor	18	2.5	6	1	1.5
	L. Incisor	18	3	7	2	1.5
	Canine	20	9	16	7	3.25
	1st Molar	12–15.5	5.5	12	5	2.25
	2nd Molar	12.5–18	10	20	9	3

*C, central; L, lateral

Table 7.2   Chronology of permanent tooth formation and eruption

Tooth		Mineralization Begins*	Enamel Complete (years)*	Emergence (years)+	Eruption Sequence	Root Complete (years)*
Maxillary	C. Incisor	3–4 m	M 3.7 / F 3.3	M 8.3 / F 7.4	5	M 10.6 / F 9.3
	L. Incisor	10–12 m	M 4.0 / F 3.8	M 9.1 / F 8.1	6	M 11.1 / F 9.7
	Canine	4–5 m	M 4.9 / F 4.1	M 11.0 / F 9.4	8	M 13.7 / F 11.9
	1st Premolar	1.5–1.75 y	M 5.8 / F 5.1	M 11.1 / F 9.7	9	M 13.5 / F 11.8
	2nd Premolar	2.2–2.25 y	M 6.3 / F 5.9	M 11.6 / F 10.6	11	M13.8 / F 12.6
	1st Molar	Birth	M 2.7 / F 2.6	M 7.8 / F 7.2	3	M 10.1 / F 9.2
	2nd Molar	2.5–3 y	M 6.7 / F 6.3	M 12.4 / F 11.8	13	M 14.6 / F 13.6
	3rd Molar	7–9 y	M 13.3 / F 12.8	M 17.4 / F 17.8	16	M 18.2 / F 18.8

(Continued)

Table 7.2   (*Continued*)

Tooth		Mineralization Begins*	Enamel Complete (years)*	Emergence (years)+	Eruption Sequence	Root Complete (years)*
Mandibular	C. Incisor	3–4 m	M 3.6 F 3.3	M 7.3 F 6.7	1	M 9.2 F 8.1
	L. Incisor	3–4 m	M 4.0 F 3.7	M 8.1 F 7.3	4	M 9.9 F 8.8
	Canine	4–5 m	M 4.8 F 4.1	M 10.9 F 9.2	7	M 13.5 F 11.4
	1st Premolar	1.75–2 y	M 5.6 F 5.0	M 11.2 F 9.9	10	M 13.3 F 11.9
	2nd Premolar	2.25–2.5 y	M 6.3 F 5.9	M 11.9 F 10.6	12	M 14.0 F 12.8
	1st Molar	Birth	M 2.7 F 2.6	M 7.8 F 7.2	2	M 10.0 F 9.2
	2nd Molar	2.5–3 y	M 6.7 F 6.3	M 12.5 F 11.8	14	M 14.8 F 13.8
	3rd Molar	8–10 y	M 13.3 F 12.8	M 17.4 F 17.7	15	M 18.5 F 18.3

*m, months; y, years

+M, male; F, female

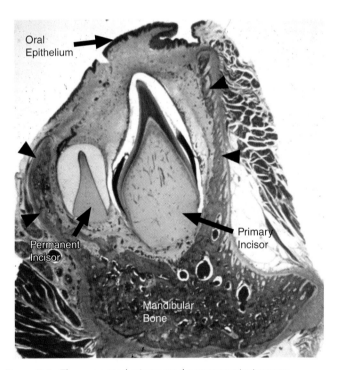

Figure 7.4   The unerupted primary and permanent incisors are developing in the same bony crypt (arrowheads) of the mandible. The late bell stage permanent incisor is located on the lingual side of the primary incisor. Some enamel matrix remains in the cervical region of the crown of the primary incisor, and its root has begun to form. As the root elongates and the tooth continues its eruption, a bony septum will form between the root and the developing permanent tooth, providing an attachment site for periodontal ligament fibers and enclosing the permanent tooth in its own crypt. (From Moss-Salentijn, L. (1972) *Orofacial Histology and Embryology: A Visual Integration.* Reproduced by permission of F.A. Davis Company, Philadelphia, PA.)

movements. The cause and purpose of these movements are unknown, but may be related to the growth of the jaws. As the jaws increase in size, additional pre-eruptive movements serve to position the forming permanent premolar and molar tooth germs in optimal positions for their subsequent eruption. The premolar tooth germs become positioned between the roots of the primary molars; the maxillary molar tooth germs, whose occlusal surfaces originally face in a distal direction, become more vertical; and the mandibular molar tooth germs, which initially are tipped mesially, also assume an upright orientation.

Eruptive tooth movement

Intraosseous phase

Upon completion of the crown, the initial growth of the root causes some resorption of the basal bone. Subsequently, resorption of bone occurs coronally to create an eruption pathway. The rate of eruption during the **intraosseous phase** is slow, between 1 and 10 μm/day. Elongation of the root occurs as the tooth erupts (Fig. 7.4). If root formation does not keep pace with eruption, bone is formed apically. The main sites of bone deposition are in the interradicular areas and at the alveolar crest, the latter increasing the height of the alveolar process.

Supraosseous phase

Once the crown reaches the alveolar crest, the rate of eruption increases, up to about 75 μm per day. Most of the root growth occurs during **supraosseous phase**, and completion of the root also requires resorption of basal bone. Eruption to the occlusal plane requires continued root growth along with bone formation apically and at the alveolar crest and interradicular septum. However, root growth slows as the apical foramen narrows, and is very slow thereafter.

The speed of eruption is closely coordinated with bone resorption and formation. During the intraosseous phase, the rate of coronal bone resorption determines the eruption speed. During the supraosseous phase, the rate of apical bone formation and the rate of root elongation determine eruption speed. The periodontal ligament also may have a role in the supraosseous phase of eruption.

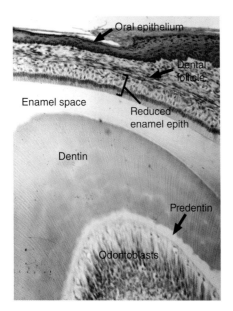

Figure 7.5   The enamel (space) of the incisor is covered by the reduced enamel epithelium and the dental follicle. A layer of columnar-shaped reduced ameloblasts is immediately adjacent to the enamel (space). The reduced enamel epithelium will fuse with the oral epithelium to create an opening through which the tooth will erupt.

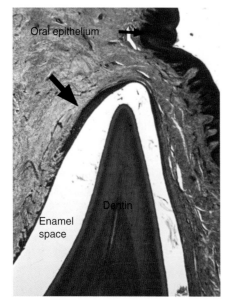

Figure 7.6   The reduced enamel epithelium near the cusp tip has proliferated and thickened (arrow) in advance of fusion with the oral epithelium. (From Moss-Salentijn, L. (1972) *Orofacial Histology and Embryology: A Visual Integration.* Reproduced by permission of F.A. Davis Company, Philadelphia, PA.)

The periodontal ligament does not form and the root is not attached to alveolar bone until the tooth is in the supraosseous phase.

Prior to emergence into the oral cavity, the reduced enamel epithelium covering the crown of the tooth and the basal layer of the oral epithelium undergo localized proliferation (Figs. 7.5 and 7.6). The two epithelia fuse, and the central region of the fused epithelia degenerates, creating an epithelium-lined pathway. In some cases a thin, nonvital membrane, the **enamel cuticle**, remains on the enamel surface, but is rapidly worn away after the tooth emerges into the oral cavity.

Posteruptive tooth movement

Root growth continues after emergence into the oral cavity and is not complete until the apical foramen has narrowed (Figs. 7.7 and 7.8). Eruption slows considerably as the tooth nears the occlusal plane. Slow eruption continues throughout life as the tooth functions in contact with its neighbors and the opposing teeth. This small movement allows the tooth and the periodontium

> Teeth develop within bony crypts in the jaws and require an eruption pathway and a driving force in order to erupt. During the intraosseous phase, coronal bone resorption creates the eruption pathway; apical bone formation and elongation of the root provide the main driving force during the intraosseous and supraosseous phases. Formation of the periodontal ligament during the supraosseous phase also may contribute to eruption.

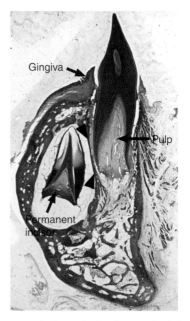

Figure 7.7   The erupted primary incisor has reached the occlusal plane, but its root is still elongating and the pulp canal is very wide. The permanent incisor is enclosed within its own bony crypt, with a thin septum of bone (arrowheads) separating it from the root of the primary tooth. The enamel of the permanent incisor is undergoing maturation, and its root is just beginning to form. (From Moss-Salentijn, L. (1972) *Orofacial Histology and Embryology: A Visual Integration*. Reproduced by permission of F.A. Davis Company, Philadelphia, PA.)

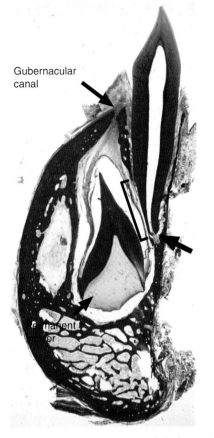

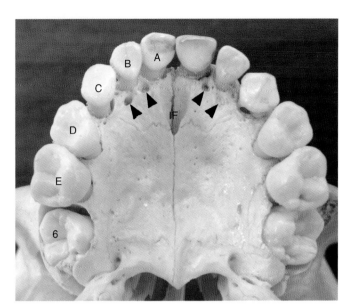

Figure 7.9   Photograph of the hard palate and maxillary teeth of the skull of a 5- to 5-1/2 year-old. None of the primary teeth (A–E) have exfoliated. The first permanent molars (6) are in the supraosseous phase of eruption. The openings of the gubernacular canals (arrowheads) are located on the lingual side of the primary incisors. Incisive foramen (IF).

Figure 7.8   The root of the primary incisor is fully formed and has a narrow apex (arrow). The enamel of the permanent tooth is almost completely mature, and root formation is underway. Eruptive movement of the permanent tooth in both occlusal and facial directions has resulted in resorption of the bony septum between the two teeth, and partial resorption of the lingual surface of the primary tooth root (bracket). The gubernacular canal opens at the crest of the alveolar process lingual to the primary tooth. (From Moss-Salentijn, L. (1972) *Orofacial Histology and Embryology: A Visual Integration.* Reproduced by permission of F.A. Davis Company, Philadelphia, PA.)

to adapt to the functional demands of occlusion, to compensate for wear of the crown and to maintain facial height.

Eruption of the permanent teeth

The process of eruption of the permanent teeth (**successional** or **succedaneous teeth**) that replace the primary teeth is similar to the eruption of the primary teeth, except that the root(s) of the primary teeth also must be resorbed. The initial eruption pathway of the permanent tooth is formed by enlargement of the **gubernacular canal** (Fig. 7.8). The gubernacular canal contains the remnants of the epithelial dental lamina, from which the enamel organ of the permanent tooth develops, and collagenous connective tissue that surrounds the epithelial cord and is continuous with the dental follicle and the lamina propria of the oral mucosa. The gubernacular canals open on the alveolar bone on the lingual side of the

primary teeth (Fig. 7.9). As the permanent teeth continue their eruption in the occlusal and facial directions, resorption of the primary tooth root(s) occurs. **Odontoclasts**, cells similar in structure and function to osteoclasts and formed by fusion of bone marrow-derived precursor cells, resorb the cementum and dentin of the primary tooth roots (Fig. 7.10). This enlarges the eruption pathway for the permanent tooth, and destroys the attachment of the primary tooth, eventually leading to its loss (**exfoliation**). Resorption of coronal dentin from the pulpal surface also may occur. Occasionally this may extend into the enamel (Fig. 7.10), demonstrating that odontoclasts are capable of resorbing each of the three mineralized tissues of the teeth.

The permanent tooth emerges into the oral cavity a short time after exfoliation of the primary tooth. At this stage the root of the permanent tooth is incompletely formed; it will continue to elongate and the root canal and apex will narrow to their final dimensions (Fig. 7.11). In the incisor region, the permanent teeth occasionally may emerge lingual to the primary teeth, prior to their exfoliation. Continued eruption of the permanent tooth in the occlusal and facial directions will eventually lead to the loss of the primary tooth.

> Successional permanent teeth develop on the lingual (palatal) side of the primary teeth. Their initial eruption pathway is created by the gubernacular canal, but continued occlusal and facial eruptive movement requires resorption of the root of the primary teeth by odontoclasts.

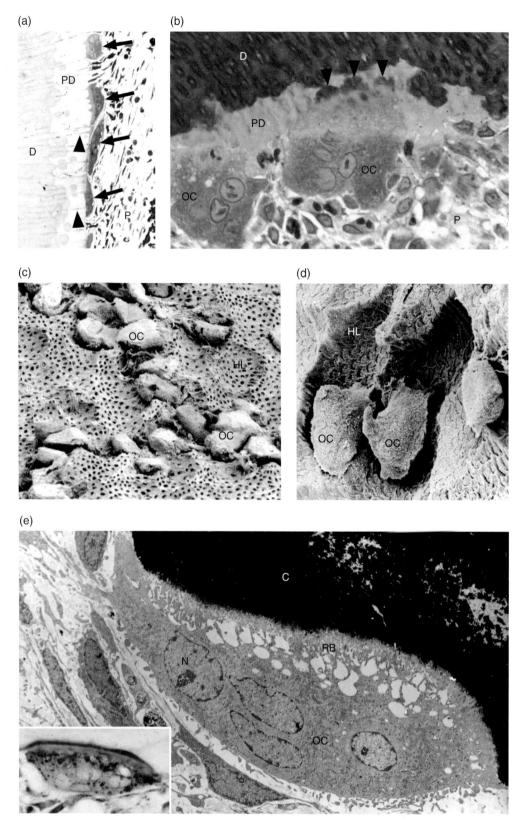

Figure 7.10 Odontoclasts resorbing dentin, enamel, and cementum of human deciduous teeth. (a) Several odontoclasts (arrows) are present at the pulpal surface of the dentin. Cytoplasmic processes of the odontoclasts are present in dentinal tubules (arrowheads). Pulp (P); predentin (PD); dentin (D). (b) Multinucleated odontoclasts (OC) resorbing predentin and mineralized calcospherites (arrowheads). (c) Scanning electron micrograph of odontoclasts on the surface of dentin. The small dark dots are dentinal tubules. Howship's lacuna (HL). (d) Scanning electron micrograph of odontoclasts resorbing enamel. Enamel rods and interrod enamel are visible in the Howship's lacunae. (e) Transmission electron micrograph of a multinucleated odontoclast resorbing cementum (C) on the external root surface. Nucleus (N); ruffled border (RB). The inset is a light micrograph of a similar odontoclast; the magenta stain indicates activity of tartrate-resistant acid phosphatase (TRAP), an enzymatic marker for osteoclasts and odontoclasts. (a and b), from From Sahara, N. et al. (1994). Odontoclastic resorption of the superficial nonmineralized layer of predentine in the shedding of human deciduous teeth. *Cell and Tissue Research*, 277(1), 19–26. Reproduced with kind permission from Springer Science and Business Media. (d), from From Sahara, N. et al. 1998) Ultrastructural features of odontoclasts that resorb enamel in human deciduous teeth prior to shedding. *Anatomical Record*, 252(2), 215–228. Reproduced with permission from John Wiley and Sons. (c) and (e), Courtesy of Dr. Noriyuki Sahara, Shiojiri, Japan).

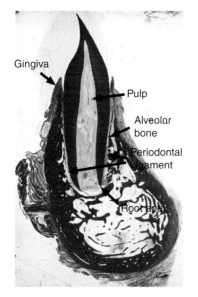

Figure 7.11   The permanent incisor has reached the occlusal plane. Its root will continue to elongate, and the apex eventually will narrow to create an apical foramen of 0.3- to 0.6-mm diameter. (From Moss-Salentijn, L. (1972) *Orofacial Histology and Embryology: A Visual Integration*. Reproduced by permission of F.A. Davis Company, Philadelphia, PA.)

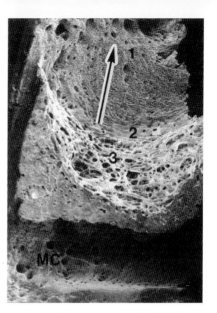

Figure 7.12   Scanning electron micrograph of the bony crypt of an erupting premolar of a dog. The tooth was erupting in the direction of the arrow. Bone resorption was occurring around the crown of the tooth, indicated by the scalloped surface (1). The smooth middle area (2) indicates a resting or inactive bone surface. The apical region (3) shows newly formed bone, indicated by the bony trabeculae. Mandibular canal (MC). (From Marks, S.C., Jr. & Schroeder, H.E. (1996) Tooth eruption: theories and facts, *The Anatomical Record*, 245(2), pp. 374–393. Reproduced by permission of John Wiley and Sons.)

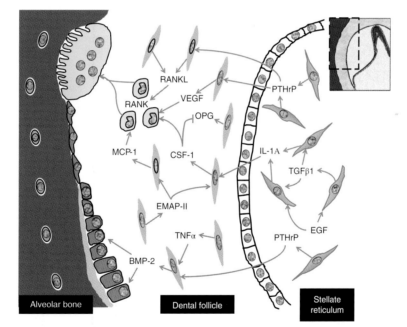

Figure 7.13   Diagram illustrating the regulation of bone resorption and bone formation during tooth eruption by factors produced by the dental follicle and the stellate reticulum of the enamel organ. The area enclosed by the dashed line in the inset at the upper right indicates the approximate region shown in the diagram. The curved row of white cells is the outer enamel epithelium. The coronal portion of the dental follicle produces factors that regulate the formation of osteoclasts. Bone marrow-derived monocyte precursors (small yellow cells) of osteoclasts (large yellow cell) are recruited to the dental follicle by CSF-1 and MCP-1. Endothelial monocyte-activating polypeptide II (EMAP-II) upregulates the production of CSF-1 and MCP-1, and also may help in recruiting monocytes to the dental follicle. The fusion of monocytes to form osteoclasts is promoted by the interaction of RANK on their membranes with RANKL. The expression of RANK on the osteoclast precursors is upregulated by CSF-1. CSF-1 downregulates the expression of OPG, the soluble decoy receptor for RANKL, thus decreasing the amount of this inhibitor of osteoclast formation. Not shown is the downregulation of another inhibitor of osteoclast formation, secreted frizzled-related protein-1, by CSF-1 and tumor necrosis factor-α (TNF-α). The expression of genes that promote bone formation is upregulated in the apical half of the dental follicle. TNF-α increases the expression of BMP-2 in dental follicle cells. BMP-2 expression is correlated with the increase in alveolar bone formation by osteoblasts (green cells). The stellate reticulum also has an important role in tooth eruption. IL-1α is expressed by stellate reticulum cells, and its receptor is expressed in the dental follicle. EGF increases the expression of both IL-1α and its receptor, and also increases TGF-β1 expression in the stellate reticulum. TGF-β1 enhances the expression of IL-1α and its receptor, and IL-1α signaling increases CSF-1 and MCP-1 expression in the dental follicle. The stellate reticulum produces PTHrP, and its receptors are present on dental follicle cells. PTHrP enhances the formation of osteoclasts directly by upregulation of RANKL expression by dental follicle cells, and indirectly by upregulation of vascular endothelial growth factor (VEGF), which promotes RANK expression by osteoclast precursors. PTHrP also upregulates BMP-2 expression by dental follicle cells.

Cellular and molecular mechanisms of tooth eruption

As described earlier, the teeth develop in bony crypts in the maxilla and mandible. In order to erupt into the oral cavity, an eruption pathway must be created by resorption of the bone overlying the crown of the tooth (Fig. 7.12). Formation of bone in the apical region of the erupting tooth also must occur. As demonstrated by experimental studies in rodents and other species, the dental follicle plays a critical role in regulating coronal bone resorption and apical bone formation during tooth eruption.

The coronal portion of the dental follicle produces factors that regulate the formation of osteoclasts (Figure 7.13). Bone marrow-derived monocyte precursors of osteoclasts are recruited to the dental follicle by **colony stimulating factor-1 (CSF-1)** and **monocyte chemotactic protein-1 (MCP-1)**. Fusion of the monocytes to form osteoclasts is promoted by the interaction of **receptor activator of nuclear factor kappa B (RANK)** on their membranes with **RANK ligand (RANKL)**, which is produced by dental follicle cells. Downregulation of the expression of inhibitors of osteoclast formation, **osteoprotegerin (OPG)** and **secreted frizzled-related protein-1,** further promotes osteoclast formation. The expression of genes that promote bone formation is upregulated in the apical half of the dental follicle. **Bone morphogenetic protein-2 (BMP-2)** is expressed at higher levels in the apical half of the dental follicle than in the coronal half, and the increase in its expression is correlated with the increase in alveolar bone formation. Thus, the dental follicle creates an environment conducive to osteoclast formation and bone resorption coronally, and bone formation apically.

The enamel organ, specifically the stellate reticulum, also plays an important role in tooth eruption. **Epidermal growth factor (EGF)** increases the expression of **interleukin-1 alpha (IL-1α)** and **transforming growth factor-β1 (TGF-β1)** expression in the stellate reticulum. TGF-β1 also enhances the expression of IL-1α, and IL-1α signaling increases CSF-1 and MCP-1 expression in the dental follicle. Stellate reticulum cells also produce **parathyroid hormone-related protein (PTHrP)**, which enhances osteoclast formation and upregulates BMP-2 expression in dental follicle cells. Thus, **paracrine signaling** by molecules expressed in the stellate reticulum affects the expression of molecules regulating bone resorption and bone formation in the dental follicle.

> The dental follicle and the stellate reticulum of the enamel organ produce a variety of factors that recruit osteoclast precursors and promote osteoclast formation, resulting in coronal bone resorption to create the eruption pathway. They also secrete factors that promote osteoblast differentiation and stimulate apical bone formation.

Structure and formation of the dentogingival junction

The components of the **dentogingival junction** include the enamel and/or the cementum of the tooth, the **junctional epithelium,** the **sulcular epithelium,** the **gingival epithelium**, and the connective tissue supporting these epithelia (Fig. 7.14). The junctional epithelium is formed from the reduced enamel epithelium when the latter merges with the oral epithelium during eruption of the tooth, and is firmly attached to the enamel (or cementum when gingival recession has occurred). The stratified squamous non-keratinized sulcular epithelium is immediately coronal to the junctional epithelium, and is thicker than the junctional epithelium but is not attached to the tooth surface. The space between the sulcular epithelium and the tooth surface is the **gingival sulcus** or **crevice**. The sulcular epithelium is continuous with the gingival epithelium at the free gingival margin. The gingival epithelium includes that of the free gingivae and the attached gingivae. The gingival tissues are fully described in Chapter 9.

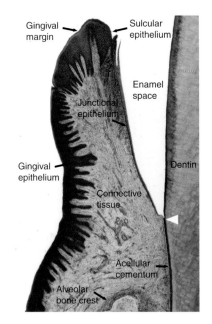

Figure 7.14 Dentogingival junction. The junctional epithelium is a thin, multilayered epithelium attached to the tooth surface. The gingival sulcus is lined by a thicker, stratified squamous non-keratinized epithelium. The gingival epithelium is a thick, stratified squamous (para)keratinized epithelium, with prominent epithelial ridges (rete pegs). The supporting connective tissue exhibits signs of slight inflammation, even in a clinically healthy individual. The white arrowhead indicates the cemento-enamel junction. (From Bosshardt, D.D. & Lang, N.P. (2005) The junctional epithelium: from health to disease. *Journal of Dental Research*, 84, 9–20. Copyright International and American Associations for Dental Research. Reprinted by permission of SAGE Publications.)

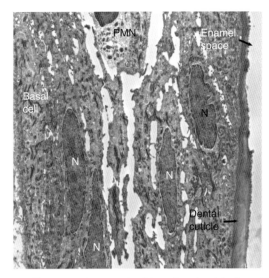

Figure 7.15   Electron micrograph of junctional epithelium. The innermost layer of cells (at the right), derived from the reduced ameloblasts, are directly attached to the tooth surface, or in this case, to a "dental cuticle" of unknown composition on the enamel surface. The suprabasal epithelial cells are flattened, with fluid-filled intercellular spaces. The basal cells (left) attach to the connective tissue through a typical basal lamina. A portion of a polymorphonuclear neutrophilic leukocyte (PMN) is seen in the intercellular space. Nuclei of junctional epithelial cells (N). (From Bosshardt, D.D. & Lang, N.P. (2005) The junctional epithelium: from health to disease. *Journal of Dental Research*, 84, 9–20. Copyright International and American Associations for Dental Research. Reprinted by permission of SAGE Publications.)

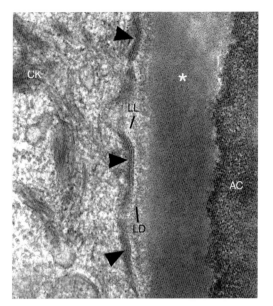

Figure 7.16   Electron micrograph of the attachment of the junctional epithelium to the tooth surface from a clinically healthy site but with gingival recession. The epithelial cell is attached to the internal basal lamina via hemidesmosomes (arrowheads). A "dental cuticle" (*) is present between the basal lamina and acellular cementum (AC). Cytokeratin filaments (CK); lamina lucida of the basal lamina (LL); lamina densa of the basal lamina (LD). (From Bosshardt, D.D. & Lang, N.P. (2005) The junctional epithelium: from health to disease. *Journal of Dental Research*, 84, 9–20. Copyright International and American Associations for Dental Research. Reprinted by permission of SAGE Publications.)

The junctional epithelium is a multilayered epithelium composed of non-keratinizing squamous cells oriented parallel to the tooth surface (Fig. 7.15). At its coronal end, the junctional epithelium is 15 to 30 cell layers thick, but only 1 to 3 cell layers thick at its apical end. The basal cell layer faces connective tissue and is attached to it by a typical basal lamina. The basal cells and the cells of the adjacent 1 to 2 suprabasal layers are cuboidal or slightly flattened in shape. The cells of the remaining suprabasal layers are flattened, and the innermost layer of cells is attached to the tooth surface (enamel or cementum) via hemidesmosomes and the specialized basal lamina (the **internal basal lamina**) initially formed following the secretory stage of amelogenesis (Fig. 7.16). The composition of the internal basal lamina differs from that of basal laminae at the interface between epithelia and connective tissue. It lacks type IV collagen, but contains laminin 5 as well as the unique components, amelotin and ODAM, initially incorporated during amelogenesis. Adjacent junctional epithelial cells are attached to one another by desmosomes, which are fewer in number than in other stratified squamous epithelia, and by occasional gap junctions. The intercellular spaces are wider than those in the sulcular and gingival epithelia. In a healthy periodontium, the interface between the junctional epithelium and the underlying connective tissue is relatively smooth, as is that of the sulcular epithelium. This contrasts with the gingival-connective tissue interface, which exhibits prominent epithelial rete pegs and connective tissue papillae (Fig. 7.14).

The junctional epithelium is a dynamic tissue that is continually remodeled. It has a high turnover rate; the epithelial cells, including those attached to the tooth surface, migrate in a coronal direction and are exfoliated at the base of gingival sulcus. The epithelium is maintained by division of the basal and suprabasal cells, which have a high rate of proliferation. The junctional epithelium is capable of rapid repair after minor trauma, such as occurs during clinical probing to determine sulcus or pocket depth. Even after surgical removal of the junctional epithelium during gingivectomy, a new junctional epithelium forms from the basal cells of the oral epithelium in about three weeks.

The connective tissue supporting the junctional epithelium differs from that of the lamina propria beneath the sulcular and gingival epithelia as well as the epithelium in other areas of the oral mucosa. It is considered deep connective tissue, which is believed to limit the ability of the junctional epithelium to mature, keeping it in a relatively undifferentiated state. Although the lamina propria beneath the sulcular epithelium permits this epithelium to differentiate, an inflammatory cell infiltrate is always present, even in clinically normal situations. Mononuclear leukocytes and polymorphonuclear neutrophilic leukocytes

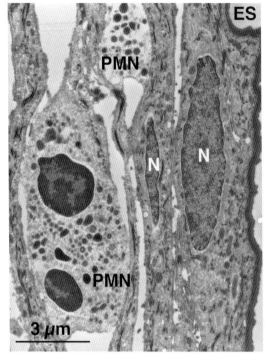

Figure 7.17   Electron micrograph of polymorphonuclear neutrophilic leukocytes (PMN) in the intercellular spaces of the junctional epithelium from a clinically healthy tooth. Nuclei of epithelial cells (N); enamel space (ES). (From Bosshardt, D.D. & Lang, N.P. (2005) The junctional epithelium: from health to disease. *Journal of Dental Research*, 84, 9–20. Copyright International and American Associations for Dental Research. Reprinted by permission of SAGE Publications.)

(PMNs) are normally found between the cells (Fig. 7.17). These inflammatory cells traverse the junctional epithelium, enter the gingival sulcus and eventually reach the oral cavity. Even in a clinically healthy periodontium, a large number of these cells, estimated at 30,000 per minute, enter the oral cavity from around all of the teeth. An increase in the number of inflammatory cells migrating through the epithelium occurs during gingivitis and periodontitis. A variety of cytokines and antimicrobial substances produced by the inflammatory cells and the junctional epithelial cells, and derived from blood and tissue fluid, also pass through the epithelium into the gingival sulcus. It is thought that the constant presence of inflammation in the lamina propria prevents keratinization of the sulcular epithelium.

> The junctional epithelium is derived from the reduced enamel epithelium, and forms a tight attachment to the enamel and/or cemental surface. The sulcular epithelium forms from the gingival epithelium, but is non-keratinized and separated from the tooth surface by the gingival sulcus. The junctional epithelium turns over rapidly, and is highly permeable, allowing tissue fluid and inflammatory cells to enter the gingival sulcus.

Blood vessels supplying the junctional and sulcular epithelia form a flattened network in the lamina propria, paralleling the epithelium-connective tissue interface (Fig. 7.18). At the apical extent of the junctional epithelium these vessels are continuous with the vessels of the periodontal ligament. However, if

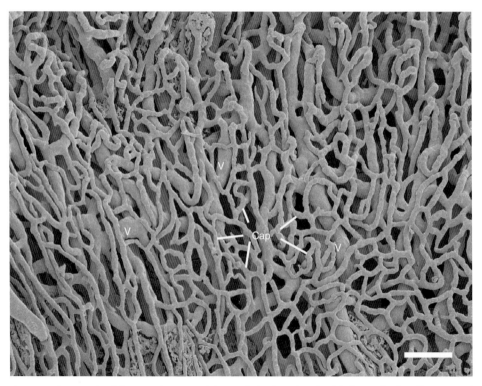

Figure 7.18   Scanning electron micrograph of the vascular network beneath the junctional epithelium of a dog. The network consists of a flattened mesh of capillaries (Cap), with deeper gingival veins (V). Scale bar = 100 um. (From: Matsuo, M. & Takahashi, K. (2002) *Microscopy Research and Technique,* 56(1), 3–14. Reprinted by permission of John Wiley and Sons.)

periodontal inflammation persists for a long period and/or is sufficiently severe, the arrangement of the blood vessels is altered. The junctional and sulcular epithelia proliferate in response to the inflammation. The junctional epithelium grows along the root surface in an apical direction, extending the depth of the gingival sulcus and creating a periodontal "pocket." The sulcular epithelium forms cellular extensions deep into the connective tissue. These extensions create "papillae" of connective tissue; blood vessels extend into the papillae and form loops similar to the typical arrangement of vessels in the papillae of the attached gingivae. These epithelial extensions, the connective tissue papillae, and the changes of the vascular network appear to be permanent alterations. A return to the normal architecture does not occur even if the inflammatory condition is resolved.

Clinical correlations

Delayed eruption or failure of eruption

The speed and timing of eruption is critical for proper tooth positioning. Delays in the eruption process can result in **ankylosis,** or fusion of the root cementum to the alveolar bone, and failure of eruption. Ankylosis may occur in either primary or permanent teeth, and most often affects the molars.

The most common cause of delayed or failed tooth eruption is mechanical interference. Supernumerary teeth, crowding, soft tissue or bony impaction, and odontogenic tumors and cysts can prevent a tooth from reaching its normal position in the mouth. Third molars and maxillary canines are the teeth most commonly affected by impaction. Impacted third molars often are surgically removed. Impacted canines frequently may be surgically exposed and orthodontically guided into position in the arch. If impacted teeth are allowed to remain submerged within the jaw, there is a potential for cyst formation, neoplastic change, infection, and damage to adjacent teeth. However, guidelines developed by expert panels and issued by various agencies and professional groups generally recommend that removal of impacted third molars should be limited to patients with evidence of local pathology and patients with certain medical or surgical conditions (e.g., organ transplants, radiation therapy), or if the tooth is in a fracture line or impedes reconstructive jaw surgery or tumor removal. Asymptomatic impacted teeth should be monitored on a regular basis. Published data also suggest that prophylactic removal of impacted third molars in adolescents to prevent future crowding of incisor teeth is not justified.

Failure of eruption can occur as an isolated condition or as part of a syndrome, such as cleidocranial dysplasia. **Primary failure of eruption** is a clinical condition in which, in the absence of local mechanical obstruction, permanent teeth fail to completely erupt and do not respond to orthodontic treatment. Eruption may be halted in either the intraosseous or supraosseous phase. Primary failure of eruption differs from ankylosis in that there is no fusion of the tooth to the alveolar bone. It predominantly occurs in posterior teeth, affecting all teeth posterior to the most anterior affected tooth, and resulting in posterior open-bite malocclusions. These patients also exhibit a high incidence of **Class III malocclusions** as a result of improper forward and downward growth of the maxilla. Primary failure of eruption has been associated with mutations in the genes for runt-related transcription factor 2 (Runx2), TNF receptor associated factor (TRAF) 6, and fibroblast growth factor receptor (FGFR) 1–3. About 45% of cases are familial. This form of primary failure of eruption has been associated with mutations in the parathyroid hormone receptor-1 (PTHR1) gene, with autosomal dominant inheritance.

The pathologic condition **osteopetrosis** is characterized by abnormal bone remodeling and increased bone density resulting from defective osteoclast resorption. Osteoclast function may be impaired, or osteoclast formation may be affected. The failure of or reduction in bone resorption delays or prevents tooth eruption. Mutations in several genes have been identified as causes of various forms of osteopetrosis. These include the cellular form of carbonic anhydrase (CAII), which provides H^+ ions to the vacuolar (V)-type proton ATPase that acidifies the extracellular space; T-cell, immune regulator 1 (TCIRG1), which codes for the proton pump; chloride channel 7 (CLCN7), which transports Cl^- ions to lysosomes and the extracellular space to maintain electroneutrality; and cathepsin K (Ctsk), a cysteine protease that degrades extracellular matrix components. Mutations in other genes, including RANKL, have been associated with less frequent types of osteopetrosis.

Cleidocranial dysplasia is a genetic skeletal dysplasia characterized by hypoplasia of the clavicles and deficient ossification of the anterior fontanel, resulting in an enlarged forehead, **hypertelorism**, and hypoplasia of the midface region. Dental abnormalities include supernumerary teeth (hyperdontia), crowding, malocclusion, retention of the primary teeth, and delayed eruption of the primary and permanent teeth. Cleidocranial dysplasia is caused by mutations of the RUNX2 gene, and is inherited in an autosomal dominant pattern.

> Delayed or failed tooth eruption occurs most frequently as a result of mechanical obstruction. When teeth are delayed in eruption, ankylosis may occur. Several gene mutations also may cause failure of eruption, either as an isolated condition or as part of a syndrome.

References

1. Bosshardt, D.D. & Lang, N.P. (2005) The junctional epithelium: from health to disease. *Journal of Dental Research,* 84, 9–20.
2. Marks, S.C. Jr. & Schroeder, H.E. (1996) Tooth eruption: theories and facts. *Anatomical Record,* 245(2), 374–393.
3. Rhoads, S.G., Hendricks, H.M., & Frazier-Bowers, S.A. (2013) Establishing the diagnostic criteria for eruption disorders based on genetic and clinical data. *American Journal of Orthodontics and Dentofacial Orthopedics,* 144(2), 194–202.
4. Wise, G.E. (2009) Cellular and molecular basis of tooth eruption. *Orthodontics and Craniofacial Research,* 12(2), 67–73.
5. Wise, G.E., Frazier-Bowers, S., & D'Souza, R.N. (2002) Cellular, molecular, and genetic determinants of tooth eruption. *Critical Reviews in Oral Biology and Medicine,* 13(4), 323–334.
6. Wise, G.E. & King, G.J. (2008) Mechanisms of tooth eruption and orthodontic tooth movement. *Journal of Dental Research,* 87(5), 414–434.

Glossary

Ankylosis: Fusion of the tooth root to the alveolar bone by a bony bridge.

Bone morphogenetic protein-2 (BMP-2):   A member of the transforming growth factor-beta (TGF-β) superfamily; induces differentiation of osteoblasts and stimulates production of cartilage and bone.

Class III malocclusion: The relationship of the maxillary and mandibular first permanent molars when the mesiobuccal cusp of the maxillary molar is positioned distal to the buccal groove of the mandibular molar when the teeth are in occlusion. The mandibular incisors thus are positioned anterior to the maxillary incisors.

Cleidocranial dysplasia: An autosomal dominant genetic disease caused by mutation of the RUNX2 gene.

Colony stimulating factor-1 (CSF-1):   A growth factor produced by bone marrow stromal cells, osteoblasts, endothelial cells, fibroblasts, and some epithelial cells. CSF-1 is required for the differentiation of progenitor cells into osteoclasts, regulation of osteoclast function, and osteoclast survival. Also called macrophage colony stimulating factor (M-CSF).

Dentogingival junction: The junction of the erupted tooth and the oral mucosa, consisting of the junctional epithelium and the epithelium of the gingival sulcus.

Enamel cuticle: Remnants of the fused reduced enamel epithelium and the oral epithelium that adhere to the tooth upon eruption but are rapidly worn away during function.

Epidermal growth factor (EGF):   A growth factor that promotes cell proliferation, differentiation, and growth; EGF is produced by several cell types and is present in saliva, milk, plasma, and urine.

Exfoliation: The process of loss or shedding of the primary (deciduous) teeth. Also refers to the loss of surface cells from a stratified epithelium, such as the skin or oral mucosa.

Gingival epithelium: The stratified squamous keratinized or parakeratinized epithelium covering the oral surface of free and attached gingivae.

Gingival sulcus (crevice):   The (potential) space between the free gingivae and the tooth surface, lined by non-keratinized stratified squamous epithelium that is not adherent to the tooth and is continuous with the gingival epithelium.

Gubernacular canal: A connective tissue-lined canal through the alveolar bone, containing the remnants of the dental lamina of the developing permanent tooth, and opening on the maxilla or mandible lingual to the primary teeth, establishing an eruption pathway.

Hypertelorism: A development defect characterized by an abnormally large distance between two organs, frequently referring to the orbits (eyes).

Interleukin-1 alpha (IL-1α):   A cytokine produced by a variety of cells that promotes inflammation.

Internal basal lamina: The basal lamina through which the junctional epithelium attaches to the tooth surface.

Intraosseous phase: The first phase of eruption, when the developing tooth is enclosed in its bony crypt; the rate of eruption is slow and requires both apical bone formation and coronal bone resorption.

Junctional epithelium: The junctional epithelium is formed by the reduced enamel epithelium upon eruption of the tooth, seals the base of the gingival sulcus, and attaches the gingival tissues to the tooth surface.

Mixed dentition: The period in which both primary and permanent teeth are present in the mouth; from the time of eruption of the first permanent tooth (~6 years) until the exfoliation of the last primary tooth (~12 years).

Monocyte chemotactic protein-1 (MCP-1):   A chemokine that regulates migration of monocytes/macrophages, memory T- lymphocytes, and natural killer (NK) cells, and their infiltration into tissues.

Odontoclast: A large multinucleated cell that resorbs tooth structure (cementum, dentin, or enamel); formed by fusion of bone marrow-derived precursors, similar or identical to osteoclasts.

Osteopetrosis: A bone disease characterized by abnormal bone remodeling and increased bone density resulting from defective osteoclast resorption; caused by mutations in genes critical for osteoclast function or formation.

Osteoprotegerin (OPG):   A protein secreted by dental follicle cells, osteoblasts, and other cells that is a "decoy receptor" for RANK ligand, preventing monocyte fusion to form osteoclasts.

Paracrine signaling: Cell-cell communication between neighboring cells via the release of soluble factors that diffuse through the surrounding extracellular space or connective tissue and interact with receptors on the target cells.

Parathyroid hormone-related protein (PTHrP):   A paracrine hormone produced by the stellate reticulum important for coronal bone resorption and apical bone formation during tooth eruption.

Primary failure of eruption: A clinical condition in which permanent teeth fail to erupt completely, associated with mutations in the genes for Runx2, TRAF6, FGFR1-3, and PTHR1; occurs in the absence of local mechanical obstruction, and does not respond to orthodontic treatment.

RANK ligand (RANKL):   A transmembrane protein produced by dental follicle cells, osteoblasts, and other cells that binds to RANK on osteoclast precursors, promoting osteoclast formation.

Receptor activator of nuclear factor kappa B (RANK):   A cell surface receptor on osteoclast precursors that, when activated by RANKL, promotes cell fusion and formation of osteoclasts.

Secreted frizzled-related protein-1:   A negative regulator of Wnt signaling, expressed in numerous tissues including the dental follicle; inhibits formation of osteoclasts.

Successional (succedaneous) teeth: The permanent teeth that form in association with the primary precursors and replace them after exfoliation.

Sulcular epithelium: The non-keratinized stratified squamous epithelium lining the gingival sulcus.

Supraosseous phase: The phase of tooth eruption once part of the crown is above the crest of the alveolar bone, until the tooth reaches its functional position.

Transforming growth factor-β1 (TGF-β1):   A protein produced by most tissues that regulates cell growth, proliferation, differentiation, and death.

Chapter 8 Temporomandibular Joint

Felipe Porto

Department of Oral Health and Diagnostic Sciences, School of Dental Medicine, University of Connecticut

The temporomandibular joint (TMJ) is the joint where the mandible articulates with the cranium (Fig 8.1). The following characteristics make the TMJ a complex and unique joint:

1. It is classified as a **compound joint** even though it does not include three bone structures in the articulation. However, the **articular disc**, which is interposed between the condylar head of the mandible and the squamous portion of the temporal bone, is considered as a third bone (even though it is not a bone, but a dense fibrous connective tissue).

2. It is considered a **ginglymoarthrodial joint** due to the fact it combines hinge (pivoting) and gliding (sliding) movements.

3. The TMJ on one side cannot work independently from the joint on the other side.

As mentioned, the TMJ includes the temporal bone, the mandible, and an articular disc composed of fibrous connective tissue. Before discussing details of the function of the TMJ, it is important to describe the structure of the components of this joint.

Structure of the TMJ

Temporal bone

The areas of the temporal bone that are of interest for the TMJ are the **mandibular fossa** and the **articular eminence**. The mandibular fossa, also called the articular fossa or glenoid fossa, is a concave area in the **squamous portion (squama)** of the temporal bone, limited anteriorly by the articular eminence and posteriorly by the **postglenoid process**, which is localized immediately anterior to the external acoustic meatus. The articular eminence

is a convex bar of bone upon which the articular disc slides during mandibular function (Fig 8.2).

Mandible

The mandible is a horseshoe-shaped bone which holds the lower teeth. It is largely formed from an intramembranous ossification. The condylar process, the anterior border of the coronoid process, and the mental process are formed by endochondral ossification. The mandible is stabilized only by soft tissue (including mainly muscles and ligaments) and it has no direct bony connections to the skull.

The area of the mandible that is of direct interest of the TMJ is the condylar head or **condyle**, which articulates with the temporal bone.

On the coronal plane the condyle is observed to have two poles, the lateral pole and the medial pole; the latter is more prominent, extending farther beyond the neck of the condyle (Fig 8.3). On a transverse plane the medial pole is positioned slightly more posterior than the lateral pole, and therefore when a long axis line connecting the two poles is drawn it will be medially directed to the anterior border of the foramen magnum (Fig 8.4). The anterior surface of the condyle is concave while the posterior surface is convex.

Articular disc

The articular disc is interposed between the condyle and the mandibular fossa. It is composed of a dense fibrous connective tissue (type I collagen), and it is only innervated on its periphery. Behind the disc, however, there is a well-vascularized and innervated tissue called **retrodiscal tissue**, which when loaded can

Fundamentals of Oral Histology and Physiology, First Edition. Arthur R. Hand and Marion E. Frank.
© 2014 John Wiley & Sons, Inc. Published 2014 by John Wiley & Sons, Inc.

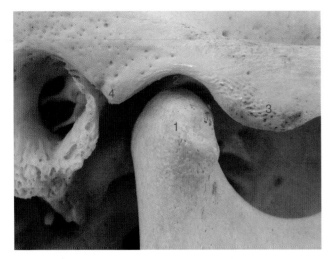

Figure 8.1   Bony structures of the TMJ (right side): (1) Condyle; (2) mandibular fossa; (3) articular eminence; (4) postglenoid process.

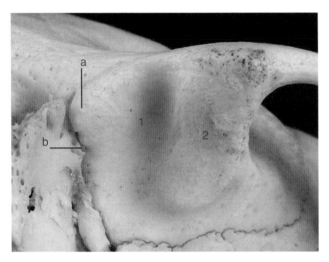

Figure 8.2   Inferior view of the mandibular fossa (1) and the articular eminence (2). Also note the postglenoid process (a) and the squamo-tympanic fissure (b).

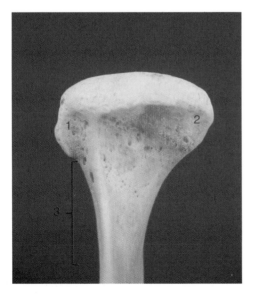

Figure 8.3   Right condyle (anterior view): (1) lateral pole; (2) medial pole; also note the neck of the condyle (3).

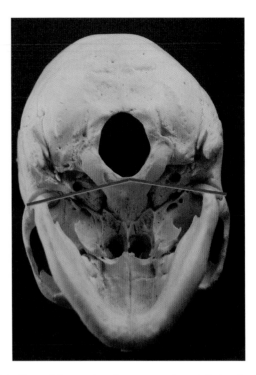

Figure 8.4   Base of the cranium (transverse plane, inferior view), showing that the imaginary lines connecting the medial and lateral poles of the condyles are posteriorly and medially directed toward the anterior border of the foramen magnum.

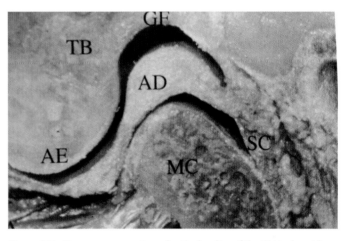

Figure 8.5   Bony components and articular disc of the TMJ: glenoid or mandibular fossa (GF), temporal bone (TB), articular disc (AD), articular eminence (AE), mandibular condyle (MC), and synovial capsule (SC). Note the three portions of the disc—the condyle is positioned on the intermediate zone. (From: Wadhwa, S. & Kapila, S. (2008) TMJ disorders: future innovations in diagnostics and therapeutics. *Journal of Dental Education*, 72, 930–947.)

elicit pain. On the sagittal plane the disc can be divided into three distinct regions: the posterior region, which is the thickest one; the central region or intermediate zone, which is the thinnest area; and the anterior region. Ideally the condyle should be positioned on the intermediate zone (Fig 8.5).

The disc is attached posteriorly to the retrodiscal tissue, which is bordered superiorly by the **superior retrodiscal lamina** (SRL), and inferiorly by the **inferior retrodiscal lamina** (IRL). The SLR

(a)

(b)

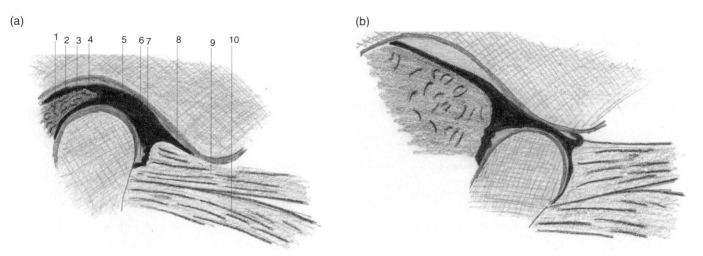

Figure 8.6   TMJ on the sagittal plane view: (a) closed-mouth and (b) open-mouth. (1) Retrodiscal tissue, (2) superior retrodiscal lamina, (3) inferior retrodiscal lamina, (4) superior joint cavity, (5) articular disc, (6) inferior joint cavity, (7 and 8) anterior capsular ligament, (9) superior lateral pterygoid muscle, and (10) inferior lateral pterygoid muscle.

Table 8.1   Attachments of the articular disc

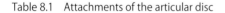

Attachment	Localization	To
Superior retrodiscal lamina	Posterior superior	Squamotympanic fissure
Inferior retrodiscal lamina	Posterior inferior	Periosteum of the neck of the condyle
Retrodiscal tissue	Posterior	—
Anterior capsular ligament (superior portion)	Anterior superior	Anterior margin of the articular surface of the temporal bone
Anterior capsular ligament (inferior portion)	Anterior inferior	Anterior margin of the articular surface of the condyle
Superior Lateral Pterygoid	Anterior	Infratemporal surface of the greater sphenoid wing
Lateral discal ligament	Lateral	Lateral pole of the condyle
Medial discal ligament	Medial	Medial pole of the condyle

consists of connective tissue with many elastic fibers. Both the IRL and SRL attach to the articular disc. Unlike the SRL, the IRL is formed by collagenous and nonelastic tissue.

The **anterior capsular ligament** attaches the disc anteriorly to the anterior margin of the articular surface of the temporal bone (superiorly) and to the anterior margin of the articular surface of the condyle (inferiorly). In between the superior and inferior portions of the anterior capsular ligament, the disc is also attached to the **superior lateral pterygoid muscle** (Fig 8.6).

Finally, the disc is also attached to the lateral and medial pole of the condyle through the **lateral discal (or collateral) ligament** and **medial discal (or collateral) ligament**, respectively (Table 8.1).

As mentioned, the disc is completely surrounded by attachments, therefore creating two separated spaces: the **superior articular space** (or superior joint cavity), where the translation between the disc and the mandibular fossa/articular eminence occurs; and the **inferior articular space** (or inferior joint cavity), where the rotation between the condyle and the disc occurs (Fig 8.6). The superior space is delineated by the mandibular fossa and by the superior surface of the articular disc. The inferior space is delineated by the inferior surface of the articular disc and the mandibular condyle. The **synovial fluid** fills both articular spaces (Fig 8.7 and Fig 8.8).

Only the periphery of the articular disc is innervated, but the tissue attached to the disc posteriorly (the retrodiscal tissue) is well innervated and vascularized, and if loaded can cause pain.

Synovial fluid

Synovial fluid is secreted by cells of the synovial lining, and it serves not only as a lubricant minimizing friction upon articular movement but also supports the metabolic exchange among the capsule, the articular tissues, and the synovial fluid itself.

The synovial fluid lubricates the TMJ by two different mechanisms: **boundary lubrication** and **weeping lubrication**.

Boundary lubrication occurs when the joint is moved, thereby forcing the synovial fluid to relocate from one area of the joint to another. This mechanism prevents friction in the moving joint.

The second mechanism of lubrication is called weeping lubrication. The weeping lubrication is related to the ability of the articular surfaces to absorb a small volume of synovial fluid. Upon function, compressive force occurs on the articular surfaces of the joint, forcing the small volume of synovial fluid to be released. It is important to note that prolonged compressive forces to the articular surfaces will deplete the small amount of synovial fluid.

The boundary lubrication is related to joint movements while the weeping lubrication is related to compressive forces on the articular surfaces of the joint.

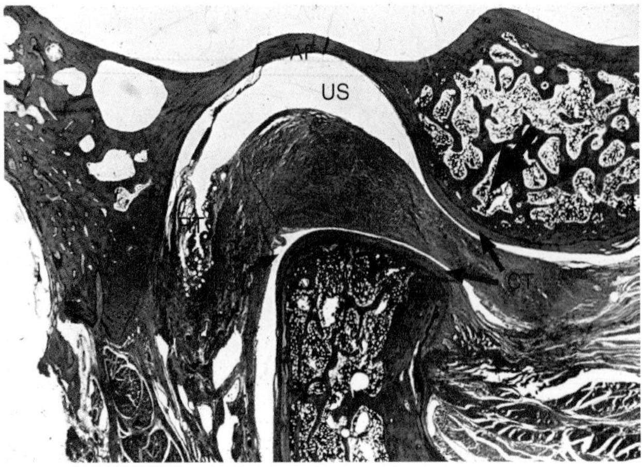

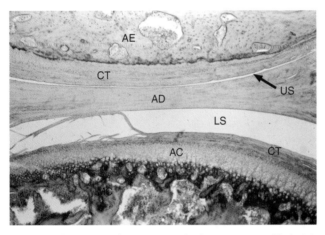

Figure 8.7   Very low-power photomicrograph of the temporomandibular joint sectioned in a sagittal plane. The articular fossa (AF) and articular eminence (indicated by the blue arrow) are visible above, and the head of the condyle (MC) below. The articular disc (AD)—an extension of the fibrous capsule surrounding the joint—separates the two bony surfaces. Notice that a layer of dense connective tissue (CT) covers the surfaces of both the temporal bone and the condyle. The condyle is approximately in its physiological position, riding on the posterior slope of the articular eminence rather than in the depth of the articular fossa. Only a thin layer of bone separates the articular fossa from the cranial cavity. Note the retrodiscal tissue (RT) located posterior to the condyle. (From Moss-Salentijn, L. (1972) *Orofacial Histology and Embryology: A Visual Integration.* Reproduced with permission from F.A. Davis Company, Philadelphia, PA.)

Figure 8.8   A low-power photomicrograph of a temporomandibular joint from an adolescent monkey. The bone and covering connective tissue (CT) of the articular eminence (AE) are above, the disc (AD) near the center, and the condyle (MC) below. The dense CT covering the articular cartilage (AC) of the condyle is quite thick. Some alignment of the cartilage cells into columns is visible in the cartilage, although a continuous layer of bone appears to cover its lower surface, indicating that growth in this joint is just now ceasing. Upper joint space (US) and lower joint space (LS).

The synovial fluid contains **hyaluronic acid** (HA), which is important to maintain the lubrication capability of the synovial fluid. The hyaluronic acid is easily degraded under inflammatory conditions, and when degraded it does not prevent lysis of the **phospholipids** by **phospholipase A2 (PLA2)**. The phospholipids cover the articular surfaces facilitating the sliding movement,

therefore when they are broken down the friction between the articular surfaces increases.

> The lubrication of the TMJ occurs by two different mechanisms: boundary lubrication and weeping lubrication.

Capsule and ligaments

A fibrous nonelastic membrane called the capsule or capsular ligament surrounds the TMJ. The capsule of the TMJ serves to resist any forces that tend to separate the articular surfaces (Fig 8.9). The capsule also retains the synovial fluid. Even though some authors recognize the disc as an extension of the capsule, the capsule is well innervated, unlike the disc that is almost completely devoid of nerve supply (except for its periphery). The inner surface of the capsule is lined by synovial membrane.

Two other functional ligaments support the TMJ: the **discal** or **collateral ligaments** and the **temporomandibular ligament**.

The discal ligaments, as mentioned previously, attach the medial and lateral edge of the disc to the respective poles of the condyle (Fig 8.10). The discal ligaments do not stretch since they are composed of connective tissue fibers, but they allow the articular disc to slide anteriorly and posteriorly on the articular surface of the condyle. Like the capsule, the discal ligament is innervated and vascularized and can cause pain when injured.

The temporomandibular ligament consists of two portions: an outer oblique portion (OOP) and an inner horizontal portion (IHP). Both originate at the outer surface of the articular eminence and zygomatic process. The OOP extends posteroinferiorly to the outer surface of the condylar neck, and the IHP extends backward to the lateral pole of the condyle and posterior portion of the disc (Fig 8.11).

The directions of the ligament's portions help one to remember their functions:

- The OOP resists excessive inferior displacement of the condyle and limits the amount of rotation that the condyle can undergo in a fixed point, forcing the condyle to start the translation movement if wider opening is needed.

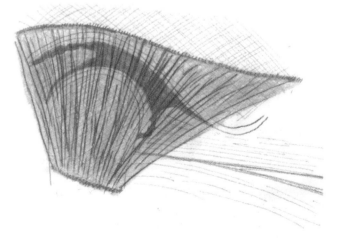

Figure 8.9   Capsule.

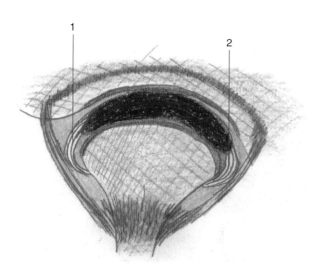

Figure 8.10 Discal ligaments (anterior view): (1) lateral discal ligament and (2) medial discal ligament.

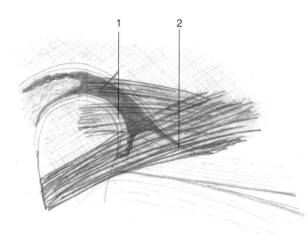

Figure 8.11 Temporomandibular ligament (lateral view): (1) Inner horizontal portion and (2) outer oblique portion.

- The IHP restricts posterior displacement of the condyle–disc complex, protecting therefore the retrodiscal tissue.
- Finally, since both TMJs work simultaneously the temporomandibular ligament prevents lateral dislocation of one joint and medial dislocation of the opposite joint.

The TMJ also has two accessory ligaments: the **sphenomandibular ligament** and the **stylomandibular ligament**. The sphenomandibular ligament attaches the spine of the sphenoid bone to the lingula on the ramus of the mandible, while the stylomandibular ligament runs from the styloid process to the angle of the mandible.

Innervation and vascularization of the temporomandibular joint

The innervation of the TMJ is provided mainly by the auriculotemporal nerve, however, two other nerves also innervate the TMJ: the deep posterior temporal nerve and the masseteric nerve. The majority of nerve endings in the TMJ are **free nerve endings**, but **Ruffini's nerve endings, Golgi-Mazzoni corpuscles**, and **Pacinian corpuscles** also are present.

The blood supply of the TMJ is more complex than the innervation. Many vessels supply the TMJ: the superficial temporal artery, internal maxillary artery, meningeal artery, deep auricular artery, anterior tympanic artery, and ascending pharyngeal artery. It is important to note that the vascular supply of the condyle comes from its marrow spaces (via the inferior alveolar artery) and via feeder vessels originating from larger vessels.

> The auriculotemporal nerve is the main nerve providing sensory innervation to the temporomandibular joint. Therefore an auriculotemporal nerve block might help to identify whether the TMJ is the source of a patient's facial pain.

TMJ histology

Four layers constitute the articular surfaces of the condyle and the posterior slope of the articular eminence: the **articular zone, proliferative zone, fibrocartilaginous zone**, and **calcified cartilage zone** (Fig 8.12).

The articular zone is the most superficial layer. This zone is able to dissipate the frictional loads during jaw function due to the fact it contains **superficial zone proteins** (SZP), which also are present at the superficial layer of the disc. The SZP are synthesized and secreted in the synovial fluid, which is responsible for boundary lubrication. This articular layer of the condyle and the posterior slope of the articular eminence is composed of dense fibrous connective tissue in contrast to most of the synovial joints, which are composed of hyaline cartilage. This characteristic is beneficial to the TMJ, since the dense fibrous connective tissue supports more loading than the hyaline cartilage, is less

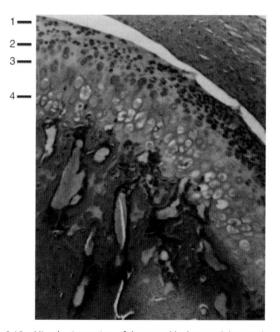

Figure 8.12 Histologic section of the mandibular condylar cartilage showing the four distinct zones: (1) articular zone, (2) proliferative zone, (3) fibrocartilaginous zone, and (4) calcified cartilage zone. (From: Wadhwa, S., & Kapila, S. (2008) TMJ disorders: future innovations in diagnostics and therapeutics. *Journal of Dental Education*, 72, 930–947.)

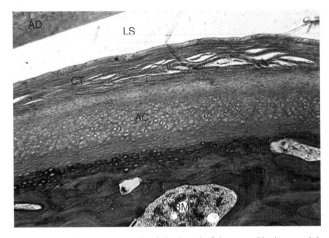

Figure 8.13 Photomicrograph of the head of the mandibular condyle. The bone (MC) is covered by a layer of cartilage (AC), and the cartilage is covered by a layer of dense, irregular fibrous connective tissue (CT). This is an adult condyle and no evidence of growth is visible. Articular disc (AD), lower joint space (LS), and bone marrow (BM). (From Moss-Salentijn, L. (1972) *Orofacial Histology and Embryology: A Visual Integration.* Reproduced with permission from F.A. Davis Company, Philadelphia, PA.)

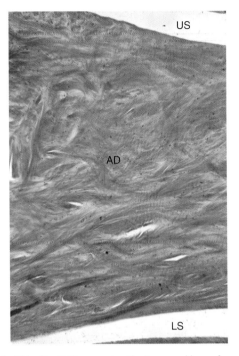

Figure 8.14   This disc (AD) separates the temporal bone from the condyle of the mandible, dividing the joint space into upper (US) and lower (LS) compartments. It is comprised of avascular, dense, irregular, and collagenous connective tissue. (From Moss-Salentijn, L. (1972) *Orofacial Histology and Embryology: A Visual Integration.* Reproduced with permission from F.A. Davis Company, Philadelphia, PA.)

susceptible to breakdown, and presents better capability for repair (Fig 8.13). At the mandibular fossa level this fibrous layer is thinner than at the posterior slope of the articular eminence.

The second zone is a very cellular layer called the proliferative zone. Even though this zone is mainly cellular, there is no organization or arrangement of the cartilage cells in this zone. It contains the undifferentiated mesenchymal tissue, which is responsible for the proliferation of articular cartilage. This proliferation happens as a natural response to loading of the articular surfaces. **Sox-9 protein** is expressed in this zone, but there is no expression of collagen type II.

The third zone is the fibrocartilaginous zone or chondroblastic zone. The characteristics of this zone are: the bundle arrangement of the collagen fibrils, which are disposed in a crossing pattern, and the random orientation of cartilage, forming a tridimensional network that offers resistance against compressive and lateral forces. In this zone, the cartilage cells are extremely mature, but they are still capable of proliferation. There is expression of Sox-9, **Indian hedgehog protein** and collagen types I and II in this layer.

The deepest zone is called calcified cartilage zone or hypertrophic zone. This fourth layer contains hypertrophic cartilage cells (chondrocytes) that overlie a layer of mineralized cartilage, which overlies an area of subchondral bone known as a bone formation zone. The hypertrophic chondrocytes die, their lacunae are invaded by blood vessels and osteoprogenitor cells from the medullary space, and osteoblasts differentiate and deposit bone on the remaining cartilage framework. This zone is also characterized by remodeling activity, which is possible since the cartilage extracellular matrix serves as a scaffold while endosteal bone growth continues. In this zone, the cells are characterized by the expression of Indian hedgehog, **osteopontin**, and collagen type X.

The articular disc of the TMJ is formed mainly by collagenous fiber bundles and scattered cells (Fig 8.14). The TMJ disc cells are primarily chondrocyte-like cells surrounded by faint halos. At the medial and lateral regions of the disc the collagen fibers are predominantly anteroposteriorly disposed, while in the posterior band those fibers run mediolaterally. However, the anterior band contains more anteroposteriorly oriented collagen fibers than mediolateral fibers. The anteroposterior fibers in the anterior band of the disc are reinforced by fibers from the superior lateral pterygoid muscle. The transverse fibers that run in the central portion of the disc blend with the lateral and medial discal ligaments. Collagen fibers in the TMJ disc are almost completely formed by collagen type I.

In contrast with most of the other synovial joints, the articular layer that covers the articular surfaces of the condyle and mandibular fossa is composed of dense fibrous connective tissue instead of hyaline cartilage.

Function (biomechanics) of the TMJ

The main characteristic of TMJ function is that it is physically impossible to move the TMJ of one side independently from the other. Any movement on one side will generate some movement on the opposite side. The mandibular condyle's movements include rotation and translation; a combination of those movements can make the mandible open or close, move laterally, and move forward (protrusive movement) and back to its original position.

In an ideal scenario, during those mandibular movements the articular disc should remain interposed between the condyle and the fossa/articular eminence, with the condyle resting on the intermediate zone of the disc. The articular disc remains in place during function due to its morphology and the pressure between the articular surfaces. The ligaments of the TMJ limit the range of mandibular movement. The same happens with the ligaments of the articular disc, which passively limit extreme movements of the disc. It is important to remember that ligaments do not stretch and they do not actively participate in normal function or serve as guides; their only purpose is to limit extreme movements.

> The morphology of the articular disc and the pressure between the articular surfaces are responsible for maintaining the disc in place.

Rotational movement occurs in the inferior space between the condyle and the articular disc, while translation occurs in the superior space, between the condyle–disc complex and the mandibular fossa /articular eminence. The mandibular condyle, the articular disc, and the mandibular fossa (and/or articular eminence, depending on the stage of the movement) are constantly in close contact regardless of whether the joint is moving or in rest position. In rest position this close contact is only possible because the masticatory elevator muscles keep a constant mild contraction, known as tonus.

During mouth opening the first 20–30mm is accomplished with rotation of the mandibular condyles. Beyond this point the condyle–disc complex slides on the posterior slope of the articular eminence to a point slightly anterior to the crest of the articular eminence; this sliding movement is called translation. A normal range of mouth opening is considered to be 40 mm or greater. This distance is measured from the edge of the lower central incisors to the edge of the maxillary central incisors (interincisal distance), but the patient's overbite needs to be added to this measurement; if the patient presents an anterior open bite, this open bite distance needs to be subtracted from the measurement.

As previously mentioned, the superior retrodiscal lamina (SRL) is composed of elastic connective tissue. This characteristic of the SRL is critical during TMJ function. When the mouth is closed, traction on the disc by the SRL is minimal. When the condyle starts to move forward, sliding on the posterior slope of the articular eminence, the SRL stretches, causing the articular disc to rotate posteriorly on the superior surface of the condyle. However, it is important to stress that what maintains the disc in place is not the SRL or the superior lateral pterygoid muscle, which is attached to the anterior border of the disc. The articular disc is maintained in place by its morphology along with the interarticular pressure.

The superior lateral pterygoid muscle plays another important role during jaw function. While the **inferior lateral pterygoid muscle** is responsible for moving the condyle forward (protraction), the superior lateral pterygoid only works in combination with the elevator muscles during mouth closing

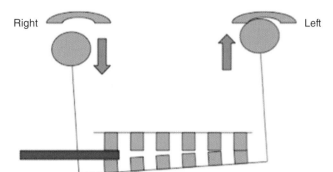

Figure 8.15 Diagram showing an increase in interarticular pressure on the left-hand side and a decrease in interarticular pressure on the right-hand side when biting on the right-hand side. Remember, however, the articular surfaces (which include the articular surfaces of the discs) on both sides remain in constant contact. On the right-hand side, the posterior border of the disc would be positioned in between the condyle and the mandibular fossa, thereby preserving the contact between articular surfaces.

or chewing. In other words, during mouth opening the superior lateral pterygoid is inactive. When chewing food on one side, the food will work as a fulcrum, and the TMJs will not be uniformly loaded. When that happens, the interarticular pressure in the TMJ on the biting side (ipsilateral side) decreases, while the pressure on the contralateral joint increases (Fig 8.15). Therefore, one might think this process would create a space in between the articular surfaces on the TMJ corresponding to the side where the food is being chewed. However, this does not happen because, during power strokes of the mandible, the superior lateral pterygoid contracts, pulling the articular disc forward as much as its morphology permits. This brings the thicker part of the disc (posterior border) to the top of the condyle, which keeps the articular surfaces of the TMJ in constant contact. During this function, the fibers of the superior lateral pterygoid that are attached to the neck of the condyle pull the condyle against the posterior slope of the articular eminence.

During lateral movements, the TMJ on one side works differently from the opposite side. If the mandible is moved toward the right side, the left condyle translates on the posterior slope of the articular eminence, while the right condyle remains in the mandibular fossa. In other words, during lateral excursive movements, the condyle that translates the most is the one contralateral to the movement (Fig 8.16). The normal range of lateral movement is 8 mm, measured from the maxillary dental midline to the mandibular dental midline. If the superior and inferior dental midlines are not coincident, that difference needs to be added or subtracted, depending on the side toward which the patient is moving the mandible.

> Movement of the TMJ on one side always causes movement of the TMJ on the opposite side.
> The articular surfaces of the TMJ are maintained in constant contact.

(a)

(b)

(c)

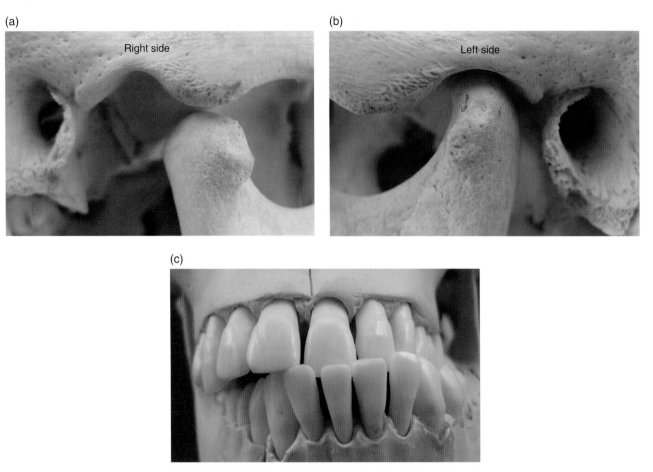

Figure 8.16   During lateral movement toward the left-hand side (c), the condyle on the right-hand side (a) translates on the posterior slope of the articular eminence, while the left condyle (b) remains in the fossa.

Clinical correlations

Disc displacement

Disc displacement is a very common **temporomandibular disorder** (TMD). Usually the disc is displaced anteriorly, staying in front of the mandibular condyle. Using the anatomical information previously mentioned, it is possible to conclude that when the articular disc is anteriorly displaced the retrodiscal tissue will be pulled to the area previously occupied by the disc. Compression of the retrodiscal tissue can elicit pain since this area, in contrast to the articular disc, is well innervated.

Disc displacement can occur with and without reduction. In a disc displacement with reduction the disc reassumes its position on the top of the condyle upon function of the mandible. When that happens, it frequently generates sound (usually reported as clicking or popping sounds). This clicking sound upon mouth opening is called "opening click" and can happen at any time during the movement, depending on the traction of the superior lateral pterygoid muscle, traction of the SRL, and mainly on the disc–condyle morphology. However, the opening click most frequently happens toward the end of the condylar rotation and beginning of the condylar translation. A second clicking sound might be present during mouth closing. It is called "closing click" or "reciprocal click", and generally occurs when the teeth are close to occlusion (intercuspal position).

Clinicians need to be aware, however, that not all TMJ sounds are related to displacement of the disc. Structural incompatibility of the articular surfaces as well as **subluxation** of the condyle also can generate TMJ sounds. In contrast to disc displacement, the opening and closing click sounds due to morphologic changes of the condyle, disc, or fossa are consistent with regard to presence and location. Therfore, both clicks happen at the same interincisal distance.

A useful diagnostic tool is to ask the patient to protrude his/her mandible immediately after the opening click and ask him/her to continue opening and closing the mouth, keeping the mandible in a protruded position. If during this procedure no more TMJ sounds are noticed, a possible diagnosis is disc displacement with reduction.

Another procedure used during the clinical exam to help the clinician diagnose a disc displacement with or without reduction is to observe the path followed by the patient's mandible during opening and closing movements.

If the patient has a disc displacement, he/she might present a deviation or deflection of the mandible during mouth opening and closing. Deviation happens when upon mouth opening the mandible moves out of the normal midline and then goes back to the midline and remains there until maximal mouth opening. Deflection happens when upon mouth opening the mandible goes out of the midline and remains out (moving even farther) until maximal mouth opening (Fig 8.17).

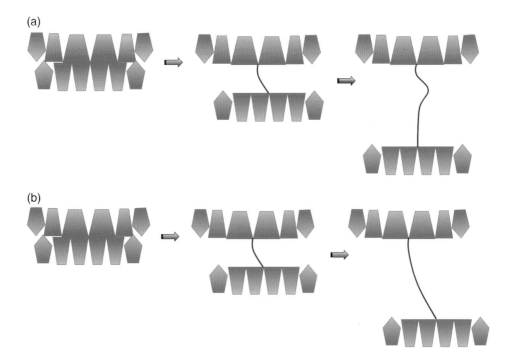

Figure 8.17   Diagram representing (a) deviation of the mandible during mouth opening and (b) deflection of the mandible during mouth opening.

Deviation is mostly related to disc displacement with reduction, while deflection is most often related to unilateral disc displacement without reduction. However, it is important to emphasize that deviations and deflections are also associated with other articular and/or muscle disorders. When those deviations or deflections are observed, further investigation is necessary in order to identify the cause. The clinical exam and/or panoramic x-ray image are not conclusive of a final diagnosis of disc displacement. Magnetic resonance imaging (MRI) technique is the gold standard to diagnose this condition, as well as to determine if the disc reduces or not upon mandibular function (Fig 8.18). If the deviation or deflection is linked to a disc displacement, the mandible will deviate or deflect toward the affected side upon mouth opening. This can be explained because the condyle on the unaffected side moves faster than the one where the disc is displaced, since the disc, when in a displaced position, prevents the normal movement of the condyle (Fig 8.19).

Measuring the mandibular lateral movements also adds important information to identify if the patient has TMD. In a patient with an acute disc displacement without reduction the lateral movement of the mandible toward the contralateral side is limited. Remember that in order to laterally move the mandible toward one side the condyle of the opposite side is the one that translates on the posterior slope of the articular eminence, while the condyle on the side to where the mandible is moving remains in the mandibular fossa (Fig 8.16). Therefore, if a patient presents with an acute left disc displacement without reduction, he/she will present with deflection of the mandible toward the left side upon mouth opening, and lateral movement limitation toward the right side. With chronic disc displacement, the patient might present with normal mandibular function. Understanding the TMJ's biomechanics helps the clinician associate the pattern of movements with the correct disorder (Fig 8.19).

Arthritides of the TMJ

In this condition destructive bony changes are seen in the TMJ (Fig 8.20). Osteoarthritis is the most common arthritides. When destructive bony changes occur on the condyle, for example, the condyle will become shorter, but no space will appear between the articular surfaces, because as was previously mentioned the articular surfaces of the TMJ remain in constant contact. Also, any movement of one TMJ will induce some movement of the opposite TMJ. Therefore, if the patient presents with osteoarthritis of one TMJ causing bony destruction of the mandibular condyle, the whole mandible will shift position and occlusion will be disrupted. In this scenario, the clinician needs to understand that the malocclusion is a consequence of the disease and not the cause. An occlusal treatment will likely not eliminate the pain and stiffness that may be associated with this joint disorder.

> TMJ sounds do not only occur as a result of disc displacement with reduction. Therefore a final diagnosis of a disc displacement cannot be obtained based on TMJ sounds, but only with a MRI.

TMJ dislocation

During normal function of a healthy TMJ, the condyle translates up to the crest of the articular eminence (or slightly anterior). If the condyle moves too far beyond this point, it can get confined in front of the articular eminence, and the patient may be unable to reposition it back to the mandibular fossa (Fig 8.21). This condition is called **temporomandibular joint dislocation**.

When a patient is describing this condition, he/she will mention that his/her mouth is locked open.

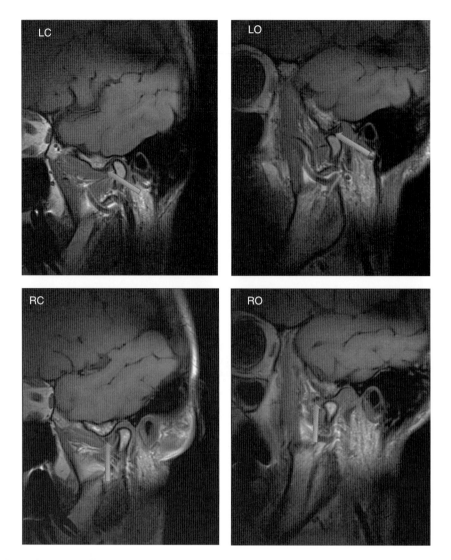

Figure 8.18   T1-weighted MRI of the TMJs of a 60-year-old female with bilateral anterior disc displacement: with reduction on the left-hand side and without reduction on the right-hand side. (LC) left TMJ with closed mouth, (LO) left TMJ with open mouth, (RC) right TMJ with closed mouth, and (RO) right TMJ with open mouth. Note the disc on the left-hand side is reduced at the top of the condyle, following opening of the mouth, and the disc on the right-hand side remains anteriorly displaced following opening of the mouth. The disc has a low signal on a T1 MRI (dark image in front of the arrow). (Courtesy Dr Alan Lurie, University of Connecticut.)

> Even though a mouth opening of 40 mm or more is considered normal, the clinician must always consider the patient's history. Patients normally might open much more than 40 mm, and therefore even when experiencing a restricted mouth opening they might be able to open at least 40 mm.

Histology association

The TMJ is the only synovial joint in the body in which the cartilage of the joint surface is covered by collagenous connective tissue. Several peculiarities of the pathologies of this joint result from this situation. One is that the cartilage is capable of growing by surface apposition throughout the life of the individual. Thus, tumors of the pituitary gland which secrete excess growth hormone will stimulate growth of the jaw while having only a minor influence on the long bones of the extremities.

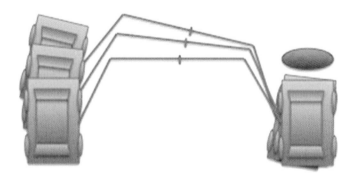

Figure 8.19   This diagram is an analogy to the mandibular movement in a patient with unilateral disc displacement. The cars, which are representing the condyles, are firmly connected to each other. The connection represents the body of the mandible. In red is an obstacle representing a displaced disc. Note that the car on the left–hand side of the diagram keeps moving forward, since it has no obstacle, whereas the car on the right cannot move forward. Since the two cars are connected, the whole system (cars + connection) starts to deviate toward the side with the obstacle.

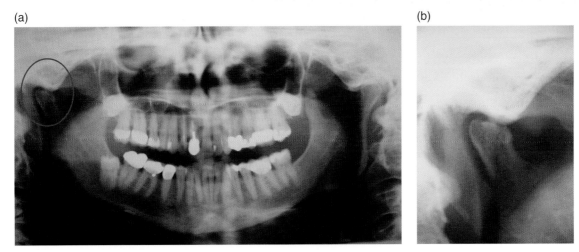

Figure 8.20   Osteoarthritis on the right TMJ. (Courtesy Dr Marcelo Medeiros, Brazil.)

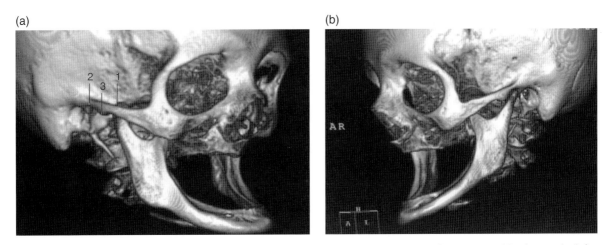

Figure 8.21   TMJ dislocation on the right-hand side: Note that the right condyle is in front of the articular eminence (a), whereas the left condyle is well positioned in the mandibular fossa (b). Condyle (1), mandibular fossa (2), and articular eminence (3).

Clinical case

A 20-year-old female visits her new dentist complaining of limited mouth opening. When taking the history, the dentist learned that the patient has experienced this limited range of mandibular movement for the past seven days, following a trauma to the left side of her chin while she was playing soccer. The patient said she experienced some discomfort for a couple of days, but ibuprofen was able to control the pain. The patient also mentioned that a couple of years ago she had experienced trauma to the same area. She remembered that she experienced a severe sharp pain in the right pre-auricular area; she also remembered that on the following day an acute posterior open bite had developed on the contralateral side of the trauma. According to the patient this malocclusion only lasted for a few days, and she could then notice very repeatable clicking sounds of her right TMJ upon jaw function. She also mentioned that she remembered clearly that her dentist at that time determined that the clicking sounds occurred at about 25mm of mouth opening, and a second click, which was noticeable upon mouth closing, occurred at about 5mm. According to the patient, since that first trauma she has not experienced any problem other than the "annoying clicking" of the right TMJ up to the time she had the second trauma.

During the clinical evaluation, the dentist noticed:

- The patient could only open 27mm, with a deflection to the right side

- Lateral movement limitation to the left side
- No TMJ sounds upon function.

The dentist then explained to the patient what possibly was happening. Based on her history, it seemed that, even though both traumas were similar, what she might have experienced on the first occasion was an abrupt posterior lateral movement of the right condyle due to the trauma on the left side of her chin. This acute movement may have resulted in an intracapsular inflammation, in which the intracapsular effusion forced a slight downward movement of the condyle, causing the posterior open bite on the right side. Also, due to this acute condylar movement, the disc could have been displaced anteriorly and was being reduced upon function (disc displacement with reduction). Following the second trauma, however, the disc possibly was no longer being reduced, and the patient probably was experiencing a disc displacement without reduction of the right TMJ. Even though the history and the clinical evaluation led the dentist to the diagnosis of disc displacement without reduction, he was very careful to use the words *possibly, may,* and *probably* when explaining everything to the patient, because he was knowledgeable enough to know that only magnetic resonance imaging (MRI) could confirm his working diagnosis.

References

1. Benjamin, M. & Ralphs, J.R. (2004) Biology of fibrocartilage cells. International Review of Cytology, 233, 1–45.
2. Ten Cate, A.R. (2008) Temporomandibular joint. In: *Ten Cate's oral histology: development, structure and function* (ed. A. Nanci) 7th edn. Mosby, St. Louis, Missouri.
3. de Bont, L.G., Boering, G., Havinga, P., & Liem, R.S. (1984) Spatial arrangement of collagen fibrils in the articular cartilage of the mandibular condyle: a light microscopic and scanning electron microscopic study. *Journal of Oral Maxillofacial Surgery,* 42, 306–313.
4. de Bont, L.G., Liem, R.S., & Boering, G. (1985) Ultrastructure of the articular cartilage of the mandibular condyle: aging and degeneration. *Oral Surgery Oral Medicine Oral Pathology,* 60, 631–641.
5. Detamore, M.D. & Athanasiou, K.A. (2003) Structure and function of the temporomandibular joint disc: implications for tissue engineering. *Journal of Oral Maxillofacial Surgery,* 61, 494–506.
6. Isselhard, B. (2003) *Anatomy of Orofacial Structures,* 7th edn. Mosby, St. Louis, Missouri.
7. Lang, J. (1995) *Clinical Anatomy of the Masticatory Apparatus and Peripharyngeal Spaces,* 1st edn. Thieme, New York.
8. Milam, S.B. (2005) Pathogenesis of degenerative temporomandibular joint arthritides. *Odontology,* 93, 7–15.
9. Milam, S.B., Klebe, R.J., Triplett, R.G., & Herbert, D. (1991) Characterization of the extracellular matrix of the primate temporomandibular joint. *Journal of Oral Maxillofacial Surgery,* 49, 381–391.
10. Mills, D.K., Fiandaca, D.J., & Scapino, R.P. (1994) Morphologic, microscopic, and immunohistochemical investigations into the function of the primate TMJ disc. *Journal of Orofacial Pain,* 8, 136–154.
11. Minarelli, A.M., del Santo, M., Jr., & Liberti, E.A. (1997) The structure of the human temporomandibular joint disc: a scanning electron microscopy study. *Journal of Orofacial Pain,* 11, 95–100.
12. Nitzan, D.W. (2001) The process of lubrication impairment and its involvement in temporomandibular joint disc displacement: a theoretical concept. *Journal of Oral Maxillofacial Surgery,* 59, 36–45.
13. Nitzan, D.W., Benoliel, R., Heir, G., & Dolwwick, F. (2008) Pain and dysfunction of the temporomandibular joint. In: *Orofacial Pain and Headache.* (eds. Y. Sharav & R. Benoliel) 1st edn. Mosby Elsevier, Philadelphia.
14. Nitzan, D.W., Nitzan, U., Dan, P., & Yedgar, S. (2001) The role of hyaluronic acid in protecting surface-active phospholipids from lysis by exogenous phospholipase A_2. *Rheumatology* (Oxford), 40, 336–340.
15. Okeson, J. P. (2005) *Management of Temporomandibular Disorders and Occlusion,* 6th edn. Mosby Elsevier, St. Louis, Missouri.
16. Robinson, P. D. (1993) Articular cartilage of the temporomandibular joint: can it regenerate? *Annals of the Royal College of Surgeons of England,* 75, 231–236.
17. Rosenbaum, R.S., Friction, J.R., & Okeson, J.P. (2001) Orofacial pain emerging as a dental specialty. *Journal of Massachusetts Dental Society,* 49, 36–38.
18. Sakuda, M., Tanne, K., Tanaka, E., & Takasugi, H. (1992) An analytic method for evaluating condylar position in the TMJ and its application to orthodontic patients with painful clicking. *American Journal of Orthodontics and Dentofacial Orthopedics,* 101, 88–96.
19. Shibukawa, Y., Young, B., Wu, C., Yamada, S., Long, F., Pacifici, M., & Koyama, E. (2007) Temporomandibular joint formation and condyle growth require Indian hedgehog signaling. *Developmental Dynamics,* 236, 426–434.
20. Suda, N., Shibata, S., Yamazaki, K., Kuroda, T., Senior, P.V., Beck, F., & Hammond, V.E. (1999) Parathyroid hormone-related protein regulates proliferation of condylar hypertrophic chondrocytes. *Journal of Bone Mineral Research,* 14, 1838–1847.
21. Tanaka , T. T. (1992) *TMJ Microanatomy: an Approach to Current Controversies.* Clinical Research Foundation, Chula Vista, California.
22. Wadhwa, S. & Kapila, S. (2008) TMJ disorders: future innovations in diagnostics and therapeutics. *Journal of Dental Education,* 72, 930–947.

Glossary

Anterior capsular ligament: The ligament that attaches the anterior part of the disc to the anterior margin of the articular surface of the temporal bone (superiorly) and to the anterior margin of the articular surface of the condyle (inferiorly).

Articular disc: A structure composed of dense fibrous connective tissue interposed between the mandibular condylar head and the squamous portion of the temporal bone.

Articular eminence: A convex bar of bone upon which the articular disc slides during mandibular function.

Articular zone: The most superficial layer among the four layers that constitute the articular surfaces of the mandibular fossa and condyle.

Boundary lubrication: Boundary lubrication occurs when the joint is moved, forcing the synovial fluid to dislocate from one area of the joint to another.

Calcified cartilage zone: The deepest layer among the four layers that constitute the articular surfaces of the condyle and the posterior slope of the articular eminence. Also called the hypertrophic zone.

Compound joint: A joint that includes three bone structures in the articulation.

Condyle: The structure of the mandible that articulates with the temporal bone (ideally with the articular disc interposed).

Disc displacement: Term used when the articular disc is not correctly positioned on the condylar head (considered, therefore, to be out of place).

Discal (collateral) ligaments: Ligaments that attach the medial and lateral edges of the disc to the respective poles of the condyle.

Fibrocartilaginous zone: The third layer among the four layers that constitute the articular surfaces of the condyle and the posterior slope of the articular eminence. Also called the chondroblastic zone.

Free nerve endings: Afferent nerve endings, which function as thermoreceptors, cutaneous mechanoreceptors, and nociceptors.

Ginglymoarthrodial joint: A joint that has a form of ginglymus and arthrodia, allowing hinge and sliding movements.

Golgi-Mazzoni corpuscles: Encapsulated sensory nerve endings that function as mechanoreceptors.

Hyaluronic acid: A glycosaminoglycan produced by synovial tissue and important for maintaining the lubrication capability of the synovial fluid.

Indian hedgehog protein: A protein encoded by a gene of the same name, which acts in chondrocyte differentiation, proliferation, and maturation during endochondral ossification.

Inferior articular space: The space delineated by the inferior surface of the articular disc and the mandibular condyle. The rotation between the condyle and the articular disc occurs in this space.

Inferior lateral pterygoid muscle: Attaches anteriorly to the outer surface of the lateral pterygoid plate and posteriorly to the neck of the condyle.

Inferior retrodiscal lamina: A lamina of tissue formed by collagenous and nonelastic tissue, which attaches the posterior border of the disc to the posterior margin of the articular surface of the mandibular condyle.

Lateral discal (or collateral) ligament: Ligament that attaches the lateral edge of the articular disc to the lateral pole of the condyle.

Mandibular fossa: Concave area of the squamous portion of the temporal bone, which is limited posteriorly by the postglenoid process and anteriorly by the articular eminence. The condyle–disc complex articulates with this area.

Medial discal (or collateral) ligament: Ligament that attaches the medial edge of the articular disc to the medial pole of the condyle.

Osteopontins: Phosphorylated sialoproteins, which are important extracellular structural proteins of mineralized matrices of bones and teeth.

Pacinian corpuscles: Mechanoreceptors responsible for detecting vibrations and pressure changes.

Phospholipase A2 (PLA2):   An enzyme that releases fatty acid. It can catalytically hydrolyze the bond between phospholipids, releasing arachidonic acid and lysophospholipids.

Phospholipid: A class of lipids that composes all cell membranes. It has a hydrophilic portion (head) and a hydrophobic portion (tail).

Postglenoid process: Small ridge of bone positioned posterior to the mandibular fossa and anterior to the external acoustic meatus.

Proliferative zone: The second most superficial layer among the four layers that constitute the articular surfaces of the condyle and the posterior slope of the articular eminence.

Retrodiscal tissue: Tissue localized immediately behind the articular disc, which is well vascularized and innervated.

Ruffini's nerve endings: Slowly adapting mechanoreceptors which register mechanical deformation, continuous pressure, and warmth.

Sox-9 protein: A protein encoded by a gene of the same name, which acts during chondrocyte differentiation.

Sphenomandibular ligament: A TMJ accessory ligament which is attached to the spine of the sphenoid bone and to the lingula of the mandible.

Squamous portion (or squama) of the temporal bone: One of the four portions of the temporal bone. The other portions are: mastoid portion, petrous portion, and tympanic portion.

Stylomandibular ligament: A TMJ accessory ligament, which is attached to the styloid process of the temporal bone, and to the angle and posterior border of the ramus of the mandible.

Subluxation: Term used when an incomplete joint dislocation happens. On the TMJ it is noticeable when the lateral pole of the condyle jumps forward to the maximally open position. Subluxation is not pathology, but an anatomical feature usually associated with the articular eminence.

Superficial zone proteins: Large proteoglycans synthesized by chondrocytes and synoviocytes and found in the synovial fluid. Also known as lubricin.

Superior articular space: The space delineated by the mandibular fossa and the superior surface of the articular disc. Translation between the disc and the mandibular fossa–articular eminence occurs in this space.

Superior lateral pterygoid muscle: Attached anteriorly to infratemporal surface of the greater sphenoid wing and posteriorly to the capsule, articular disc, and neck of the condyle.

Superior retrodiscal lamina: A lamina of tissue formed by connective tissue with many elastic fibers, which attaches the posterior border of the disc to the tympanic plate.

Synovial fluid: Fluid secreted by the cells of the synovial membrane present in all synovial joints. It reduces the friction between the articular surfaces, helps as a shock absorber, and also supports metabolic exchange between the capsule, the articular tissues, and the synovial fluid itself.

Temporomandibular disorder: Defined by Dr. Jeffrey Okeson as being "a collective term embracing a number of clinical problems that involve the masticatory musculature, the TMJ and associated structures, or both."

Temporomandibular joint dislocation: Occurs when the mouth is opened beyond its normal limit, causing the condyle to be positioned (and trapped) in front of the crest of the articular eminence.

Temporomandibular ligament: One of the main ligaments that support the function of the TMJ; it consists of an outer oblique portion (OOP) and an inner horizontal portion (IHP).

Weeping lubrication: Weeping lubrication is related to the ability of the articular surfaces to absorb a small volume of synovial fluid. Upon function, compressive force on the articular surfaces of the joint forces release of the small volume of synovial fluid.

PART IV
MUCOSAL STRUCTURE AND FUNCTION

Chapter 9 Oral Mucosa and Mucosal Sensation

Ellen Eisenberg, Easwar Natarajan, and Bradley K. Formaker

Department of Oral Health and Diagnostic Sciences, School of Dental Medicine, University of Connecticut

Oral mucosa is the moist soft tissue membrane that lines the oral cavity. In the course of a single day, the oral mucosa is subject to a host of intrinsic and external environmental stimuli, irritants, and stressors, both physiologic and potentially pathological in nature. Such stimuli include the teeth, denture prostheses, foods, beverages, therapeutic and nontherapeutic foreign objects, chemical agents, extreme fluctuations in both temperature and hydration, and a vastly diverse microbial flora. Yet, despite the constant stimulation, provocation, and punishment it sustains, oral mucosa is remarkably resilient. Indeed, maintenance of oral mucosal integrity is essential for comfort, protection, tactile, thermal, and taste sensation, speech, initiation and animation of the cascade of reflexes involved in the process of preparing foods and liquids for swallowing and digestion, and reflexes, like gagging, associated with the elimination of noxious substances. Among the mechanisms that ensure preservation and optimal function of the oral mucous membrane as a whole are (1) the microstructure of the oral surface epithelium; (2) the intricate apparatus that attaches the naturally avascular epithelium to the underlying stromal tissues that provide it with critical vascular, neural, nutritional, and immunological support; (3) the mechanical strength provided by a supportive extracellular matrix; and (4) secretions from both the major salivary glands and, in particular, a multitude of submucosal minor salivary glands that serve to lubricate the oral surface, contribute to the digestive process, facilitate speech and taste sensation, and take part in various other functions essential to homeostasis.

> Functions of the oral mucosa include: physical, reflexive, and immunological protection, sensation (taste, tactile and temperature), and preparation of the food bolus which includes initiation of both deglutition and the digestive process.

The oral cavity - anatomy

The oral cavity is the gateway to the **alimentary** canal and a portal to the upper respiratory tract, and the lips mark the entry way into the oral cavity. The lips are comprised of three anatomic subdivisions, two of them external and one internal. The external or "dry" subdivisions include the skin of the lips, with dermal appendages, and the highly vascular vermilion ("red") borders of the lips which, in contrast, lack dermal appendages (Figures 9.1a, 9.1b, 9.2). The **vermilion border** is sharply demarcated from the skin of the lips. Its surface is characterized by skin markings and uniform coloration (Figure 9.1a). The internal "wet" portion of the lip, the labial mucosa, demonstrates prominent vascular markings. A rich complement of submucosal minor salivary glands provides the labial mucosa with secretions that are expressed onto the mucosal surface. The secretions lubricate the soft tissues and teeth and provide comfort and protection (Figure 9.1b).

The external portions of the lips are exposed to extrinsic environmental stimuli and irritants, particularly fluctuations in wetting and drying and traumatic injury, especially from the

Fundamentals of Oral Histology and Physiology, First Edition. Arthur R. Hand and Marion E. Frank.
© 2014 John Wiley & Sons, Inc. Published 2014 by John Wiley & Sons, Inc.

(a)

(b)

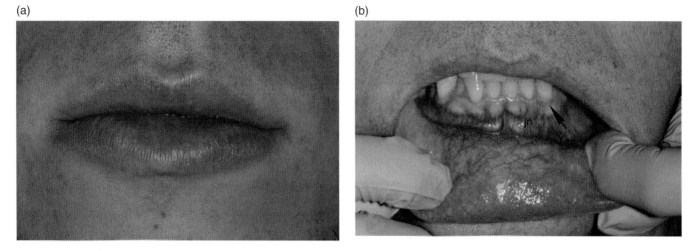

Figure 9.1   Parts of the lip. (a) External segments of the upper and lower lips. Note that the skin of the lips has hair shafts and other skin append-ages. In contrast, the vermilion borders are evenly -colored, hairless, sharply demarcated from the adjacent skin, and demonstrate subtle vertical skin markings. (b) The labial mucosa is the moist internal portion of the lip. Underlying vasculature is readily discernible on the labial mucosa and the contiguous vestibular mucosa (v) and the alveolar mucosa. The junction between the pale-appearing attached gingiva (arrow) and the alveolar mucosa is the mucogingival junction (jn).

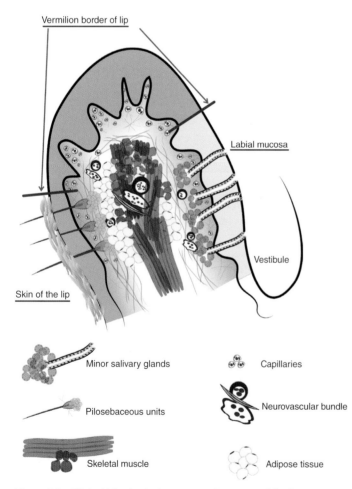

Figure 9.2   Clinical-histological representation, parts of the lip.

teeth. In comparison to the upper lip, which resides in the shadow of the nose, the external portion of the lower lip is in a more prominent anatomic position. This is significant because over time, chronic exposure of the vermilion border and skin of

the lower lip to ultraviolet light places it at particular risk for **actinic** (sun-related) damage. Chronic actinic-related alterations include collagen degeneration, atrophy of the epithelial surface, **precancerous** epithelial changes, and squamous cell carcinoma (lip cancer).

> The skin and vermilion borders of the external lips are dry tissues that are not covered by oral mucosa. Oral mucosa begins at the junction between the dry vermilion border of the lips and the moist labial mucosa.

As a discrete anatomic region, the oral cavity begins where the oral mucosa begins, that is, at the junction of the vermilion border and the labial mucosa. It extends posteriorly to the **palatoglossal folds**, the more anterior of two arch-like soft tissue structures that mark the entrance to the **oropharynx**. The more posteriorly positioned of these arches are the **palatopharyngeal folds** at the opening of the oropharynx. The palatoglossal and palatopharyngeal folds together form the **tonsillar pillars**. On clinical examination, nodular, lobulated lymphoid tissue masses, the palatine tonsils, can be seen bilaterally in the **tonsillar fau-ces**, the concave tissue recesses between the palatoglossal and the palatopharyngeal folds (Figure 9.3). Along with the palatine tonsils, other smaller aggregates of oral mucosa-associated lym-phoid tissues distributed in the posterior oral cavity comprise **Waldeyer's ring**. They include the lingual tonsils on the posterior dorsal-lateral surfaces of the tongue, and small, raised, orange-pink colored papules on the soft palate, the posterior pharyngeal wall, and occasionally the floor of the mouth (Figure 9.4).

The maxillary and mandibular alveolar ridges and teeth subdivide the oral cavity internally into its two major regional components, the outer of which is termed the **oral vestibule**; the inner portion is the **oral cavity proper**. The oral vestibule is bounded by the **buccal** mucosa and labial mucosa (inner cheeks and lips, respec-tively) (Figure 9.5). The deep troughs that mark the inferior and

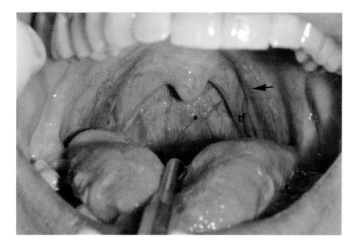

Figure 9.3   Soft palate, uvula, and palatoglossal folds. Clinical photograph demonstrates the bilateral, arch-like palatoglossal folds (anteriorly) (black arrow) and the palatopharyngeal folds (more posteriorly) (green arrow). In the depression in between these arches is the tonsillar fauces (tf) where the relatively large palatine tonsils, a component of Waldeyer's ring of lymphoid tissue (not visible in this photograph), reside. The uvula projects down ward from the soft palate and is seen in the midline. The posterior wall of the pharynx contains several small orange-pink aggregates of lymphoid tissue (*).

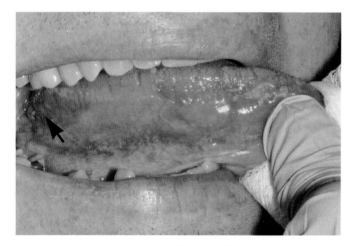

Figure 9.4   Lateral-ventral surfaces of tongue, foliate papillae. The lateral-ventral tongue surfaces are nonkeratinized. Note the transition from the relatively thick, rough and heavily keratinized dorsal surface superiorly to the smoother lateral and ventral surfaces of the tongue, inferiorly. The lingual veins are readily seen through the nonkeratinzed ventral tongue surface. Lingual tonsils (lymphoid tissue of Waldeyer's ring) and foliate papillae (arrow) reside on the most posterior lateral-ventral surface of the tongue. The lingual tonsils are small, orange-pink nodules and lie posterior and dorsal to the foliate papillae.

superior limits of the buccal and labial mucosae are the maxillary and mandibular **vestibules**. Both vestibules reflect onto and are contiguous with the alveolar mucosa that overlies the upper and lower alveolar ridges. The mucosal tissue directly below the crowns of the mandibular teeth, above the crowns of the maxillary teeth and bound down to their respective underlying alveolar bone is the **attached gingiva** ("gum"). The clinically evident boundary that distinguishes the flexible, thin alveolar mucosa with its

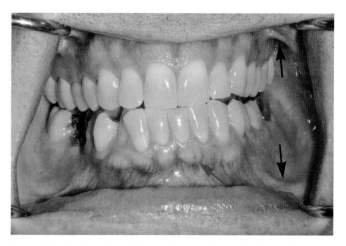

Figure 9.5   Oral vestibule. The maxillary and mandibular vestibules (troughs) are the superior and inferior boundaries, respectively, of the buccal and labial mucosae. Note the arc-like connective tissue attachments (frena or frenula) (black arrows) that traverse the vestibules and link the buccal and labial mucosae with the alveolar mucosae. Because of their thinner, nonkeratinized epithelial surfaces, underlying vasculature is visible in the vestibular and alveolar mucosae, in contrast to the denser, keratinized mucosa of the pale-pink attached gingiva. As also seen in Fig. 9.1, the mucogingival junction (green arrow) is the boundary that separates the attached gingiva from the alveolar mucosa.

visibly redder coloration from the immobile, more pale or pink stippled-appearing attached gingiva is the **mucogingival junction**.

> The oral cavity is subdivided into the oral cavity proper and the oral vestibule.

The oral cavity proper is bounded by the hard and soft palates superiorly, the palatoglossal folds posteriorly, the maxillary and mandibular alveolar processes laterally and anteriorly, and the floor of the mouth inferiorly. The oral portion (or body) of the tongue projects upward and forward into the oral cavity from the floor of the mouth. It comprises the anterior two-thirds of the tongue, which ends at the **terminal sulcus**, a V-shaped groove on the dorsal tongue surface just posterior to and parallel with the circumvallate papillae (Figure 9.6). At the apical convergence and most posterior point of the V of the terminal sulcus is the **foramen cecum**, which lies immediately anterior to the base of the tongue. The base of the tongue marks the entrance to the oropharynx.

> The posterior boundary of the oral cavity proper is at the terminal sulcus of the dorsal tongue. This marks the junction between the oropharynx and the oral cavity.

The oral cavity as a whole is indeed a distinct anatomic region of the body, and should be regarded separately from the skin and vermilion borders of the external lips and the oropharynx. Keeping this in mind, students and clinicians should be aware that epidemiological and statistical data concerning various pathological conditions of the vermilion borders and skin of the

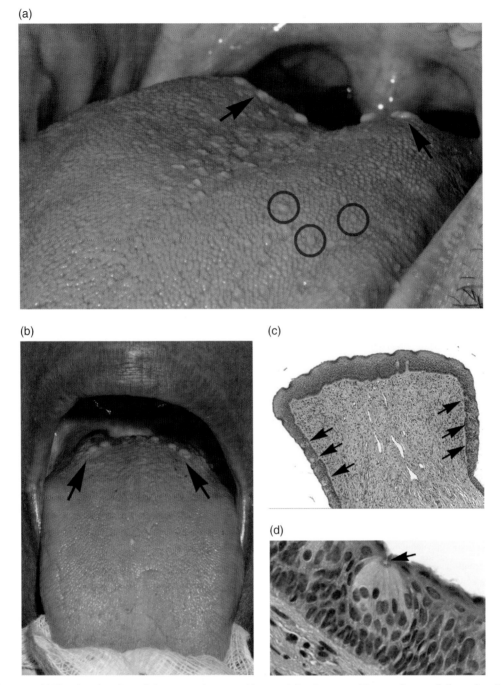

Figure 9.6 Dorsal tongue. (a) The dorsal surface of the tongue is covered by specialized mucosa. The roughness of the surface is attributable to the abundant, small hair-like filiform papillae that cover much of the anterior two- thirds of the tongue, and lack taste buds. The less numerous, small, round, white-red, papular fungiform papillae are distributed over the dorsal surface (center of grey circles). On the most posterior one third of the oral portion of the tongue are the 8 to 12 large circumvallate papillae (arrows) that are lined up in a V-formation and converge at the foramen cecum. (b) This view of the dorsal tongue demonstrates the arrangement of circumvallate papillae in a V-shaped configuration at the junction of the anterior two-thirds and the posterior one-third (arrows). (c) Taste buds (arrows) are present in the epithelium of the lateral surfaces of the circumvallate papilla. (d) An individual taste bud within the epithelium of the papillary trough. The orifice (taste pore) (arrow) of the taste bud opens into the lateral wall of the circumvallate papilla, allowing for taste sensation to be received by the taste bud.

external lips, the oral cavity, and the oropharynx are frequently pooled together and reported as a single statistic. However, it is improper and potentially misleading to combine information concerning these three disparate anatomic regions. Presenting such aggregated data as equally representative of these disparate regions collectively can and has resulted in serious misconceptions concerning their individual vulnerability to various disease processes. Combining data can and has led to the erroneous impression that there are no differences among the external lips, the oral cavity, and the oropharynx relative to various tissue responses and specific disease susceptibility and experience. However, the oral cavity and its lining tissue, the oral mucosa, are indeed unique and deserve consideration independent and distinct from their nearest neighbors, the external lips anteriorly and the oropharynx posteriorly.

Oral mucosa

The general structure of oral mucosa

The entire oral mucosal surface is lined by **stratified** (layered) **squamous** (scale-like) **epithelium**, an avascular, highly organized, and semipermeable ectodermal tissue that varies in thickness and

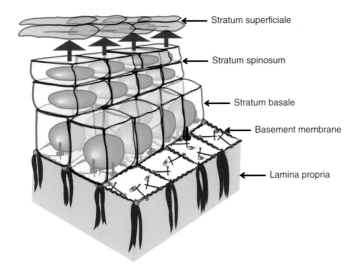

Figure 9.7   Representation of stratified squamous epithelium. Demonstration of the layers of stratified squamous epithelium as they proceed to maturation and desquamation at their apical domain. The epithelium resides on a basement membrane which overlies the lamina propria.

surface keratinization according to its location in the mouth and the functional demands of that location. Oral stratified squamous epithelium replenishes itself relatively frequently. The roughly 14 to 21 days of epithelial turnover time is necessarily rapid because of the considerable challenges oral mucosa is subjected to, functional and otherwise, throughout the waking hours and during sleep (Figures 9.7, 9.8).

> Oral mucosal epithelium varies in thickness according to functional demand and location. Because they are constantly being stimulated in the course of function, oral epithelial cells have a relatively rapid turnover time (14–21 days).

The basal-most portion of stratified squamous epithelium is arranged in undulating projections termed **rete pegs**. The rete pegs are part of the mechanism of attachment of the squamous epithelium to the basement membrane, which separates it from several layers of underlying stromal connective tissue. The most superior and widest layer is the **lamina propria** (Figures 9.8a, 9.8b). The lamina propria in turn is subdivided into two layers, the **papillary** layer and the reticular layer (Figures 9.8b, 9.8c). In some locations within the oral cavity the transition between these two layers may be subtle, making their distinction from one another difficult to recognize. The relatively loose papillary layer of the lamina propria is the more superficial segment, which lies immediately inferior to the epithelium. Here a thin, delicate fibrocollagenous tissue **stroma** contains vascular channels, fibroblasts, elastic fibers, and peripheral nerves. Some unmyelinated axonal endings of the stromal neural elements project upward and penetrate the overlying epithelium to function as sensory receptors, while others terminate in **Meissner's corpuscles** in the lamina propria (see "Oral Sensation" section). Additionally, efferent autonomic nerve fibers innervate blood

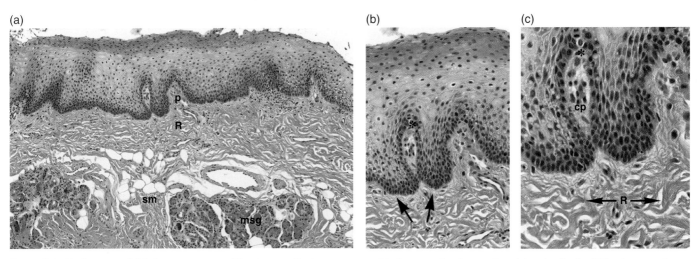

Figure 9.8   Oral mucosa. (a) At low power magnification stratified squamous epithelium overlies the papillary (p) and reticular (R) lamina propria and submucosa (sm), with adipose tissue and lobules of minor salivary glands (msg). (b) Downward, undulating epithelial rete pegs (arrows) interdigitate with the apical (upper most) (*) aspect of the papillary lamina propria. (c) Note the regimented-appearing epithelial basal cells. Stem cells reside within the basal layer at the apex of the papillary lamina propria (*). Small blood vessels (cp) and delicate collagen fibers are present in the papillary lamina propria, as contrasted with the thicker collagen fibers of the reticular lamina propria (R with arrows) that run parallel to the epithelial surface.

(a)   (b)

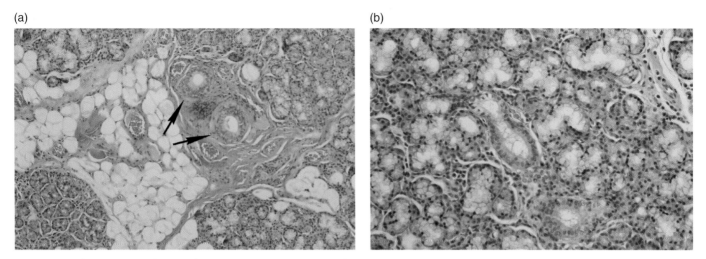

Figure 9.9   Submucosa. (a) Submucosal adipose tissue, minor salivary glands and blood vessels. Two large excretory ducts are seen centrally (arrows). (b) Minor salivary gland lobules. Mucous acini with serous demilunes, and intralobular ducts (d).

(a)   (b)

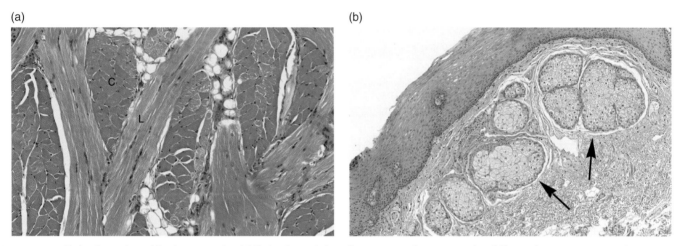

Figure 9.10   Skeletal muscle and Fordyce granules. (a) Skeletal muscle bundles, tongue. Fibers oriented in different directions are cut in longitudinal (L) and cross-section (C). Note the intervening adipose tissue. (b) Buccal mucosa, nonkeratinized epithelium. Ectopic sebaceous glands in the lamina propria (Fordyce granules) (arrows).

vessels and minor salivary glands located in the lamina propria and submucosa.

Underlying the papillary layer is the reticular layer of the lamina propria (Figures 9.8a, 9.8b). The collagen bundles of the reticular layer are generally more concentrated and denser than the more slender and loose collagen fibers of the papillary layer. The reticular layer's collagen and elastic fibers are woven together in a lattice-like network or **reticulum**. With the exception of the attached gingiva and the anterior portion of the hard palate and raphe, which are fixed directly to the underlying alveolar bone as a muco-periosteum, in all regions of the oral cavity there is a **submucosal** layer beneath the lamina propria. The submucosal layer consists of broad bands of fibrocollagenous and elastic tissue containing blood vessels and nerves. Depending on its specific anatomic location in the oral cavity, the submucosa may also contain minor salivary gland lobules (Figures 9.8, 9.9) whose excretory ducts are contiguous with and exit onto the mucosal surface (Figure 9.2) (labial mucosa, buccal mucosa, hard and soft palates), lymphoid tissue (posterior-lateral tongue, soft palate and uvula, floor of the

mouth), skeletal muscle (tongue, lips, buccal mucosa, soft palate, floor of mouth) (Figure 9.10a) and varying amounts of adipose tissue (Figure 9.9), of which there is an abundance in the buccal mucosa and soft palate. In the buccal mucosa and the vermilion borders of the lips there also may be **ectopic** sebaceous glands (**Fordyce granules**, or **Fordyce spots**) (Figure 9.10b).

- Rete-pegs are the downward, undulating projections of the oral epithelium that interdigitate with the upward papillary projections of the superficial lamina propria. They increase the surface area and strengthen the attachment of the epithelium to the underlying stroma.

- The lamina propria is divided into a superficial (papillary) segment and a deeper (reticular) segment. Inferior to the lamina propria lies the submucosa.

- The attached gingiva lacks a submucosal layer. It is attached directly to the underlying bone as a mucoperiosteum.

Stratified squamous epithelium – general principles and differentiation

Epithelium – general principles

Epithelium is the tissue that invests most external and internal body surfaces (e.g., skin, GI tract, respiratory tract, urinary tract). Also, specialized epithelial tissue is central to the function of several organs. In addition to its critical role in providing a protective barrier (skin, mucosa), specialized epithelial cells play a role in exocrine secretory function (e.g., mucous glands, exocrine pancreas), transport (e.g., respiratory epithelial cilia), filtration (e.g., renal podocytes), metabolism (e.g., hepatocytes) and thermal regulation (e.g., sweat glands). Some epithelial cells function expressly as special sensory receptors (smell, taste, vision, hearing, etc.). Regardless of the type of epithelium, they all share the fundamental characteristics enumerated below. Epithelial cells:

- reside in close apposition and adhere to one another via adhesion molecules that create cell junctions
- exhibit polarity, both in terms of function and form. Various functions correlate with morphologic surface domains (a free surface or **apical domain**; a basal domain; and a lateral domain) that are dictated by membrane proteins. The classification of various epithelia is based on the specific specialization or morphology of the apical (uppermost) domain
- attach to an underlying protein and polysaccharide-rich, non-cellular **basement membrane** at their basal-most surface.

Stratified squamous epithelium – strata, features, and differentiation

Stratified squamous epithelium invests the oral mucosa. It conforms to all of the general principles described above and is defined by the presence of squamous (scaly) epithelial cells at its apical portion and a basal domain bound down to a basement membrane. At the base, the epithelial–connective tissue interface is an undulating arrangement of epithelial projections, the rete pegs that dovetail with the connective tissue papillae of the superficial lamina propria. Similar to their counterparts in the epidermis of the skin, keratinocytes of oral mucosal epithelium are arranged in layers of cells that progress from the basal-most inferior layer upward to the surface where they assume a flattened, squamoid (scaly) morphology (Figure 9.7). Squamous epithelial cells are **keratinocytes**. As is characteristic of most epithelial cells, squamous cells contain predominantly an abundance of **cytokeratins**, intermediate filament proteins of differing molecular weights; this is in addition to actin and other filamentous proteins. The constellation of specific cytokeratins particular to each keratinocyte's maturational stage is responsible for that cell's individual shape and structure and its adhesion to neighboring keratinocytes. The whole program that dictates the squamoid morphology of apical cells is initiated in the basal layer.

> The differentiation of stratified squamous epithelium is a highly regulated process. It proceeds from the stratum basale upward to climax at the stratum superficiale where mature cells are ultimately desquamated.

Stratum basale/stratum germinativum/basal layer

The basal-most cell layer, the **stratum basale** (basal layer, **stratum germinativum**), consists of a single layer of basal keratinocytes (**epithelial basal cells**). Morphologically, basal cell nuclei tend to be round, basophilic, and large (relative to their cytoplasmic volume); the cytoplasm is cuboidal and basophilic (~ 10–$12\,\mu m$) (Figures 9.8, 9.11). The basal cells rest on a basement membrane, the interface zone between the epithelium and the underlying connective tissue. Individual basal cells are attached to the basement membrane by **hemidesmosomes**. Hemidesmosomes are the defining transmembrane linkers or "integrators" of stratified squamous epithelium (Figure 9.12). They are composed of an intricate complex of proteins that are centered around a transmembrane **heterodimer**, specifically **integrin** $\alpha 6\beta 4$. Within the cytoplasm the $\alpha 6\beta 4$ integrin is connected to bundles of intermediate filaments and actin via intracellular linking proteins, bullous pemphigoid antigens (BP230 and BP180). The extracellular domain binds to **laminin** 5 (a ligand for several integrins), a glycoprotein that is one of several extracellular matrix proteins that make up the basement membrane.

The defining characteristic of basal cells, in addition to their morphology, is their proliferative capacity (thus the alternative designation, stratum germinativum). Keratinocytes originate in the basal-most layer from a population of stem cells that undergo mitotic division. Stem cells are generally concentrated in the basal regions around the apices of the papillary lamina propria (Figures 9.8b, 9.8c). This population of stem cells undergoes division, with one daughter cell remaining behind in this region. The other daughter cell moves sideways and inferiorly towards the tips of the rete pegs to form committed **transit amplifying cells (TACs)**. The TACs are highly proliferative (thus the designation "amplifying") and are normally restricted to one to two basal cell layers. Upon completion of mitotic division, they progress to terminal differentiation in a highly orchestrated manner. The cells that are destined for differentiation undergo critical changes in their hemidesmosomal attachment ($\alpha 6\beta 4$ to $\alpha 3\beta 1$ integrins) that results in the cessation of cell division and almost immediate morphological changes as they transit upward into the spinous layer.

Stratum spinosum/spinous layer

Once the migrating basal keratinocytes transit into the immediately suprabasal region of the several cells-wide **stratum spinosum** they assume the appearance of spinous cells. Larger than basal cells and with a progressively lower nucleus-to-cytoplasm ratio, spinous cells are ovoid or stellate rather than cuboidal in shape. On conventionally stained sections (hematoxylin and eosin), they demonstrate abundant eosinophilic cytoplasm with a progressively shrinking nucleus as they approach the surface (Figures 9.8, 9.11a). In addition, they are

(a)

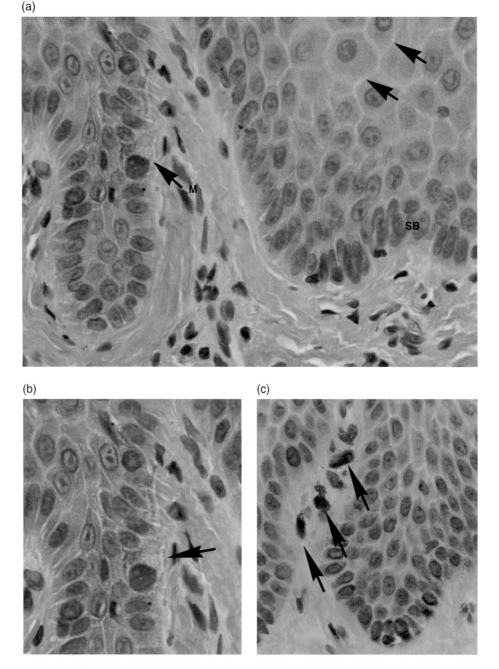

Figure 9.11   Stratified squamous epithelium; rete pegs, melanocytes, and melanin incontinence. (a) Rete pegs. The cells of the stratum basale (SB) are cuboidal and regimented with relatively large nuclei as compared to the spinous cells. Note the intercellular bridges (spines) between the polyhedral-appearing spinous cells (arrows). Among the cells of the stratum basale, a melanocyte with its dendritic projections and pigment is seen (M with arrow). (b) Melanocyte within the basal cell layer (arrow). (c) Melanin incontinence. In some chronic inflammatory processes, melanin (brown granular pigment) which is normally transported into adjacent basal cells may be spilled into the lamina propria where it is engulfed by *macrophages* ("melanophages") (arrows).

characterized by distinctive spine-like projections (prickles, **acanthe**) on the surfaces of their respective plasma membranes. The spines represent extensions into the intercellular space of cell processes bearing **desmosomes**, the elaborate, tufted biochemical and mechanical attachment apparatus that links individual keratinocytes to adjacent keratinocytes. Desmosomes are intracytoplasmic **placodes** comprised of proteins (desmoplakins and plakoglobin) located on the inner aspect of the plasma membrane (Figure 9.12). Within

the cytoplasm, a braid-like weave of intermediate keratin filaments attaches itself to the desmosome. From the intracytoplasmic placode **desmoglein** and **desmocollin** (paddle-like proteins from the cadherin family of attachment proteins) penetrate the intercellular space. They form Velcro-like linkages with their counterparts on the surface of neighboring cells to create robust intercellular bonds. This attachment apparatus creates the intercellular bridges visible on light microscopy (Figure 9.11).

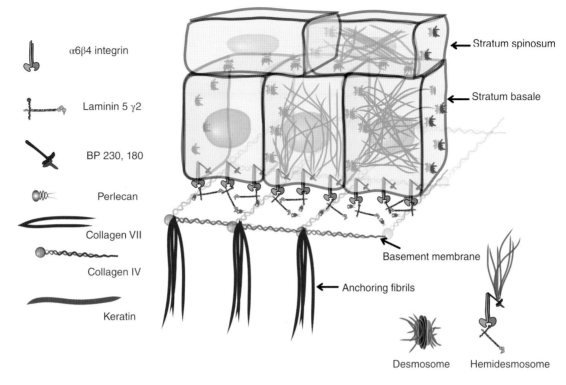

α6β4 integrin

Laminin 5 γ2

BP 230, 180

Perlecan

Collagen VII

Collagen IV

Keratin

Stratum spinosum

Stratum basale

Basement membrane

Anchoring fibrils

Desmosome   Hemidesmosome

Figure 9.12   Ultrastructure of epithelial-basement membrane arrangement. Epithelial basal cells rest on a *basement membrane*. The basement membrane is comprised of a complex of collagen IV, Laminins, and a meshwork of various other extracellular matrix proteins (perlecan, nidogen, entactin, etc.). Anchoring fibrils attach the basement membrane to the lamina propria. Basal cells are bound to Laminin 5 via hemidesmosomes that are anchored intracellularly to filamentous proteins in the cytoplasm. Epithelial cells are attached to one another via desmosomes. They are attachment complexes comprised of placodal proteins that link with the keratin cage within the cytoplasm.

Spinous cells are, by definition, post-mitotic and nonprolifera-tive at this point. The changes in morphology described above are accompanied by and a direct result of (1) the accumulation of a constantly changing range of keratin filaments, (2) change in the nature of basal domain attachment, (3) activation of apop-totic mechanisms, (4) loss of cell organelles, (5) chromatin condensation/breakdown (**pyknosis/karyorrhexis**), and (6) protein crosslinking across cell membranes (keratin and involu-crin complexes). This spectrum of change ultimately eventuates in exfoliation as keratotic debris (Figure 9.7) within the **stratum superficiale**.

Stratum superficiale/stratum corneum/cornified layer/keratin layer

The stratum superficiale (cornified layer/keratin layer) is the defining apical domain and the maturational end-point of stratified squamous epithelium. It is characterized morphologically by the presence of flattened epithelial cells. This layer can vary both in width and degree of surface kerati-nization (nonkeratinized, parakeratinized, or orthokerati-nized), depending upon anatomic location, the degree of stimulation from friction, or both. Cells may be anuclear or contain highly condensed "pyknotic" nuclei (Figure 9.13). At this point the cells have lost most cytoplasmic organelles and have accumulated predominantly cytokeratins, forming a dense protein-rich meshwork with tight intercellular junctions. Prior to the cells being shed into the oral cavity, it is these tight intercellular junctions that provide critical water resistance and protection. These cells also provide a surface for coating with protective salivary proteins.

Stratum superficiale – nonkeratinized, orthokeratinized, parakeratinized

By light microscopy the stratum superficiale in the oral cavity can be classified as being nonkeratinized, orthokeratinized, or parakeratinized (Figure 9.13). Irrespective of the degree of keratinization, there is considerable variation in the width of the stratum superficiale among various oral mucosal locations. Oral mucosal surfaces like the attached gingiva and the hard palatal mucosa as well as the dorsal tongue are covered by a dense layer of surface keratin. These locations are subjected to considerable frictional force and stimulation during the process of mastica-tion, and are consequently referred to as "keratinized" oral mucosa. In contrast, the remaining oral mucosal surface epithe-lium, which comprises the lining mucosa, is referred to as "nonkeratinized" mucosa.

Nonkeratinized squamous epithelium lines the greatest surface area of the oral mucosa, and includes the buccal and labial mucosae, the alveolar and vestibular mucosae, soft pal-ate, tonsillar pillars, floor of the mouth, and ventral and lat-eral surfaces of the tongue (Figure 9.13). The epithelium covering the fungiform, foliate, and circumvallate papillae (three of the four types of specialized dorsal tongue mucosae) is similarly described. The designation of these epithelia as

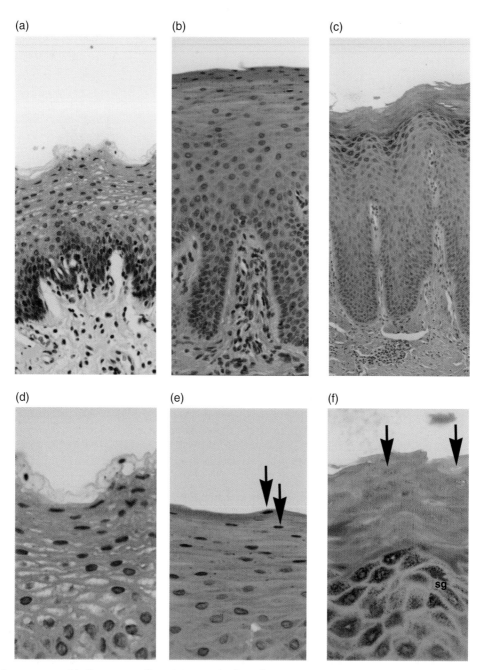

Figure 9.13   Stratified squamous epithelium, types of keratinization. (a, d) Nonkeratinized epithelium. (b, e) Parakeratinized epithelium. Pyknotic nuclei (arrows) are retained within the stratum corneum. (c, f) Orthokeratinized epithelium. Dense, eosinophilic, non-nucleated keratin with a few "ghost" nuclei (arrows) comprises the stratum corneum. A prominent granular cell layer (stratum granulosum; sg) is seen immediately inferior (f). Note the prominent blood vessels in the papillary lamina propria (a, b, c).

"nonkeratinized" is misleading, given that all keratinocytes contain abundant intracytoplasmic keratin filaments. As oral squamous cells differentiate and mature in their migration from the stratum basale upward and through more superficial layers, the composition of the keratin filaments unique to the keratinocytes in each epithelial stratum changes. When compared to their "keratinized" counterparts, keratinocytes from "nonkeratinized" mucosal surfaces contain sparsely distributed and less fasciculated bundles of **tonofilaments**. On electron microscopy, the **tonofibrils** in keratinocytes from keratinized surfaces are tightly bound and dense. Additionally, the cells within the superficial layers tend to be much larger in nonkeratinized mucosae. The composition of the glycolipid rich membrane-coating granules of keratinized versus nonkeratinized epithelium is different. As the membrane-coating granules fuse with the cell membranes of both keratinized and nonkeratinized mucosal epithelium, they release their contents into the intercellular spaces to produce a dynamic membrane. This controls the permeability of water soluble substances through the superficial keratin (cornified) layer. In keratinized mucosa, this is a more effective barrier against water loss and ingress of various chemicals, including noxious substances. Therefore, while tissue sections from keratinized and nonkeratinized tissues demonstrate morphological differences, their respective designations are misleading. In reality nonkeratinized epithelium actually is "keratinized," but to a significantly lesser degree than keratinized epithelium.

Orthokeratin is a term used to designate keratin that stains deeply with eosin and consists of flat dehydrated cells that lack nuclei or retain ghost-like nuclear remnants (Figure 9.13). It often has a basket-woven appearance and is the keratin that is seen on epidermal surfaces. Within the oral cavity, orthokeratinized epithelium is seen primarily on attached mucosal surfaces. In addition to the surface characteristics, it has a conspicuous granular cell layer, the **stratum granulosum**, just below the stratum superficiale. Stratum granulosum cells appear flatter than spinous cells, with ovoid nuclei and conspicuous basophilic keratohyalin granules that occupy their cytoplasms (Figure 9.13). The appearance of these globular granules, composed of **filaggrin** and **trichohyalin**, signals the initiation of the final stage of squamous **apoptosis**. It results from a rapid drop in pH (7.17 to 5.0), with consequent desmosomal degradation and complete breakdown of nuclear structures and organelles (Figure 9.7).

Parakeratin describes a keratotic surface in which nuclei are retained and appear shrunken, spindly, and dark (pyknotic) (Figures 9.13, 9.25). On H & E staining, parakeratinized epithelium is paler and relatively more eosinophilic than orthokeratin. Additionally, in parakeratinized epithelium there is no stratum granulosum evident on light microscopy (Figures 9.13, 9.25). Parakeratinized epithelium is seen surfacing the filiform papillae, vermilion border of the lip, dorsal tongue, and in areas where there is relatively rapid turnover of epithelium.

Oral stratified squamous epithelial cells:

- in the stratum basale are attached to the basement membrane by hemidesmosomes. They are cuboidal, proliferate by mitotic division, and migrate upward.
- in the stratum spinosum are attached to one another by desmosomes. They are larger than basal cells, nonproliferative, and proceed toward the stratum superficiale.
- in the stratum granulosum contain basophilic cytoplasmic granules. Nonkeratinized and parakeratinized epithelium lack a stratum granulosum.
- in the stratum superficiale have reached maturity. They are flat, nonproliferative, and will ultimately be shed from the surface into the oral cavity.

The epithelial-stromal interface

The basal-most layer of epithelial cells is attached to a basement membrane, an interface zone that separates the epithelium from the papillary layer of the lamina propria, where the capillary-rich, loose, thin fibrocollagenous tissue is arranged in papillary (finger-like) upward projections that interdigitate with the epithelial rete pegs (Figure 9.8). Because squamous epithelium itself is avascular, this intimate hand-in-glove relationship between the epithelium and the connective tissue immediately beneath it provides for the greatest possible surface area for nutrient exchange and waste elimination, intercommunication, dispersion of mechanical forces that are exacted on the epithelial surface, immunologic protection, and sensation. The length, width, and number of rete pegs vary with respect to oral location and the functional demands exacted on the mucosa in that site. For example, there are more rete pegs per unit area in attached gingival and hard palatal mucosa (masticatory mucosa) than in the buccal mucosa (lining mucosa).

The basement membrane is the complex interface zone between the overlying squamous epithelium and the underlying connective tissue stroma.

On light microscopy the basement membrane appears as an uncomplicated line of demarcation between the overlying epithelium and the underlying lamina propria. This apparent simplicity is deceptive: electron microscopy reveals an elegantly organized and complex construction, the **basal lamina**. The basal lamina consists of two layers, an electron-lucent **lamina lucida** adjacent to the basal membrane of the epithelial cells, and the **lamina densa**. The lamina densa is a distinct, coarse, electron-dense web of filaments comprised of a meshwork of extracellular matrix proteins that forms an anchoring substrate for the hemidesmosomes of the overlying cells. This foundation consists primarily of laminins (laminin 5), type IV collagen, perlecan, and several other glycoproteins and proteoglycans (Figure 9.12).

The hemidesmosomes in stratified squamous epithelium are composed of a heterodimer, α6β4 integrin that links the intermediate filament **cytoskeleton** to the basement membrane meshwork. As described above, linking proteins like BP230 and BP180 (collagen XVII) tether the integrins to the actin/keratin cytoskeleton within the cytoplasm. The extracellular domain of the hemidesmosome binds to the laminin 5 heterotrimer, which in turn is bound down to the underlying collagen IV and perlecan substrate (Figure 9.12). Inferior to the lamina densa and attached to it in a series of loops are the vertically oriented collagen VII anchoring fibrils. They are bound down to horizontally oriented collagen I fibers within the superficial lamina propria. These in turn are threaded and woven into the collagen of the underlying reticular lamina propria. This complex macro- and microscopic attachment apparatus provides a resilient, flexible base capable of responding to and resisting shearing forces.

Non-keratinocytes

In addition to the normal population of keratinocytes, there are other non-keratinocytic specialized cells that reside within the epithelium. Among them are the melanocytes, the Langerhans cells, and Merkel cells. In addition to the aforementioned non-keratinocytes, lymphocytes, and other inflammatory cells may migrate transiently into the epithelium.

Melanocytes

Melanocytes are dendritic cells derived from the neural crest, and are responsible for the elaboration of melanin pigment. During embryonal development they migrate into the basal-most layer of the epithelium, where they are distributed among the basal keratinocytes and attach themselves to the basement membrane (Figures 9.11a, 9.11b). Although melanocytes have the appearance of clear cells among the basal keratinocytes on light microscopy, they actively produce melanin in Golgi-derived structures called **premelanosomes**, by the oxidation of tyrosine to 3, 4-dihydroxy-phenylalanine (DOPA) via tyrosinase. As more melanin is produced the premelanosome eventually matures into a mature melanin granule, the **melanosome**. Transfer of pigment-carrying melanosomes to neighboring keratinocytes is accomplished through the process of phagocytosis, whereby the tips of the melanocytic **dendrites** are phagocytized by keratinocytes. The melanin obtained in this manner can be dispersed among other keratinocytes in more distant layers. Irrespective of skin color, the number of melanocytes per unit area is unchanging so that darker pigmentation is a function of increased melanin production and decreased melanin degradation rather than an increase in the number of pigment producing cells. In some inflammatory conditions, melanocytes and melanin-containing keratinocytes within the epithelium can become disrupted and spill melanin pigment into the lamina propria region where it is phagocytized and contained within **melanophages**. This phenomenon is termed inflammatory melanin incontinence (Figure 9.11c).

Langerhans cells

Langerhans cells are immunologically active, dendritic cells that originate from myeloid precursors in the bone marrow. They migrate into the oral mucosal epithelium and remain in the stratum spinosum (Figure 9.14). They survey the local environment and present antigen to subpopulations of T-cells that in turn act in response to cytokines secreted by the epithelial cells. In this manner, Langerhans cells are key functionaries in the process of immune-surveillance and in essence link the oral mucosa with the entire immune system.

Merkel cells

Independent of keratinocytes and the non-keratinocytic dendritic cells, **Merkel cells** are a self-maintaining population believed to have neurosecretory properties associated with the special sense of pressure perception. Once thought to be derived from the neural crest, it is now known that Merkel cells arise from an epithelial progenitor cell during development. They

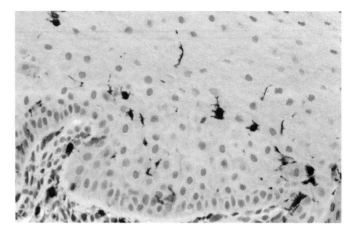

Figure 9.14   S-100 immunohistochemistry, Langerhans cells. Immunohistochemistry reveals dendritic Langerhans cells (brown stain) within the stratified squamous epithelium.

reside among the epithelial basal cells in close proximity to terminal axons in the lamina propria that function as neuroepithelial tactile receptors.

Non-Keratinocytes

- Melanocytes reside in the stratum basale. They are dendritic and distribute melanin pigment widely to keratinocytes. Irrespective of skin color, the number of melanocytes is constant.
- Langerhans cells reside in the stratum spinosum. They are antigen-presenting cells and participate in immune surveillance.
- Merkel cells are neurosecretory cells that play a role related to proprioception.

Types of oral mucosa

Oral mucosa is subdivided into three basic types: **moveable (or lining) mucosa, masticatory mucosa**, and **specialized mucosa**, based on anatomic location and the corresponding functional demands on that location within the mouth. Specialized mucosa is found on the dorsal tongue exclusively.

Lining (moveable) mucosa

Much of the surface area of both the oral cavity and oral vestibule is lined by lining (moveable) mucosa. As compared with masticatory mucosa, lining mucosa is surfaced by nonkeratinized stratified squamous epithelium with relatively short and broad rete pegs. Lining mucosa includes the labial and buccal mucosae, their contiguous vestibular and alveolar mucosae, the soft palate, uvula and tonsillar pillars, floor of the mouth, and lateral and ventral surfaces of the tongue, locations where the oral mucous membrane is pliable, moveable, and not attached to underlying bone. The submucosal layers of the labial and buccal mucosae and the ventral tongue mucosa demonstrate varying amounts of minor salivary glands, adipose tissue and striated muscle (Figures 9.9, 9.10). The submucosal layers of the above areas are fixed to the epimysium of underlying striated muscle bundles and are therefore capable of stretching. As compared to the attached gingival and hard palatal mucosae, lining mucosa is less subject to frictional tear and shearing forces from direct contact with food during the process of mastication. However, the buccal and labial mucosae in particular are readily exposed to traumatic agents, including the teeth, so that their resiliency is frequently challenged.

Masticatory mucosa

The attached gingiva and hard palatal tissues comprise masticatory mucosa that is bound down to underlying alveolar bone. Masticatory mucosa is immobile and thinner and firmer than lining mucosa (Figure 9.15a). Unlike moveable mucosa, masticatory mucosa is surfaced by keratinized stratified squamous epithelium that has more numerous and longer rete pegs that interdigitate with taller papillary projections of the underlying papillary lamina propria. The clinically obvious stippled, orange peel-like appearance of normal attached gingiva is attributable to the latter epithelium–connective tissue relationship (Figure 9.15b). The lamina propria of gingival masticatory mucosa is a mucoperiosteum, comprised of coarse collagen fibers that are directly attached and essentially fixed to the periosteum of the underlying alveolar process. There is no submucosal layer in gingival masticatory mucosa, so that attached gingiva has neither adipose tissue nor submucosal glands.

With the exception of the palatal gingival mucosa adjacent to the teeth, the masticatory mucosa of the hard palate does have submucosal tissue layers, and can be subdivided into regions distinguished from one another by their respective submucosal contents. The palatal zone lying anterior and lateral to the midline palatal raphe contains abundant adipose tissue and is designated as the fatty region; by contrast, the zone posterior and lateral to the fatty region that lies between the gingiva and the palatal raphe is the so-called glandular region, with abundant submucosal glands (Figure 9.16).

Specialized mucosa

The mucosa on the dorsal surface of the tongue is designated as specialized because it contains four distinct types of surface projections, the **lingual papillae** (Figures 9.6, 9.17). Three of the four types of lingual papillae are unique in that they carry taste receptors, the taste buds. The physiology of taste is described in Chapter 10.

Filiform papillae

Filiform papillae are the most abundant of all of the lingual papillae. They cover much of the anterior two-thirds of the dorsal tongue surface, and are responsible for its typically light pink or whitish color and relatively rough, somewhat abrasive texture (Figures 9.6a, 9.6b). The latter feature plays a role in the process of chewing and preparing food for swallowing, so that functionally the dorsal tongue is also a masticatory mucosal surface. Under the microscope filiform papillae appear as rows of keratinized (cornified) chevron-like extensions of the thick surface epithelium that point in a posterior direction toward

(a)

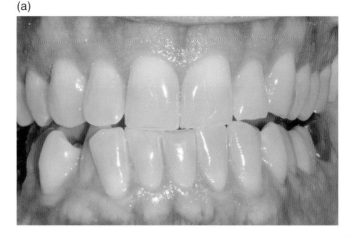

(b)

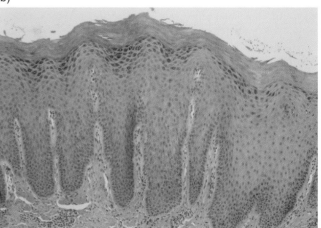

Figure 9.15   Masticatory mucosa, attached gingiva. (a) In comparison to lining (moveable) mucosa, the attached gingiva is characterized by its pale-pink color and stippled texture. (b) The latter features are attributable to the thick, undulating orthokeratin layer and the longer, more abundant rete pegs that interdigitate with the underlying connective tissue papillae, respectively.

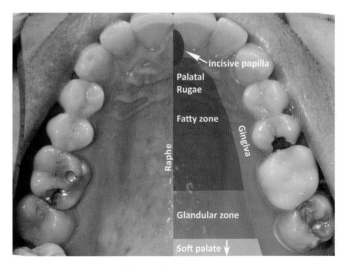

Figure 9.16   The zones of the palate.

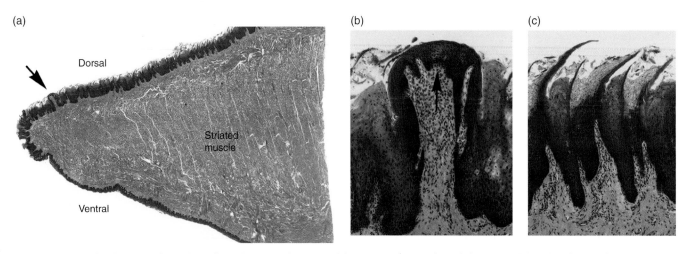

Figure 9.17   Specialized mucosa: lingual papillae. (a) A sagittal section of the tongue shows a heavily keratinized dorsal surface. Filiform papillae create a corrugated appearance. The ventral surface is nonkeratinized. Scattered amongst the filiform papillae are occasional fungiform papillae (arrow). (b) A fungiform papilla with taste bud (arrow) on the superior surface. (c) Numerous small filiform papillae, with their chevron-like parakeratotic surfaces and a thin core of connective tissue.

the oropharynx (Figures 9.17a, 9.17c). Over a period of several hours, superficial waste matter consisting of food particles, secretory material, desquamated keratin that is constantly shed into the oral cavity through natural cellular attrition, and various other debris tends to accumulate among the filiform papillae. On clinical examination this may impart a temporarily white "coated" appearance to the dorsal tongue surface. At regular intervals throughout the day, the cumulative material is naturally debrided from among the filiform papillae through normal masticatory function, and eliminated into the oropharynx through deglutition (swallowing). Unlike the other three types of lingual papillae, filiform papillae are devoid of taste buds.

Fungiform papillae

Fungiform papillae are far fewer in number than the filiform papillae. They appear as single small, round, smooth-surfaced, mushroom-like surface projections that are scattered among the filiform papillae in the tip region and anterior portion of the dorsal tongue (Figures 9.6a, 9.17a, 9.17b). Their often pink to reddish color is attributable to absence of keratin on their surfaces and a richly vascular underlying connective tissue core. On their superior surfaces, fungiform papillae bear taste buds (Figure 9.17b).

Foliate papillae

Foliate papillae are located on the far posterolateral surfaces of the oral tongue. They present clinically as a cluster of several slightly raised, pink- or orange-colored parallel surface ridges separated by grooves that run perpendicular to the long axis of the tongue (Figure 9.4). In many individuals they may be subtle, and therefore difficult to identify on clinical examination. Under the microscope, the nonkeratinized surface epithelium that lines the ridges of these papillae is punctuated by numerous taste buds whose sensory receptive endings open into the intervening grooves that separate an individual foliate papilla from its neighbor. The increased surface area allows for prolonged contact with chemical substances introduced into the oral cavity, thus enhancing their ability to stimulate taste signals.

Circumvallate (vallate) papillae

Individual circumvallate papillae are the largest of all the lingual papillae. There are on average 12 or fewer circumvallate papillae located on the posterior one-third of the dorsal tongue surface. Lined up in two obliquely oriented rows, they converge in a V-formation that runs immediately anterior to and parallel with the terminal sulcus and whose apex points toward the foramen cecum and oropharynx (Figures 9.6a, 9.6b). On protrusion of the tongue, they are readily recognizable as reddish or orange-colored, round, slightly raised nodules, each of which on closer inspection is encircled by a trough. The epithelium on the superior surface of a circumvallate papilla is covered with a thin layer of keratin. By contrast, the epithelium lining the troughs is nonkeratinized and is punctuated by numerous taste buds (Figures 9.6c, 9.6d). The excretory ducts of underlying serous-secreting minor salivary glands, **von Ebner's (lingual serous) glands**, exit into the bases of the troughs between the papillae. Chemical reactants in foods and other ingested substances enter the troughs, are dissolved in the serous secretions from von Ebner's glands, and bathe the taste receptors that open into the troughs. This anatomic arrangement also serves to enhance the mechanism of taste perception.

Specialized mucosa of the tongue

- Filiform papillae are hair-like, the most numerous, and lack taste receptors.

- Fungiform papillae are distributed on the dorsal tongue as small papules. They have taste receptors.

- Foliate papillae are located on the posterolateral surface of the tongue bilaterally. They are oriented perpendicular to the long axis of the tongue and have numerous taste receptors.

- Circumvallate papillae are located on the posterior third of the dorsal tongue. They are the largest of the lingual papillae and converge at the foramen cecum. They have circumferentially situated taste receptors on their lateral surfaces.

Oral sensation

As noted in the Introduction, the structures and tissues of the oral cavity must be able to sense a variety of stimuli, including food substances of various textures, taste, temperature, and chemical agents, and non-food objects. Additionally, the functions of mastication, swallowing, and speaking require exquisite tactile and proprioceptive information. Thus, the oral cavity, including the mucosa, teeth, and periodontal tissues, has a rich sensory innervation.

Cranial nerve V – The trigeminal nerve

Somatosensory information from the oral cavity is transmitted to the central nervous system (CNS) primarily via the fifth cranial nerve. The **trigeminal nerve** (literally, "three twins") is the largest of the twelve cranial nerves and has three main branches: the ophthalmic, the maxillary, and the mandibular (Figure 9.18). The ophthalmic and maxillary branches are wholly sensory; there are no efferent fibers in either branch. Afferent ophthalmic innervation includes the forehead, eyes, nose, and mucous membranes of the frontal sinus and nasal vestibule. Afferent maxillary fibers innervate the upper lip, upper cheek, upper jaw, upper teeth, and roof of the mouth to the palatopharyngeal arch. The mandibular branch

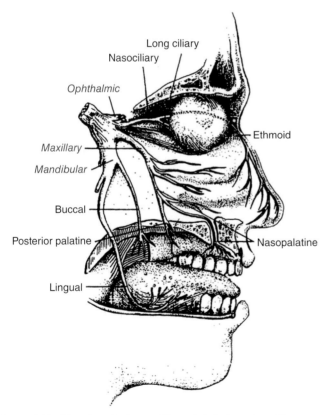

Figure 9.18   The trigeminal nerve. The ophthalmic and maxillary divisions of the trigeminal nerve provide wholly sensory information while the mandibular division contains both sensory and motor fibers. (From Finger T.E., Silver W.L., & Restrepo, D., eds. (2000). *The Neurobiology of Taste and Smell*, 2nd edn. p. 75. Wiley-Liss. Reproduced by permission of John Wiley & Sons.).

contains afferent and efferent fibers. Afferent mandibular innervation includes the lower lip, lower cheek, lower jaw, lower teeth, and anterior two-thirds of the tongue and floor of the mouth. Efferent mandibular innervation includes the muscles of mastication, the tensor veli palatini, which tenses the soft palate, the digastric muscle, which depresses the mandible, and the tensor tympani (Table 9.1).

Sensory nerve endings

There are three general types of sensory nerve endings present in the oral mucosa: free nerve endings in the lamina propria and epithelium; nerve endings associated with Merkel cells; and encapsulated nerve endings, such as Meissner's corpuscles located in the lamina propria. Trigeminal free nerve endings are present throughout the oral cavity, but are most numerous in the tongue, the anterior portion of the mouth, and the lips. Unmyelinated intraepithelial nerve fibers extend between keratinocytes to the middle or upper layers of the epithelium (Figure 9.19a and b). These fibers may respond to a variety of stimuli, including temperature, touch, and chemicals. Merkel cells, located in the stratum basale of the epithelium, contain neurosecretory granules and respond to touch. Expanded, disk-shaped unmyelinated endings of large, myelinated **Aβ nerve fibers** make contact with the Merkel cell (Figure 9.19b), forming a Merkel's disk. Meissner's corpuscles are located in the papillae of the lamina propria that indent the basal side of the epithelium (Figure 9.20). They are sensitive to low-frequency touch stimuli. They consist of unmyelinated endings of large, myelinated Aβ fibers that form a spiral within a capsule of flattened Schwann cells.

> The three branches of the trigeminal nerve provide the general sensory innervation for the oral cavity. The main types of sensory endings in the oral mucosa are free nerve endings, Merkel's disks, and Meissner's corpuscles.

Temperature sensation and TRP channels

The term **chemesthesis** describes sensations that occur as a result of chemicals activating receptor mechanisms for senses other than gustation or olfaction, usually somatosensation (i.e., pain, touch, and temperature). In the face, eyes, nose, and oral region chemesthesis involves activation of **transient receptor potential (TRP) channels** located on epithelial and mucosal trigeminal free nerve endings. Although the receptor mechanisms involved in astringency remain unknown, the "heat" of hot chili peppers and the "cool" sensation of peppermint are mediated via TRP channel activation.

TRP channels play critical roles in the response to every sensory stimulus, including light, sound, chemicals, temperature, and touch. All TRP channel proteins have 6 transmembrane domains, share various degrees of sequence homology, and are permeable to cations. Depending on channel specificity, TRP channels allow Na^+, K^+, and/or Ca^{++} to enter the cell and alter the membrane potential. Thermo-TRP

Table 9.1   Sensory and motor innervation within the three major divisions of the trigeminal nerve

Ophthalmic (V$_1$) General Somatic Afferent	Maxillary (V$_2$) General Somatic Afferent	Mandibular (V$_3$) General Somatic Afferent

Frontal
    Supraorbital: frontal sinus, forehead, scalp
    Supratrochlear: medial conjunctiva, side of nose, medial upper eyelid, forehead
 	
Nasociliary
    Anterior & posterior ethmoidal: ethmoidal air sinuses
    Internal nasal: anterior nasal septum
    External nasal: skin of the dorsum, apex of nose
    Infratrochlear: lacrimal sac, caruncle, conjunctiva, medial canthus skin
    Long ciliary: ciliary body, iris, cornea
    Short ciliary: globe of the eye
 	
Lacrimal: lateral conjunctiva, lateral upper eyelid, skin near lacrimal gland
 	
Tentorial (Meningeal): tentorium cerebelli, dura of cavernous sinus, sphenoid wing, anterior fossa, petrous ridge, Meckel's cave, posterior falx cerebri, dural venous sinuses
	Zygomatic
	    Zygomaticotemporal: side of forehead skin, lateral angle of orbit
	    Zygomaticofacial: prominence of the cheek skin
	
	Infraorbital
	    Inferior palpebral: lower eyelid skin, conjunctiva
	    External nasal: side of nose
	    Superior labial: upper lip
	    Superior alveolar
	        Posterior: maxillary sinus, maxillary molars, gums and cheek
	        Medial: maxillary premolars
	        Anterior: maxillary incisors & canines
	
	Pterygopalatine
	    Orbital: orbital periosteum
	    Greater palatine: upper gingivae, hard palate
	    Lesser palatine: soft palate, uvula, tonsils
	    Posterior superior nasal: superior and middle nasal conchae, posterior septum
	    Posterior inferior nasal: inferior nasal conchae
	    Pharyngeal: nasopharynx
	
	Meningeal: dura of middle cranial fossa
		Buccal: buccal mucous membranes, cheek skin
		
		Auriculotemporal: side of head & scalp
		    Anterior auricular: helix & tragus skin
		    External acoustic meatus: external acoustic meatus skin, tympanic membrane
		    Articular: temporomandibular joint
		    Superficial temporal: temporal region skin
		
		Lingual: anterior 2/3 of the tongue (not taste), floor of mouth, mucous membrane of mouth and mandibular gingivae
		
		Inferior alveolar: mandibular molars & premolars
		    Mandibular incisive: mandibular canines & incisors
		
		Special Visceral Efferent*
		
		Masseteric: masseter muscle
		Deep temporal: temporalis muscle
		Lateral pterygoid: lateral pterygoid muscle
		Medial pterygoid: medial pterygoid muscle, tensor palatini, tensor tympani
		Mylohyoid: mylohyoid and anterior belly of digastric muscle

*The mandibular division (V$_3$) is the only major branch to contain both efferent and afferent fibers.

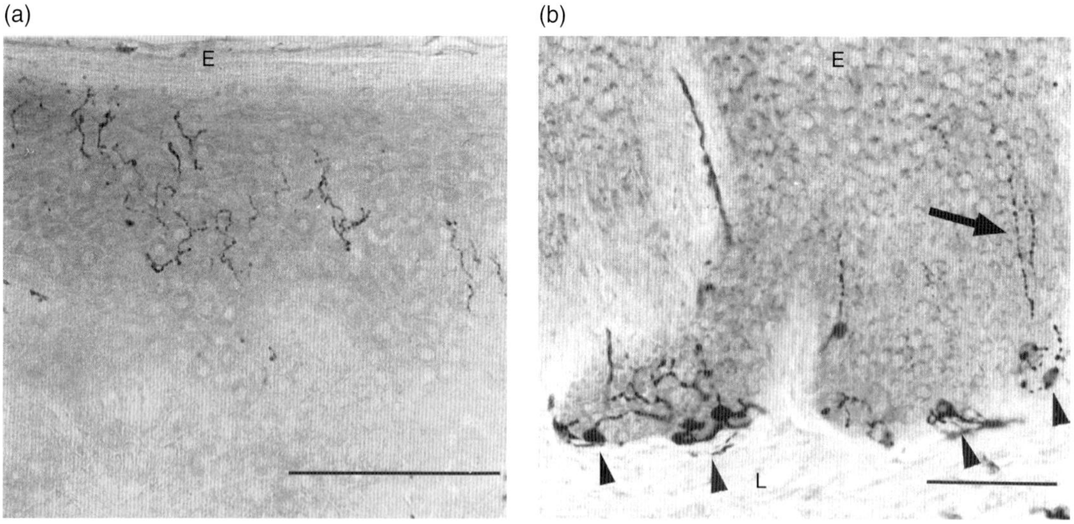

Figure 9.19   Mucosal innervation, free nerve endings, and Merkel's disks. Innervation of the oral mucosa demonstrated by immunohistochemical localization of protein gene product 9.5 (PGP 9.5), a neuronal marker. (a) Free intraepithelial nerve fibers in the alveolar mucosa reach the superficial layers of the epithelium (E). (b) Merkel cells (arrowheads) in the basal layer of the gingival epithelium are innervated by PGP 9.5-reactive nerve fibers. Free intraepithelial fibers (arrows) also are present. Scale bars = 50 μm. (From Ramieri, G. et al. (1990) The Iinnervation of Human teeth and gingival epithelium as revealed by means of an antiserum for protein gene product 9.5 (PGP 9.5). *American Journal of Anatomy* 189(2), pp. 146–154. Reproduced by permission of John Wiley and Sons.)

channels exist on the free nerve endings of myelinated **Aδ fibers** and unmyelinated **C fibers**.

The TRP genetic superfamily is divided into two groups, and thermoreceptors are members of three group 1 subfamilies: TRPV, TRPM, and TRPA (Figure 9.21). Warm receptors respond to temperatures between 25° C (77° F) and 45° C (113° F) while cool receptors respond to temperatures between 12° C (54° F) and 35° C (95° F). Responses to temperatures above 45° C or below 12° C are mediated by pain receptors called **polymodal nociceptors**. The terms "warm" and "cool" are relative to the receptor environment and thus, relative to epithelial body temperature, around 34° C or 93° F). Increases in temperature will activate warm receptors and inhibit cold receptors; conversely, decreases in temperature will activate cold receptors and inhibit warm receptors. The rate of response in the nerve fiber is proportional to the rate and degree of temperature change, and perceptions of cold or warmth depend upon the relative overall activation of these fibers to the central nervous system.

Capsaicin, the active ingredient in hot chili peppers, is perceived as hot even though no thermal heat transfer occurs. Capsaicin

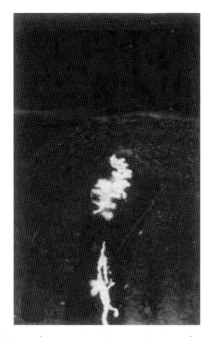

Figure 9.20   Mucosal innervation, Meissner's corpuscle. Immunofluorescent localization of PGP 9.5 in a Meissner's corpuscle (arrow) in the papillary layer of the gingival lamina propria. Scale bar = 50 µm. (From Hilliges, M. et al. (1996) Protein gene product 9.5-limmunoreactive nerves and cells in human oral mucosa., *Anatomical Record,* 245(4), pp. 621–632. Reproduced by permission of John Wiley and Sons.)

> ### Box 9.1 Adequate and inadequate sensory stimuli
>
> Generally speaking each sensory receptor responds particularly well to one type of stimulus. The stimulus to which a receptor is best tuned is called the adequate stimulus. The term adequate describes the relationship between the receptor and the stimulus that best activates it. Thermo-TRP channels are special cases of polymodal receptors; their adequate stimuli include changes in thermal energy and specific chemicals (e.g., **TRPV1** and capsaicin). In the case of auditory receptors, sound is an adequate stimulus and in the case of visual receptors, light is an adequate stimulus. Inadequate stimuli also activate sensory receptors, but require much greater strength to do so and are not tuned to the receptor *per se.* For example, the lingual branch of the trigeminal nerve will respond to 1 M NaCl. This is twice as strong as seawater and a thousand times more concentrated than what is necessary to stimulate the gustatory system. Therefore, NaCl is considered an inadequate trigeminal stimulus, but an adequate gustatory stimulus.

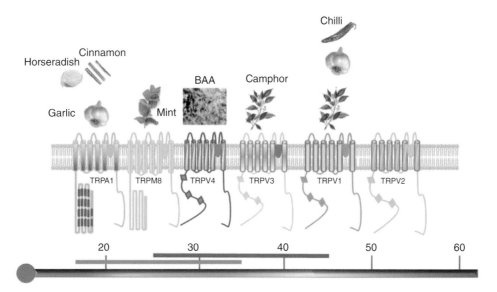

Figure 9.21   Transient receptor potential (TRP) channels. An illustration of six temperature- sensitive transient receptor potential (TRP) channels. Each TRP channel has six transmembrane segments; the channel pore is between segments 5 and 6. Thermal sensitivity is indicated by the color-coded thermometer (°C) and natural examples of exogenous non-thermal chemical stimuli are illustrated above each channel. The solid blue line illustrates the range of sensitivity to cool temperatures and the red line to warm temperatures. Temperature responses beyond the blue and red lines are mediated by polymodal nociceptors. The source of BAA is *Andrographis paniculata,* a bitter Chinese herb known as "the king of bitters." (From Vay, L., Gu, C. & McNaughton, P.A. (2012) The thermo-TRP ion channel family: properties and therapeutic implications. *British Journal of Pharmacology,* 165(4), pp. 787–801. Reproduced by permission of John Wiley & Sons.)

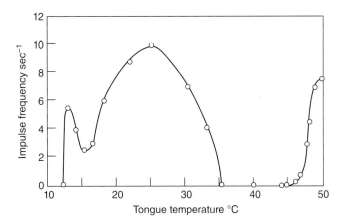

Figure 9.22 Paradoxical cold sensation. The temperature response profile of a cold-sensitive lingual nerve fiber recorded from the tongue of a cat. Impulse frequency peaks at 25° C and falls off with increasing temperature until ~35° C, when the fiber stops responding. The fiber is silent between 35 and 45° C and begins to fire again at temperatures above 45°. Humans describe the resulting sensation as "cold" regardless of stimulating temperature, thus the phenomenon known as paradoxical cold. This is a classic example of how a label-line coding system and coexpression of TRPV1 and TRPM8 on lingual free nerve endings of a single nerve fiber provides a physiological substrate for the illustrated response profile. (From Zotterman, Y. (1953) Special senses: thermal receptors. *Annual Reviews of Physiology*, 15, 357–372. Reproduced by permission of Annual Reviews, Palo Alto, CA.)

stimulates a distinct class of polymodal nociceptors and these nociceptors also respond to noxious heat stimuli, defined as temperatures greater than approximately 45° C (113° F). If a thermal fiber responds to capsaicin it also will respond to heat, but not all heat-sensitive receptors respond to capsaicin. For example, TRPV2 responds to heat (52° C or 126° F), but does not respond to capsaicin.

The receptive elements for capsaicin are located on the intracellular domain of the TRPV1 channel. Thus, capsaicin must pass through the lipid bilayer and into the cell in order to activate TRPV1. In general, the more lipophilic a chemical, the better it can penetrate the epithelia to activate thermal and nociceptive free nerve endings. TRPV1, 2, 3, and 4 all respond to various degrees of warming. In addition, TRPV3 also responds to menthol and camphor (Figure 9.21). Reports indicate that TRPV3 becomes sensitized under prolonged heat stimulation while TRPV4 becomes desensitized. TRPV4 also is activated by membrane stretch, and TRPV3 and TRPV4 are found in keratinocytes.

Just as hot polymodal nociceptors can be stimulated by capsaicin, cool receptors can be stimulated by menthol. The TRPM8 (melastatin) receptor, formerly called cool menthol receptor 1, is activated by menthol and temperature decreases below 26° C (79° F). As with TRPV1, TRPM8 is found on lingual nerve fibers innervating the tongue and lingual perigemmal fibers of fungiform taste buds. TRPM8 is also found on nerve fibers innervating tooth dentin and tooth pulp (see Chapter 5, "Dentin, Pulp, and Tooth Pain").

Some research shows that the TRPA1 channel is activated at extremely cold temperatures (<12° C (54° F)), but this result is not without controversy. TRPA1 is also activated by compounds such as cinnamon, mustard oil, and hydrogen peroxide (Figure 9.21). Thus some speculate that TRPA1 functions as a polymodal nociceptor. Experiments also show a subpopulation of trigeminal neurons in culture that respond to both menthol and capsaicin. This implies that TRPM8 and TRPV1 are coexpressed in a subpopulation of trigeminal neurons and suggests a physiological substrate for the phenomenon of **paradoxical cold**. Paradoxical cold occurs when "cool" sensitive fibers are stimulated by noxious heat (>45° C) (Figure 9.22).

In any given area of stimulation cold receptors are about 10 to 15 times more numerous than warm receptors. There are separate epithelial spots, each about 1 mm in diameter, where thermal stimulation elicits a sensation of either warmth or cold. These thermal spots correspond to the receptive fields of the free nerve endings. Trigeminal thermoreceptors have dynamic and static discharge rates. Cold and warm trigeminal fibers discharge intensely with a change in temperature and then adapt to a new steady state. Cold fibers typically respond with an initial high transient rate followed by an adaptation pattern of cyclic bursts. The larger the change in temperature the more intensely a thermal fiber responds.

> TRP channels are critical to the performance of every sensory system in the body. In the oral cavity TRP channels play a vital role in sensing thermal, stretch (touch), taste, and painful stimuli.

Clinical correlations

Illustrative case 1

Chief complaint and history: This 49-year-old Asian woman presents herself to the clinic accompanied by her teenage daughter for diagnosis and treatment of "extremely painful mouth sores" that have been progressing in severity over the past two months. The daughter says that her mother's oral pain has become so intense that for over a week she has been unable to eat any solid food or drink liquids comfortably. The patient cannot brush her teeth because the oral mucosa is so fragile that it "peels off and gets raw and painful." The daughter says that up until the onset of this problem her mother had been systemically healthy, active, and on no medications. Now, she is unable to speak clearly or sleep through the night because of the pain. On questioning, the patient denies having any open sores, blisters, or other lesions on any other mucous membranes (e.g., nasal, anogenital) or on the skin.

Examination: The oral examination reveals extensive **erythematous** (red), ragged-appearing erosions on the buccal and labial mucosae, the tongue, floor of mouth, and soft palate (Figures 9.23a, 9.23b). On gentle lateral pressure applied to areas with intact mucosa, the surface epithelium sloughs away leaving raw and painful erosions, indicating a positive Nikolsky sign. Biopsies are obtained for conventional and direct **immunofluorescence** microscopy.

Microscopy: The conventionally stained sections demonstrate intraepithelial vesicle formation due to loss of adhesion among the stratum spinosum cells (a process called "**acantholysis**")

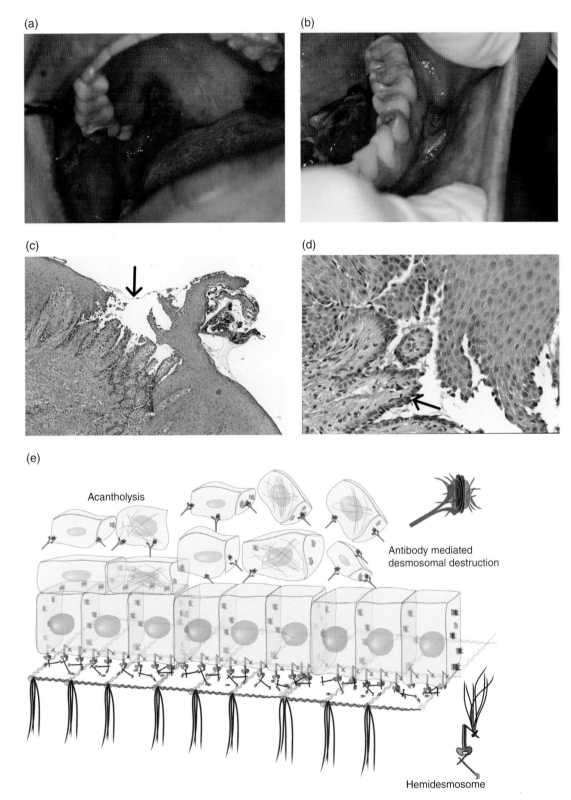

Figure 9.23   Case 1. Pemphigus vulgaris. Clinical photographs (a & b) demonstrating erythema and ulceration on (a) the buccal mucosa, soft palate, and (b) floor of mouth and mandibular buccal vestibule. Photomicrographs demonstrating (c) ruptured intraepithelial vesicle (arrow). (d) Higher magnification demonstrating suprabasal separation (acantholysis). Note that the spinous cells have separated from the *stratum basale* (arrow). (e) Schematic diagram of acantholysis, which in the case of pemphigus, is mediated by antibody directed against the desmosomes. Note that the hemidesmosomes are intact and the basal cells remain attached to the basement membrane.

(Figure 9.23c). The separation is occurring above the stratum basale, so that the basal cells remain intact and adherent to the basement membrane (Figure 9.23d). Direct immunofluorescence (DIF) reveals positive intercellular fluorescence that resembles a fishnet between the spinous cells for immune reactants (IgG and C3) bound to and attacking the desmosomes (DIF not shown).

In composite, the clinical and pathological features are diagnostic for **pemphigus vulgaris**.

Autoimmune diseases

There are several immunologically mediated dermatological conditions that may be accompanied by oral mucosal and other mucous membrane lesions. They are therefore considered **mucocutaneous** conditions. Although the underlying pathophysiologic mechanism of each mucocutaneous disease is unique, affected patients can present with a wide range of strikingly similar-appearing clinical lesions and symptoms that can create a diagnostic challenge for the clinician. Among the more serious mucocutaneous conditions with potential for involvement of the oral mucosa are **pemphigus** and **pemphigoid**, two distinct groups of chronic vesiculobullous (blistering) diseases whose names derive from the Greek word for blister, **pemphix**. Both pemphigus and pemphigoid are among the mucocutaneous diseases characterized by a positive **Nikolsky sign**. This is revealed clinically as tactile-induced fragility and/or bulla formation with resultant sloughing of the skin or mucosal surface. The Nikolsky sign is a diagnostically nonspecific clinical indication of weakness in either the desmosomal intercellular attachment between the epithelial spinous cells, or the hemidesmosomal attachment to the lamina propria at the epithelial-stromal interface.

The pemphigus group of diseases consists of four subtypes: (1) **pemphigus vulgaris**, the most common type and the one that most often involves oral mucosa; (2) **pemphigus vegetans**, frequently considered a variant of pemphigus vulgaris; (3) **pemphigus erythematosus**; and (4) **pemphigus foliaceous**. Irrespective of subtype, the underlying mechanism of disease in pemphigus is immune-mediated acantholysis, that is, loss of cell-to-cell adhesion in the stratum spinosum so that the spinous layer essentially falls apart, while the stratum basale remains intact and attached to the underlying basement membrane (Figures 9.23c, 9.23d, 9.23e). In pemphigus vulgaris the humoral arm of the immune system elaborates IgG autoantibody and C3. These immune reactants target the desmosomes, specifically desmoglein 3, a glycoprotein cadherin linked to the intermediate filaments of the cytoskeleton (Figures 9.12, 9.23). This causes the spinous cells to separate from one another, compromising the integrity of the epidermis in the skin and the epithelium in the mucosa, respectively. In clinical terms, acantholysis in pemphigus can present as cutaneous and/or mucosal blisters and fragility, desquamation (sloughing), and painful ulcerations (Figure 9.23). Untreated, pemphigus can be a devastating and even fatal disease. In about 60% of patients with pemphigus vulgaris, oral mucosal lesions antecede cutaneous lesions by months. Therefore, diagnosing the condition while it is confined to the oral mucosa and initiating appropriate treatment expediently can be effective not only for managing the oral manifestations, but for attenuating or preventing the emergence of cutaneous involvement.

There are two subtypes of pemphigoid (Table 9.2.): (1) bullous pemphigoid, which affects the skin primarily but may have accompanying mucosal lesions; and (2) mucous membrane (cicatricial, or scarring) pemphigoid, which can involve one or more mucosal tissues (i.e., oral, ocular, genital, etc.) exclusively and is neither accompanied, preceded, nor followed by cutaneous involvement. In either type of pemphigoid, **humoral** auto-immunity mediated (i.e., antibody mediated) by IgG and C3 is

Table 9.2   Important oral epithelial structures and associated oral disease

Basal keratinocyte		• Lichen planus – *(CM)*
Keratin		• White sponge nevus – *(Inh.)* • Darier-White disease – *(Inh.)*
Desmosomes		• Pemphigus – *(Ab)* • Benign familial pemphigus - *(Ab)* • Paraneoplastic pemphigus – *(CM & Ab)* • Pemphigus-like drug reaction - *(CM)*
Hemidesmosomes	Structure	Disease
	Integrins	• Mucosal pemphigoid – *(Ab)*
	BP180 BP230	• Bullous pemphigoid – *(Ab)*
	Laminin	• Junctional epidermolysis bullosa – *(Inh.)*
Basement membrane protein		Disease
Collagen VII, Laminins etc.		• Epidermolysis bullosa acquisita – *(Ab)* • Inherited epidermolysis bullosa – *(Inh.)*

CM.: Cell mediated immunological disease
Ab.: Antibody mediated immunological disease
Inh.: Inherited, genetic condition

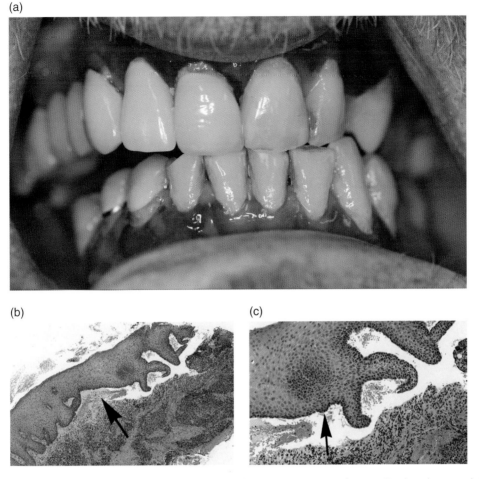

Figure 9.24   Mucosal pemphigoid. (a) Clinical photograph demonstrates classic presentation with generalized erythema and desquamation of gingiva. (b) Low- power magnification photomicrograph shows complete separation of the squamous epithelium from the underlying basement membrane resulting in a subepithelial vesicle (arrow). (c) Higher power highlights the complete separation of basal cells (arrow) from the underlying basement membrane leaving a space between the epithelium and the connective tissue. In the case of pemphigoid this results from immune-mediated destruction of the hemidesmosomal attachment.

directed against the hemidesmosomes (Figure 9.12) so that the basal cells' attachment to the basement membrane zone is disrupted, resulting in separation and "lifting off" of the entire width of the epithelium from the underlying lamina propria (Figures 9.24b, 9.24c). Clinically, oral mucous membrane pemphigoid can affect any and all oral mucosal locations, but the disease most often presents as a chronic erythematous and desquamative gingival condition that tends to wax and wane both symptomatically and in terms of clinically visible disease activity (Figure 9.24a). Although bullae may be seen on occasion, blisters in the mouth are rarely intact because they tend to rupture readily, leaving erosions or ulcerations.

In order to distinguish pemphigus from pemphigoid and from several other different conditions with similar clinical presentations, diagnosis is established by taking two representative tissue biopsy specimens of oral mucosa, of which one is submitted in formalin for conventional light microscopic examination and the other placed in a transport medium that allows for its analysis using direct immunofluorescence (DIF) technique. DIF analysis discloses (1) presence or absence of immune reactants (antibody, antibody-antigen complexes, complement, fibrin,

etc.); (2) precisely where in the tissue the immune reactants are located (e.g., intercellular within the epithelium, subepithelial, or perivascular, etc.); and (3) which particular immune reactants are identified.

Table 9.2 lists other selected important oral epithelial structures and their associated disease states.

Illustrative case 2

Chief complaint and history: The patient is a healthy 53-year-old man who admits to having a cheek- and tongue-biting habit.

Clinical examination reveals extensive, shaggy white **plaques** (slightly raised areas on the mucosa/skin caused by increase in the width of the surface epithelium) on the left and right buccal mucosae and the lateral tongue borders (Figures 9.25a, 9.25b). The white plaques do not wipe off and are not associated with any discomfort. Although the dentist assures him that the changes are suggestive of a benign, callus-like reaction of the oral mucosa to chronic friction (benign reactive hyperkeratosis or reactive epithelial hyperplasia), the patient is afraid that he has cancer and asks for a biopsy.

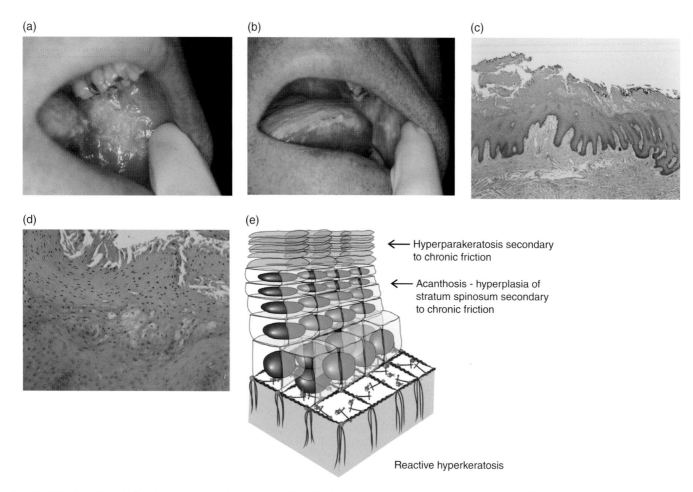

Figure 9.25 Case 2. Hyperkeratosis secondary to chronic friction. Clinical photographs demonstrating shaggy, diffuse white plaques on (a) buccal mucosa and (b) dorsolateral tongue. These asymptomatic plaques were non-wipable and distributed bilaterally. (c) Low- power photomicrograph demonstrates epithelial hyperplasia (acanthosis) with irregular -appearing, prominent thickening of the stratum superficiale (hyperkeratosis). (d) At higher magnification the stratum superficiale is characterized by hyperparakeratosis (note the intact, pyknotic nuclei within the superficial layers). (e) Schematic diagram demonstrating reactive hyperkeratosis.

Microscopy: Examination reveals hyperkeratosis (increase in width of the stratum superficiale) and epithelial hyperplasia (increase in width of the stratum spinosum, or **acanthosis**), benign reactive responses of the stratified squamous epithelium to chronic friction (Figures 9.25c, 9.25d, 9.25e).

Benign reactive epithelial hyperplasia/reactive hyperkeratosis

Among the most commonly occurring benign oral lesions are white, rough-surfaced, non-wipable plaques that arise on oral mucosal surfaces that are subjected to chronic low-grade irritation from friction. Some classic trauma- or friction-prone oral locations include the buccal and labial mucosa, where the teeth interdigitate throughout the day during both function and rest; the attached gingiva, which comes into frictional contact with foods and oral hygiene implements; and the hard palate and dorsolateral surfaces of the tongue. The white plaques are usually asymptomatic and discovered incidentally by either the patient or the dentist. In most cases the source of irritation (e.g., a sharp tooth or teeth, a fractured dental restoration, an ill-fitting dental prosthesis, an orthodontic appliance, a nontherapeutic foreign

object) is readily identifiable. The resulting white plaque, termed benign reactive hyperkeratosis or reactive epithelial hyperplasia, is analogous to a callus that develops on the palmar surface of the hand or the plantar surface of the foot. It represents an increase in either the surface keratin layer or the width of the stratum spinosum (acanthosis), or a combination of both, with otherwise normal epithelial cytomorphology and maturation (Figure 9.25e).

On oral examination, the resulting increase in surface keratinization and/or epithelial width causes the mucosa to appear white because there is a greater distance for light to pass through after it reflects off of the underlying blood vessels and back to the examiner's eye. By far the most commonly occurring example of benign reactive hyperkeratosis is linea alba, the thin, non-wipable white horizontal line that appears along the buccal mucosa, often bilaterally, in response to friction from the constant interdigitation of the teeth in function, rest, and parafunction. Benign reactive hyperkeratoses are essentially innocuous and require no treatment. The diagnosis is presumptively made from clinical examination and history, or it can be confirmed by microscopic examination of a representative biopsy specimen. If the irritant can be identified and completely eradicated, in time a benign hyperkeratotic white mucosal plaque will usually disappear. However, if the irritant persists or is reintroduced, the white plaque will likely persist or recur in response.

When a white, non-wipable oral mucosal plaque is discovered on an intraoral site that is relatively protected from most physically traumatic agents, like the ventral lateral tongue, the floor of the mouth, or the soft palate-tonsillar pillar complex, and there is no ostensible history or source of irritation to account for its presence, it can pose a diagnostic challenge. In such cases, especially if the patient has an active or past history of smoking or heavy alcohol consumption, if a presumptive local etiological agent cannot be identified or if the lesion is not clinically consistent with any of several clinically recognizable conditions that are characterized by hyperkeratosis, the diagnosis cannot be made on clinical grounds. Such white oral mucosal plaques that cannot be wiped away (i.e., are keratotic) and which cannot be accounted for or diagnosed on clinical grounds alone (i.e., no obvious inciting agent, no history of trauma, no features characteristic of other specific keratotic diseases) require a biopsy for diagnosis. A majority of non-wipable white plaques are benign. However, the clinical features of the white non-wipable plaques that are more likely to represent **epithelial dysplasia** (oral pre-cancer) or **squamous cell carcinoma** (oral cancer) include location in an oral cancer-prone site (ventral lateral tongue, floor of the mouth, soft palate–uvula–tonsillar pillar region); heterogeneous surface topography (irregular surface with ulceration or erosion, white and red color, pebbly surface character); and size equal to or in excess of 200 mm^2 (Table 9.3).

Table 9.3   White non-wipable oral mucosal plaques: features suspicious for pre-cancer (epithelial dysplasia) or cancer (squamous cell carcinoma)

1. **Location (oral cancer prone locations):**
   a. Lateral and ventral tongue
   b. Floor of mouth
   c. Soft palate, tonsillar pillars
2. **No obvious source of trauma or friction:**
   a. Persistence of lesion after elimination of suspected sources of irritation/trauma
3. **Distribution:**
   a. Unilateral
   b. Away from sources of chronic irritation
   c. Lesion larger than 200 sq. mm.
4. **Patient history:**
   a. Active or past tobacco or alcohol habit
   b. History of other carcinogen exposure (betel nut, etc.)
   c. Prior diagnosis of oral pre-cancer or cancer
   d. Persistent pain, paresthesia
5. **Clinical features and appearance:**
   a. Diffuse white, homogeneous
   b. Heterogeneous, red & white, speckled
   c. Pebbly, leathery, verrucous surface
   d. Persistent ulceration, nodularity
   e. Induration (hard), tissue immobility

References

1. Alberts, B. (2008) *Molecular Biology of the Cell.* Garland Science, New York.
2. Avery, J. K. & Chiego, D.J. (2005) *Essentials of Oral Histology and Embryology: A Clinical Approach.* Mosby Year Book, St. Louis.
3. Bjarnason, G. A., Jordan, R.C., & R. B. Sothern (1999) Circadian variation in the expression of cell-cycle proteins in human oral epithelium. *American Journal of Pathology,* 154(2), 613–622.
4. Clapham, D.E. (2003) TRP channels as cellular sensors. *Nature,* 426, 517–524.
5. Eroschenko, V. P. & DiFiore, M. S. H. (2008) *DiFiore's Atlas of Histology with Functional Correlations.* Wolters Kluwer Health/Lippincott Williams & Wilkins, Philadelphia.
6. Hiatt, J. L. & Gartner, L. P. (2001) *Textbook of Head and Neck Anatomy.* Lippincott Williams & Wilkins, Philadelphia.
7. Lesch, C. A., Squier, C. A., Cruchley, A., Williams, D. M., & Speight, P. (1989) The permeability of human oral mucosa and skin to water. *Journal of Dental Research,* 68(9), 1345–1349.
8. Lipkin, M. (1973) Proliferation and differentiation of gastrointestinal cells. *Physiological Reviews,* 53(4), 891–915.
9. Lodish, H. F. (2004) *Molecular Cell Biology.* W.H. Freeman, New York.
10. Nanci, A. (2013) *Ten Cate's Oral Histology: Development, Structure, and Function.* Mosby/Elsevier, St. Louis.
11. Natarajan, E. & Eisenberg, E. (2011) Contemporary concepts in the diagnosis of oral cancer and precancer. *Dental Clinics of North America,* 55(1), 63–88.
12. Neville, B. W. (2009) *Oral and Maxillofacial Pathology.* Saunders/Elsevier, St. Louis.
13. Orban, B. J. & Bhaskar, S. N. (1990) *Orban's Oral Histology and Embryology.* Mosby Year Book, St. Louis.
14. Regezi, J. A. & Sciubba, J.J. (2008) *Oral Pathology: Clinical-Pathologic Correlations.* Saunders, Philadelphia.
15. Robbins, S. L., Cotran, R. S. , & Kumar, V. (2010) *Robbins and Cotran Pathologic Basis of Disease.* Saunders/Elsevier, Philadelphia.
16. Ross, M. H. & Pawlina, W. (2011) *Histology: a Text and Atlas, with Correlated Cell and Molecular Biology,* 6th edn. Wolters Kluwer Health/Lippincott Williams & Wilkins, Philadelphia.
17. Siemionow, M., Gharb, B.B., & Rampazzo, A. (2011) The face as a sensory organ. *Plastic and Reconstructive Surgery,* 127, 652–662.
18. Squier, C. A. & Brogden, K. (2012) *Human Oral Mucosa: Development, Structure and Function.* Wiley-Blackwell, Oxford.
19. Squier, C. A. & Kremer, M. J. (2001) Biology of oral mucosa and esophagus. *Journal of the National Cancer Institute, Monographs,* 29, 7–15.
20. Thomson, P. J., Potten, C. S., & Appleton, D. R. (1999) Mapping dynamic epithelial cell proliferative activity within the oral cavity of man: a new insight into carcinogenesis? *The British Journal of Oral &Maxillofacial Surgery,* 37(5), 377–383.
21. Vay, L., Gu, C., & McNaughton, P.A. (2012) The thermo-TRP ion channel family: properties and therapeutic implications. *British Journal of Pharmacology,* 165, 787–801.
22. Watanabe, I.S. (2004) Ultrastructures of mechanoreceptors in the oral mucosa. *Anatomical Science International,* 79, 55–61.

Glossary

Acantholysis: loss of adhesion between the epithelial or epidermal spinous cells.

Acanthosis: increase in the width of the stratum spinosum due to increase in number of spinous cells.

Actinic: sun-related.

A-β fibers: large myelinated afferent nerve fibers, 6–12 μm in diameter, with rapid conduction velocity; associated with the sense of touch.

A-δ fibers: thinly myelinated afferent nerve fibers, 1–5 μm in diameter, with moderate conduction velocity; associated with acute (sharp) pain.

Alimentary: pertaining to the digestive tract, the process of digestion.

Apical domain: the free surface of an epithelial cell.

Apoptosis: a genetically determined process of programmed cell death.

Attached gingiva: gum tissue bound down to underlying alveolar bone.

Basal lamina: comprised of the lamina lucida and lamina densa. The lamina densa is an electron-dense web of filamentous proteins (laminins [laminin 5], type IV collagen, perlecan, other glycoproteins, and proteoglycans) that comprise a base to which the hemidesmosome of the epithelial basal cell forms an anchoring attachment.

Basement membrane: interface zone between the epithelium and papillary lamina propria. Epithelial basal cells rest upon and are attached to the basement membrane at their basal domain.

Buccal: relating to the cheek.

C fibers: unmyelinated afferent nerve fibers, 0.2–1.5 mm in diameter, with slow conduction velocity; associated with slow, burning, long-lasting pain.

Chemesthesis: sensations occurring as a result of chemical activation of somatosensory receptors

Cytokeratins: predominant intermediate filament proteins of epithelial cells.

Cytoskeleton: the internal structural framework of a cell consisting of filaments and microtubules that dictate the cell's morphology and integrity.

Deglutition: swallowing.

Dendrite: a branching extension (as in dendritic cells).

Desmocollin: transmembrane desmosomal attachment protein from the cadherin family that penetrates the intercellular space between epithelial spinous cells.

Desmoglein: transmembrane desmosomal attachment protein from the cadherin family that penetrates the intercellular space between epithelial spinous cells.

Desmosome: the intercellular bridge-like attachment apparatus that links neighboring epithelial spinous cells to one another. Desmosomes are comprised of transmembrane attachment proteins, intracytoplasmic placodes consisting of proteins (desmoplakins and plakoglobin) located on the inner aspect of the plasma membrane of the spinous cell, and keratin intermediate filaments that insert into the placodes.

Ectopic: occurring in an abnormal place or position.

Epithelial dysplasia: composite histopathological evidence of intraepithelial cytomorphological and architectural abnormalities indicative of potential for malignant progression to squamous cell carcinoma (i.e., "precancerous"/ "or preinvasive" changes).

Epithelium: lining tissue that invests most external and internal body surfaces. Provides a protective barrier (skin, mucosa). Various specialized epithelial cells play a spectrum of roles (e.g. exocrine secretory function, transport, metabolism, filtration, thermal regulation.

Erythema (erythematous): a clinical descriptive term for redness.

Filaggrin: a filament-associated protein that binds cytokeratin filaments in epithelial cells. A component of keratohyalin granules in cells of the stratum granulosum.

Foramen cecum: the most posterior point of the terminal sulcus on the dorsal tongue and immediately anterior to the base of the tongue.

Fordyce granules (Fordyce "spots"): ectopic sebaceous glands.

Hemidesmosome: attaches individual epithelial basal cells to the underlying basement membrane.

Heterodimer: a molecular complex formed by two or more non-identical macromolecules, such as proteins, that are not bound covalently.

Immunofluorescence: a laboratory technique used with the fluorescence microscope to detect presence and quantification of an antigen, antibody, or autoantibody either located in a tissue sample (direct immunofluorescence, DIF) or circulating in the serum (indirect immunofluorescence, IIF). Immunofluorescence may be used to confirm diagnoses of suspected autoimmune diseases and to monitor the patient's response to treatment of an autoimmune condition.

Integrin: these constitute a large family of transmembrane dimer proteins; they function as cell-matrix adhesion receptors or cell-cell adhesion molecules. An integrin molecule is composed of two noncovalently associated transmembrane glycoprotein subunits called α and β. Within the basal cells of epithelia they serve as a hub-like connection to bundles of intermediate filaments and actin via intracellular linking proteins, bullous pemphigoid antigens (BP230 and BP180). Specifically, α6β4 integrin in the basal cell's cytoplasm is a transmembrane linker ("integrator") of the hemidesmosome apparatus that attaches the stratified squamous epithelium to the underlying basement membrane.

Karyorrhexis: destructive fragmentation of the nucleus of a dying cell with uneven chromatin distribution.

Keratinocytes: epithelial cells that contain abundant cytokeratins; at their maturational endpoint, the oral stratified squamous epithelial cells are flattened, nonviable and shed from the surface.

Lamina propria: most superficial layers of the stroma underlying the surface epithelium. Divided into two layers, "papillary" (most superior) and "reticular," which is deep to the papillary lamina propria.

Laminin: an extracellular matrix protein (EMP); one of several EMPs that comprise the basement membrane.

Langerhans cell: dendritic, immunologically active cells responsible for antigen presentation.

Lingual papillae: surface projections on the dorsal and posteriorolateral surfaces of the tongue that comprise the "specialized" oral mucosa. The fungiform, foliate, and circumvallate papillae all contain taste receptors. The filiform papillae, which are the most numerous papillae covering much of the anterior two thirds of the dorsal tongue surface, bear no taste receptors.

Lining (moveable) mucosa: moveable, pliable, non-keratinized mucosal tissue that lines much of the oral cavity and vestibule.

Macrophage: (Gk. *macro* = big, *phagein* = eat) differentiated monocytes/ histiocytes that play a role in phagocytosis and chronic inflammatory reactions.

Masticatory mucosa: attached gingival tissue and the portions of hard palatal tissue that are fixed ("bound down") to underlying bone. The dorsal tongue mucosa, which is classified as "specialized" mucosa and which is not bound down to bone, is also considered to be masticatory mucosa. Masticatory mucosa is naturally keratinized tissue.

Meissner's corpuscle: a round or globular tactile sensory end organ comprised of encapsulated nerve endings. Touch receptors found in hairless skin and also in the oral mucosa.

Melanocyte: dendritic, non-keratinocytic cell that resides in the stratum basale and is responsible for elaboration and distribution of melanin pigment.

Melanophage: macrophage within the lamina propria that phagocytizes and contains incontinent melanin pigment spilled from disrupted epithelial cells.

Melanosome: a mature melanin granule resulting from maturation of a premelanosome. Pigment-laden melanosomes are transferred to nearby keratinocytes via phagocytosis.

Merkel cells: a sensory cell, located in the stratum basale of the epithelium, that responds to tactile stimulation; associated with unmyelinated nerve endings to form a Merkel's disk.

Mucocutaneous: pertaining to the mucous membrane and the skin.

Mucogingival junction: the clinically evident boundary between the alveolar mucosa and the attached gingiva.

Nikolsky sign: a clinical term used by both dermatologists and oral diagnosticians to describe sloughing of the skin or the oral mucosa surface on lateral pressure. A positive Nikolsky sign indicates a weakness either of cell-to-cell attachments within the epidermis or the mucosa, or between the basal cells and their attachment to the underlying basement membrane.

Oral cavity proper: the inner of the two major anatomic regions of the oral cavity.

Oral vestibule: the outer of the two major anatomic regions of the oral cavity, bounded by the buccal and labial mucosae and vestibules, and the alveolar processes of the maxilla and mandible.

Oropharynx: anatomic region immediately posterior to the oral cavity.

Orthokeratin: surface layer of keratin that lacks nuclei; the type of keratin that is present on the epidermis.

Palatoglossal folds: the more anterior of two arch-like soft tissue folds that mark the entrance to the oropharynx.

Palatopharyngeal folds: the more posteriorly positioned of the two soft tissue arches at the opening of the oropharynx.

Papillary: finger-like projections or folds.

Paradoxical cold: cold sensation occurring when cool sensitive nerve fibers are stimulated by heat greater than 45°C.

Parakeratin: flattened keratinocytes in the stratum superficiale with small, shrunken hyperchromatic (pyknotic) nuclei.

Pemphigoid: a group of autoimmune blistering mucocutaneous diseases characterized by full-thickness separation of the surface epithelium from the underlying lamina propria that is mediated by autoantibody (IgG) and C3 targeted against the hemidesmosomes.

Pemphigus: a group of autoimmune blistering mucocutaneous diseases characterized by acantholysis mediated by autoantibody (IgG) and C3 that target the epidermal and epithelial desmosomes.

Placode: a plate-like structure.

Plaque: slightly raised areas on the mucosa or skin caused by an increase in the width of the epidermis or surface epithelium with or without hyperkeratosis.

Polymodal nociceptors: sensory neurons responding to potentially damaging environmental stimuli of more than one type (modality), typically causing the perception of pain.

Precancerous: spectrum of preinvasive cellular and maturational changes in the surface epithelium of oral mucosa or epidermis of skin that reflect potential for progression to malignancy (squamous cell carcinoma).

Premelanosome: plasma membrane-bound, Golgi-derived structures in melanocytes where melanin pigment is actively produced.

Pyknosis: the irreversible condensation of chromatin in the nucleus of a cell undergoing necrosis or apoptosis. On light microscopy, pyknotic nuclei appear small, spindly or shriveled and hyperchromatic. Pyknotic nuclei are seen in parakeratinized cells within the stratum superficiale.

Rete pegs: downward undulating projections of the stratified squamous epithelium that interdigitate with the papillary lamina propria of the underlying stromal tissue.

Reticulum: lattice-like network.

Specialized mucosa: papillated tissue of the dorsal tongue comprised of four distinct papillae. Three of these papillae (fungiform, foliate, and circumvallate) carry taste receptors.

Squamous: scale like, scaly.

Squamous cell carcinoma: malignant neoplasm derived from stratified squamous epithelium. A majority of "oral cancers" are squamous cell carcinomas.

Stratified: layered.

Stratum basale (Stratum germinativum, epithelial basal cells): basal-most, single layer of cuboidal cells of the stratified squamous epithelium. Basal cells rest on a basement membrane, the interface zone between the epithelium and the underlying connective tissue.

Stratum granulosum: conspicuous granular cell layer of stratified squamous epithelium located just below orthokeratotic stratum superficiale. The granular cells' cytoplasm contains basophilic keratohyalin granules.

Stratum spinosum: the immediately suprabasal region of stratified squamous epithelium. Spinous cells have spine-like projections (prickles, *acanthe*) on the surfaces of their plasma membranes.

Stratum superficiale: the most superficial ("cornified") layer and maturational endpoint of stratified squamous epithelium. It is characterized morphologically by the presence of flattened epithelial cells. The stratum superficiale may be nonkeratinized, orthokeratinized or parakeratinized.

Stroma: the supporting connective tissue (interstitial tissue) of an organ.

Submucosa: stromal tissue inferior to the lamina propria consisting of broad bands of fibrocollagenous and elastic tissue containing blood vessels and nerves.

Terminal sulcus: the posterior boundary of the oral cavity proper on the posterior third of the dorsal tongue; the junction between the oropharynx and the oral cavity.

Tonofibrils: cytoplasmic protein structures in epithelial tissues that converge at desmosomes and hemidesmosomes.

Tonofilament: structural cytoplasmic intermediate filaments which, when bundled together form tonofibrils.

Tonsillar fauces: concave tissue recess between the tonsillar pillars where lobular lymphoid tissue masses, the palatine tonsils, are located.

Tonsillar pillars: formed by the combined palatoglossal and palatopharyngeal folds.

Transient receptor potential (TRP) channels: cation channels responding to sensory stimuli, located in axonal membranes and the plasma membranes of other cells.

Transit amplifying cells (TACs): committed, proliferative cells daughter cells derived from mitotic division of epithelial stem cells in the stratum basale. They transit upward to progress toward terminal differentiation.

Trichohyalin: a protein associated with intermediate filaments that contributes to the mechanical strength of epithelial cells. A component of keratohyalin granules of stratum granulosum cells.

Trigeminal nerve: the fifth cranial nerve, supplying somatosensory and special visceral efferent innervation to the face and oral cavity.

Vermilion border: red portion of the upper or lower external lip.

Vestibules: the deep troughs that mark the inferior and superior limits of the buccal and labial mucosae.

Von Ebner's (lingual serous) glands: exclusively serous minor salivary glands situated among the muscle fibers of the posterior portion of the tongue. The excretory ducts of von Ebner's glands exit into the troughs of the circumvallate papillae and the deep portions of the foliate papillae.

Waldeyer's ring: palatine tonsils, lingual tonsils, and other smaller aggregates of oral mucosa-associated lymphoid tissues distributed predominantly in the posterior oral cavity and the floor of the mouth.

Chapter 10 Chemoreception and Perception

Marion E. Frank

Department of Oral Health and Diagnostic Sciences, School of Dental Medicine, University of Connecticut

Oral chemoreception includes the senses of taste (gustation), smell (olfaction), and the chemical somatic senses, which will be covered in Chapter 9, "Oral Mucosa and Mucosal Sensation," and Chapter 12, "Orofacial Pain, Touch and Thermosensation, and Sensorimotor Functions." This current chapter, not solely a compilation of current knowledge on the gustatory and olfactory systems, integrates into the text experimental techniques used to develop that knowledge. Perceptual (human objective and subjective psychophysics, animal conditioned **taste aversion** and preference), physiological (receptor potential, multi- and single-neuron electrophysiology; two-photon calcium imaging in vivo, single dissociated **olfactory sensory neuron (OSN)** calcium imaging, event-related fMRI brain imaging) and morphological (light and electron microscopy) methodologies are cited.

The independent senses of taste and smell have evolved to monitor chemical environments for health and wellbeing. With them, as well as general somatosensations, distinct sources of chemosensory information, it can be decided that foods need more or less sugar or salt, whether the scent of dinner is foul or appetizing, and whether lemonade is too sharp. One of the first things learned from patients at the opening of the Connecticut Taste and Smell Clinic in 1980 was that people often confuse smells with tastes. They may feel certain that they cannot taste after an automobile accident involving head trauma but have no measurable loss of gustation. They are perfectly capable of distinguishing salt from sugar. Retronasal smelling, a recent topic of interest, helps explain the patients' confusions. Odors from the outside are sensed orthonasally during inspiration; but on expiration oral odors are sensed, retronasally. (See also *Disorders* in Glossary). Retronasal odors from the mouth, closely allied with tastes, contribute to the specific **flavor** of a food such as asparagus, which also gives urine an unusual orthonasal odor.

Tastes and smells of chemosensory compounds are attached to innate and developed preferences and aversions. Odors' primal pleasure/displeasure **dimension** (for example) is hardwired in olfactory mucosal patches of sensitivity to volatile compounds with appealing (+) or repulsive (–) odors. This is elaborated on in Box 10.1(1). Also, single chemosensory compounds may activate several chemosensory systems. For example, acetic acid has a vinegary smell, a sour taste, and painfully irritates as concentration increases. Anosmic individuals, without a sense of smell, can detect acetic acid orthonasally but only at a higher concentration than normosmic individuals. Correspondingly, individuals taste-blind for specific compounds such as phenylthiocarbamide (PTC) and related bitter compounds detect them only at high concentrations, as shown in Box 10.2(1). Moreover, chemosensory stimulus recognition is fleeting, fading with time through peripheral **adaptation** and mutual central inhibition evident in **mixture suppression** among separate neural pathways. This **coding** strategy emphasizes the **identification** of recently appearing and strong tasting or smelling chemical compounds.

In this chapter, the structure and function of the two chemosenses of taste and smell are covered in separate sections. A final section addresses clinical issues.

Taste

Fundamentals and historical perspective

Taste evaluates beneficial and dangerous water-soluble chemicals taken into the mouth to assist nutriture through the pleasure of eating and poisoning through the awfulness of tainted foods.

Fundamentals of Oral Histology and Physiology, First Edition. Arthur R. Hand and Marion E. Frank.
© 2014 John Wiley & Sons, Inc. Published 2014 by John Wiley & Sons, Inc.

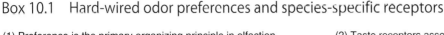

Box 10.1   Hard-wired odor preferences and species-specific receptors

(1) Preference is the primary organizing principle in olfaction.

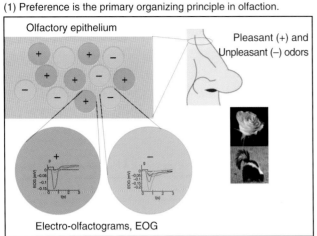

Olfactory sensory neurons (OSN) in the olfactory epithelium express odor receptors (OR). Epithelial patches respond to diverse compounds with either pleasant (e.g., phenethyl alcohol, rose) or unpleasant (e.g., butane-thiol, skunk) odors. Recordings of electrical signals (EOG) from the surface of the olfactory mucosa were obtained in awake individual humans (See also *Topographic* in Glossary), who also reported their perceptions. (From Frank, M.E. & Hettinger, T.P. (2011) An axis of good and awful in odor reception. *Nature Neuroscience*, 14, 1360–1362. Reproduced with permission from Nature Publishing.)

(2) Taste receptors associated with food items within ecological niches.

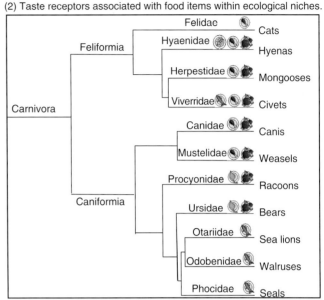

Felidae (cats) are obligate carnivores (plates: leg = carnivore, bug = insectivore, tomato + leg = ominvore, leaf = herbivore, fish = piscivore) and are indifferent to sugar. They were left without an expressed sugar receptor protein with which to identify carbohydrate sources, having lost the ability to taste sugar with pseudogenization of the *Tas1r2* gene coding for T1R2 during evolution. (From Li, X., Glaser, D., Li, W., Johnson, W.E., O'Brien, S.J., Beauchamp, G.K., & Brand, J.G. (2009) Analyses of sweet receptor gene (Tas1r2) and preference for sweet stimuli in species of *Carnivora*. *Journal of Heredity*, 100 (Supp. 1), S90–S100. Reproduced with permission from Oxford University Press.)

A century ago, Hans Henning represented the relationships between pure human taste perceptions geometrically on the surface of a tetrahedron: "**primaries**" at the four corners and mixtures of two or three taste "primaries" elsewhere on edges and faces (Fig. 10.1). In the tetrahedron drawn, compounds with each taste (sweet, salty, sour, and bitter) are positioned at corners, compounds with binary mixtures of tastes (saccharin, KCl, NH$_4$Cl) are positioned appropriately on edges between pure tastes, and a compound with a mixture of three tastes (NaSO$_4$) is positioned on a tetrahedral face. Single chemical compounds with one **taste quality**, single compounds with two or three taste qualities, and, by extension, mixtures of two or three compounds with different pure qualities are represented by the tetrahedral model.

Chemical stimuli and taste quality

Sugars, some amino acids, and artificial sweeteners such as saccharin and aspartame are sweet. Halide sodium salts NaCl and NaBr are salty. Non-sodium halide salts are salty and bitter. KCl, NH$_4$Cl, MgSO$_4$ and salts with large organic cations such as denatonium benzoate and quinine hydrochloride and zwitter-ionic amino acids as well as nonionic alkaloids (thioureas, bile acids and glycosides) are bitter, a broad category of unpleasant tastes that may include several distinct experiences. Sour-tasting acids, which are also irritants, may also have characteristic odors, such as the vinegary acetic acid. **Ethanol** is the epitome multi-chemosensory stimulus, tasting bitter and sweet and having an odor, as well as being an irritant. The non-gustatory aspects of taste stimuli were intentionally not considered in Henning's pure-taste

Box 10.2 Bitter threshold distribution and T2R38 genetics

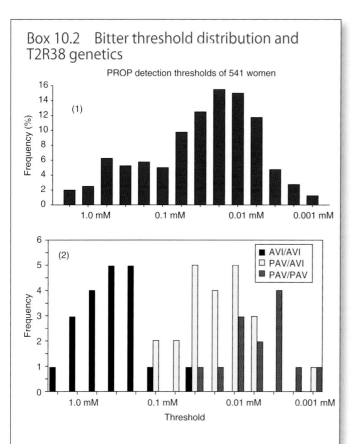

Appreciation of 6-*n*-propyl-thiouracil (PROP) bitterness predicts less alcohol intake, making non-tasters at greater risk for alcoholism. (1) Distribution of human thresholds for bitter PROP, plotted from high to low concentration, and structurally related bitter compounds has a genetic basis. (Derived from Drewnowski, A. (2003) Genetics of human taste perception. In: *Handbook of Olfaction and Gustation* (ed. R.L. Doty), 2nd edn. pp. 847–860. Marcel Dekker, New York.) (2) Three common single nucleotide polymorphisms in the gene for the bitter taste receptor T2R38 contribute to two common haplotypes PAV and AVI, associated with PROP "super-tasters" and non-tasters, respectively. In fact, PAV homozygotes are "super-tasters," AVI homozygotes are "taste blind" non-tasters, and heterozygotes are medium tasters. (A, I, P, and V are single letter codes for amino acids alanine, isoleucine, proline, and valine, respectively.) (From Duffy, V.B., Davidson, A.C., Kidd, J.R., Kidd, K.K., Speed, W.C., Pakstis, A.J., Reed, D.R., Snyder, D.J,. & Bartoshuk, L.M. (2004) Bitter receptor gene (TAS2R38), 6-n-propylthiouracil (PROP) bitterness and alcohol intake. *Alcoholism Clinical & Experimental Research*, 28, 1629–1637. Reproduced with permission from John Wiley & Sons.)

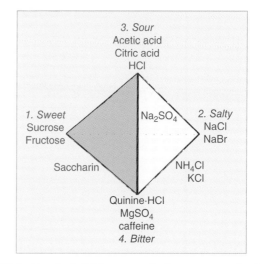

Figure 10.1 Henning's 1916 taste tetrahedron: compounds with pure taste primaries at corners (1, 2, 3, 4), mixtures on edges or faces (not in the interior because it was thought no stimulus was a mix of the four tastes). (See also *quality coding* in Glossary). Taste stimuli were dispersed on the surface of the tetrahedron according to how similar they tasted to primaries.

free fatty acids (for example, linoleic acid), glucose polymers (for example, the nutritional supplement Polycose®), and low osmolarity (water) may also be detected orally; possibly with involvement of gustatory receptors.

Species-specific taste worlds

Species differences in the gustatory quality of chemicals can be great, especially for the many compounds with bitter tastes associated with the T2R bitter genes. The variation may reflect the importance of detecting the different poisons and food items used for nourishment as habitats change and species evolve. For example, carnivorous felines are unable to taste sugar, which is consistent with pseudogenization of the T1R2 sweet-taste receptor gene during evolutionary time owing to a release from positive evolution. Conversely, ethanol (bitter-sweet and poisonous to humans at high concentrations) is primarily sweet to golden hamsters, who utilize its caloric value without inebriation poisoning when feeding on fermented grain stored in their deep burrow domiciles.

> The gustatory system detects oral chemicals that may be valuable or dangerous to health. Single chemicals taste sweet, salty, sour, bitter, and savory; five qualities for which receptors and unique perceptions are identified. There may be other tastes but gaps in knowledge of their reception and perception remain.

Studies on rodents are used as models for human taste. However, before linking human to animal taste, differences in perceptual "taste worlds" must be experimentally addressed. To this end, confusability of **taste stimuli**, quantitatively measured psychophysically in humans with **taste confusion** matrix methodology and behaviorally in animals with taste aversion generalization tests,

tetrahedron. Structures of a variety of water-soluble compounds with a broad range of tastes are shown in Fig. 10.2.

Tastes surely have four pure qualities that signal nutritious carbohydrates and minerals or harmful substances. Another taste, savory (**umami** in Japanese), has been legitimized with discovery of a receptor. It is evoked by monosodium L-glutamate (MSG), or better, a mixture of MSG and inosine monophosphate (IMP), and may signal protein sources. Other stimulus domains,

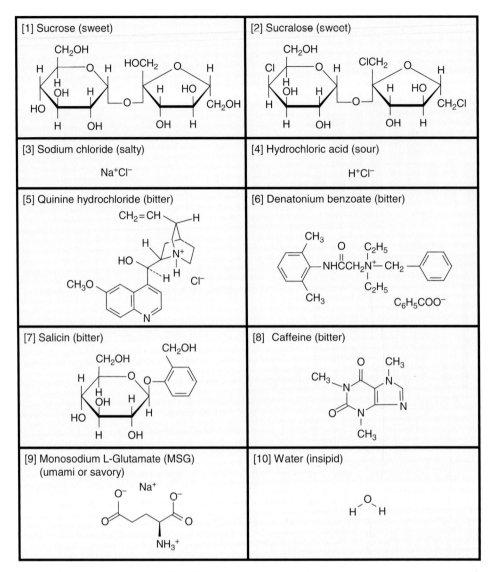

Figure 10.2   Chemicals representative of basic taste qualities. (1) Sweet sucrose occurs in sugar cane, maple sap, and many flowers and fruits; (2) sweet sucralose is an artificial sweetener derived by replacing three sucrose *OH* groups by *Cl* atoms. (3) Salty sodium chloride is the only chemical that is pure salty. (4) Sour hydrochloric acid is one of many acids producing sour H^+ ions. (5) Bitter quinine hydrochloride is a natural alkaloid from cinchona tree bark; (6) bitter denatonium benzoate is an extremely bitter synthetic chemical; (7) bitter salicin is a natural glycoside from willow tree bark and ligand of the T2R16 receptor; (8) caffeine is a weakly bitter natural alkaloid from coffee and tea. (9) Umami (savory) monosodium glutamate is a natural amino acid that is also produced synthetically. (10) Insipid (tasteless) is the taste of water, likely due to contrast with saliva. (See also *Taste Stimuli* in Glossary). (From Hettinger, T.P. (2013) Unpublished.)

reveals how taste mixtures are evaluated. Multivariate analysis of human confusions, Box 10.3(1), distributed the prototypic sweet sucrose, salty NaCl, sour citric acid, bitter quinine, and five binary taste mixtures in a **two-dimensional space**. All taste stimuli were distinct from insipid water, some mixtures fell between mixture components but some were much closer to a **dominant** component. Correspondingly, intake suppression seen in hamster generalization tests, Box 10.3(2), differed for hamsters that learned aversions to three individual compounds (sucrose, NaCl, quinine) and three binary or one ternary mixture of the compounds. Like humans, the hamsters detected components in binary mixtures, and the ability to recognize components deteriorated with the higher level ternary mixture, mixture suppression reminiscent of human tasting. (See also Fig. 10.10 under "Peripheral Nerves" below.)

Multivariate analysis of hamster taste generalizations resulted in the "taste world" shown in Fig. 10.3, which is to be compared to the human taste tetrahedron in Fig. 10.1. The quantitative multivariate analysis shows hamsters, as humans, perceive four qualities. In the hamsters' world, sweeteners and sour acids fall in distinct regions; however, the two other hamster tastes, one labeled 'Na salts' and the other 'bitter salts', differ from human tastes, demonstrating critical species variation regarding tastes of salts and bitter compounds. These differences between rodents and humans have impeded understanding of human salty and bitter tastes. Nonetheless, the multivariate taste-world model shows equivalence to Henning's tetrahedral model with four taste groupings in three-dimensional space. The objectively determined multidimensional scaling (MDS)

Box 10.3   Perceptual analysis using confusions in humans or animals

(1) Humans discriminated basic taste qualities but sometimes mistook mixture components for pure qualities.

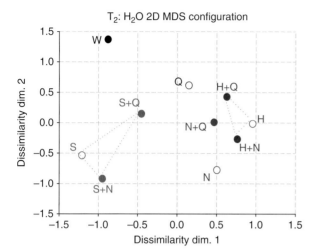

T_2: H_2O 2D MDS configuration

(2) Hamsters recognized component tastes in mixtures. (See also *Taste Aversion* in Glossary)

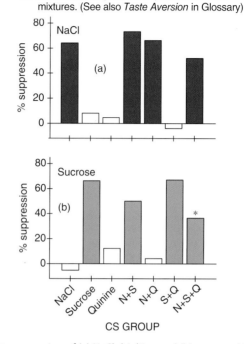

Multidimensional scaling (MDS) of pair-wise stimulus discriminability (T_2). Taste confusion matrices were obtained for 14 human subjects. Each subject identified 10 stimuli 10 times from a series of labels (such as "sugar" for sucrose and "salt" for NaCl). T_2 values (in bits of information) quantified discriminabilities (dissimilarities) among the 45 pairs of identification patterns. The dissimilarity matrix was the input for the MDS, which, by iteratively maximizing data variance accounted for, arranged the stimuli in the two dimensions (dim) shown. Dim1 distinguishes stimuli from one another and dim 2 distinguishes all taste stimuli from water. Points for stimuli that were less well discriminated fall closer to each other. Dotted lines connect points for stimuli containing sucrose (green) or citric acid (red). N = NaCl, S = sucrose, H = citric acid, Q = quinine·HCl and W = water. Neither single stimuli (open points) nor binary mixtures (filled points) were confused with water. Points for some mixtures fall between mixture components; for example, salt plus quinine falls between salt and quinine. One exception is S + N, showing salt taste is dominated by sugar taste. (From Wang, M. F., Marks, L.E., & Frank, M.E. (2009) Taste coding after selective inhibition by chlorhexidine. *Chemical Senses*, 34, 653–666. Reproduced with permission from Oxford University Press.) (See also *Identification* and *Taste Confusion* in Glossary).

Percent suppression of (a) NaCl drinking and (b) sucrose drinking was measured in groups of animals that learned aversions to the seven conditioned stimuli (CS) listed along the abscissa. Only when the CS contained NaCl (solo, mixed with sucrose, quinine, or both) was NaCl drinking suppressed. Likewise, only when the CS contained sucrose (solo, mixed with NaCl, quinine, or both) was sucrose drinking suppressed. However, the sucrose was detected less frequently in the ternary mixture than in single components or binary mixtures. N = NaCl, S = sucrose, Q = quinine. (From Frank, M.E. 2008. A perspective on chemosensory quality coding. In: *The Senses: A Comprehensive Reference*, Vol. 4 (sect. eds. D.V. Smith, S. Firestein, & B.K. Beauchamp), pp. 339–344. Academic Press, New York. Reproduced with permission from John Wiley & Sons.)

configurations are more general, with the mathematical precision to exactly position components and mixtures in one multidimensional space.

Studies of stimulus identification provide insight into real-world chemosensory processing by drawing attention to the human capacity for dynamic stimulus analysis of the shifting chemicals in complex mixtures. Table 10.1 presents an experimental protocol designed to study human dynamic chemosensory analysis in which either taste or smell stimuli are presented one after the other in pairs. The first stimulus, sampled for 5 seconds, is followed by the second stimulus to be identified. Independent stimuli, easily identified following water, are less accurately identified in a mixture due to

mixture suppression, as specified in the "not-adapted" case 1 in Table 10.1 and in Fig. 10.4, which presents results from an experiment with sucrose and sodium chloride (NaCl). Their sugar or salt tastes do not **cross-adapt**; that is, do not affect one another's identification when sequentially applied. Cases 2, 3, and 4 in Table 10.1 deal with selectively adapting individual component stimuli, which influence mixture-component identification as shown for tastes in Fig. 10.4. In essence, un-adapted extra components regain quality identity suppressed in mixtures (case 2), while adapted ambient component identities are further suppressed (case 3). When a number of stimuli are non-selectively pre-adapted together (case 4), no stimulus dominates, but all

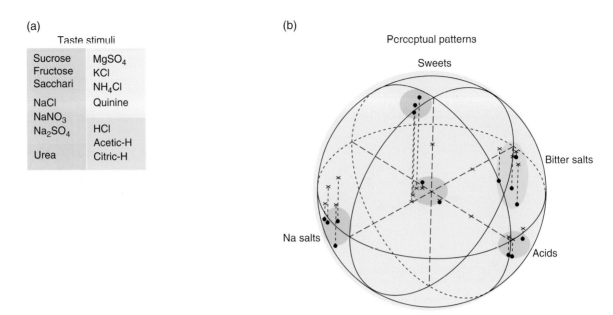

Figure 10.3   Behavioral discriminations of 14 taste compounds (a) used to identify qualitatively distinct perceptions in the hamster taste world (b). The spherical 3D multidimensional scaling (MDS) of generalizations of conditioned taste aversions (CTA), quantitatively based on percent drinking suppression values, identifies stimuli that hamsters confuse with one another, which are represented by points that are near one another. (See also *Taste Dimensions* in Glossary). Two of the points falling among Na salts represent two Na_2SO_4 concentrations. Two points at zero, the center of the sphere, represent two urea concentrations that were unaccounted for by this solution. (From Frank, M.E. & Nowlis G.H. (1989) Learned aversions and taste qualities in hamsters. *Chemical Senses*, 14, 379–394. Reproduced with permission from Oxford University Press.)

Table 10.1   Prior selective adaptation of ambient compounds aids identification of tastes or odors of extra mixture components in humans.

	Stimulus Pairs Presented			Tastes or Odors Identified
	Single Compound (A_1)	Mixture Component (A_2)		Percentage Correct (A_1 or A_2)
1		Not-Adapted		
	$0 \rightarrow A_1$	$0 \rightarrow A_2B$	$A_2 < A_1$	Mixture Component < Single Compound
2		Extra (Selectively Adapted)		
	$0 \rightarrow A_1$	$B \rightarrow A_2B$	$A_2 = A_1$	Extra Mixture Component = Single Compound
3		Ambient (Selectively Adapted)		
	$A \rightarrow A_1$	$A \rightarrow A_2B$	$A_2 < A_1$	Ambient Mixture Component < Self-Adapted Single Compound
4		Mixture (Non-Selectively Adapted)		
	$A \rightarrow A_1$	$AB \rightarrow A_2B$	$A_2 = A_1$	Mixture-Adapted Mixture Component = Self-Adapted Single Compound

Identifications of tastes or odors of binary-mixture components (A_2) are compared to identifications of single-compounds (A_1). A and B are chemical stimuli that elicit *A* and *B* independent tastes or odors; 0 = water. Identification cases 1 & 2: Single compound after water vs. mixture component after either (1) water or (2) another mixture component. Identification cases 3 & 4: Single compound after the same compound vs. mixture after (3) one component or (4) both components. (See also *Mixture Suppression* in Glossary). Data for each of the four cases are shown for a taste experiment in Fig. 10.4. (See *Adaptation* in Glossary). (Derived from data in Frank, M.E., Goyert, H.F., Formaker, B.K., & Hettinger, T.P. (2012) Effects of selective adaptation on coding sugar and salt tastes in mixtures. *Chemical Senses*, 37, 701–709; and Frank, M.E., Goyert, H.F., & Hettinger, T.P. (2010) Time and intensity factors in identification of components of odor mixtures. *Chemical Senses*, 35, 777–787.)

merely self-adapt as they do as single compounds. Apparently, mixture suppression, rather than obscuring quality information, is likely a central perceptual mechanism that adjusts effective concentrations. This process, combined with rapid sensory adaptation, makes it possible to identify single stimulus compounds detected by individual chemosensory receptors. The experimental findings, consistent with everyday experience, highlight the importance of identifiable characteristic of tastes and odors in the processing of chemosensory compounds.

Selective adaptation and mixture suppression adjust effective concentrations to make possible the identification of individual beneficial or harmful compounds in complex mixtures that are detected by independent receptors.

Peripheral activation

Taste buds detect water-soluble chemicals

About 50 taste cells (TC) reside in taste bud cellular clusters located in lingual epithelia and elsewhere in oropharyngeal mucosa. Taste cells

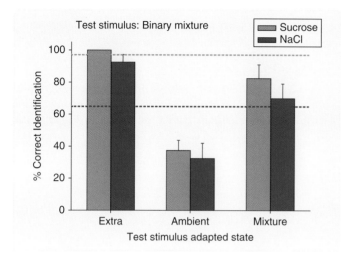

Figure 10.4   Taste mixture component identification after selective and nonselective adaptation in humans. Sucrose and NaCl have independent tastes that are perfectly (100%) identified as sugar and salt following a water rinse. However, identification of the tastes as mixture components fluctuates, as delineated in Table 10.1. Tastes of *extra* mixture components (case 2 in Table 10.1) are also identified nearly perfectly. However, tastes of selectively adapted *ambient* mixture components (case 3 in Table 10.1) are poorly identified, more so than when the mixture is preceded by the mixture (case 4 in Table 10.1). (See also *Mixture Suppression* in Glossary). Dotted lines reveal levels of identification of component tastes in the mixture preceded by water (case 1 in Table 10.1). (From Frank, M.E., Goyert, H.F., Formaker, B.K., & Hettinger, T.P. (2012) Effects of selective adaptation on coding sugar and salt tastes in mixtures. *Chemical Senses*, 37, 701–709. Reproduced with permission from Oxford University Press.)

turn over every 10 days, which reflects their epithelial origin. Fig. 10.5a is a photomicrograph of a taste bud within a fungiform papilla. Mature taste buds depend on neurotrophism; atrophied anlage remain after injury to the taste nerve. Taste-bud cells project membrane extensions, microvilli, into the gustatory pore, which contains dense mucosubstance, as pictured in the diagram in Fig. 10.5b. Type I, II, and III TC with different lineages each have unique morphologies and biochemical features, suggestive of distinct functions. Glial-like, GLAST (glutamate aspartate transporter) containing, type I dark cells with sheet-like processes intermingle among other TC, possibly serving physical and biochemical supporting roles. Type II TC (light cells) contain the biochemical necessities for taste stimulus transduction. This includes the G protein α-gustducin, T1R and T2R G protein-coupled receptors (GPCR), as well as downstream elements phospholipase C (PLCβ2) and transient receptor potential (TRP) cation channel TRPM5 necessary for TC depolarization. All must be operational for the tasting of sweet, savory and bitter compounds, which is elaborated on in the next few paragraphs. Type III TC, which project one broad apical microvillus into the gustatory pore and may be directly activated by ionic taste stimuli, are the only TC known to be synaptically associated with the axons of taste nerves at the base of the taste bud. Multiple trigeminal nerve (CN V) endings are seen apically in the papilla outside the taste bud that are capable of mediating touch, temperature and chemical irritation via TRP channels, a topic covered in Chapter 9, "Oral Mucosa and Mucosal Sensation."

Taste receptors are related to perceptual taste quality

Interactions between taste stimuli and **taste receptors (TR)** occur within gustatory pores. Nonionic taste stimuli first bind to receptor proteins in apical membranes of TC microvilli that are coupled to second-messenger systems. Members of two families of GPCR detect taste stimuli, 3 T1R and 30 T2R.

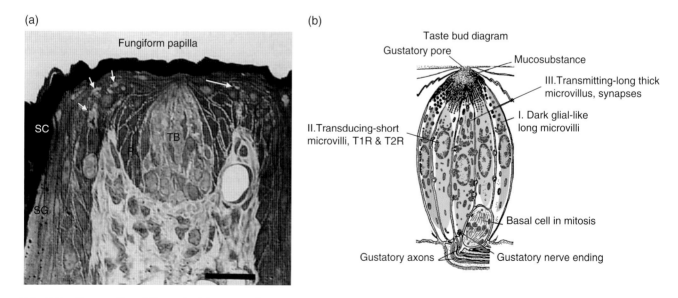

Figure 10.5   (a) Fungiform papilla and (b) taste bud diagram. In photomicrograph (a) of a toluidine- blue stained, 1-µ-thick longitudinal section through a taste bud, TB = taste bud, SC = stratum corneum, SG = stratum granulosum. Arrows point to trigeminal lingual nerve endings outside the taste bud. In diagram (b), the gustatory pore is drawn at the apical end of the taste bud where stimuli interact with receptors in microvillar membranes. Three morphological types of taste cells (I, II, III) are depicted in the body of the taste bud. At the base of the taste bud, a basal cell and gustatory nerve endings are drawn. (a): From Whitehead, M.C., Beeman, C.S., & Kinsella, B.A. (1985) Distribution of taste and general sensory nerve endings in fungiform papillae of the hamster. *American Journal of Anatomy*, 173, 185–201. (b) From Banister, L.H. (1976) Sensory terminals of peripheral nerves. In: *The Peripheral Nerve* (ed. D.N. Landon), pp. 396–463. Chapman & Hall, London. Reproduced with permission from John Wiley & Sons.)

The G protein gustducin with an α subunit quite similar to retinal rod transducin (which can substitute for gustducin) is ubiquitously involved. Sweet ligands activate the single heterodimeric GPCR T1R2/T1R3; its structure is drawn in Fig. 10.6. Umami (savory) ligands may activate heterodimer T1R1/T1R3. Each of these receptors is restricted to a distinct subset of taste cells. Structurally varied bitter ligands activate the more numerous T2R that appear together in a single TC variant. Most human T2R genes are tightly clustered on chromosomes 12 or 7. T2R38 on chromosome 7q36 is one of few human bitter receptors for which function is definitively established due to discovery and documentation of variation in tasting PTC and related compounds nearly 80 years ago. Of the two common haplotypes, PAV, found in primates, is thought to be the ancestral. (See also Box 10.2(2) above.)

Stimulus binding of ligands such as sweet sucralose and bitter salicin is associated with extracellular portions of T1R2 and T2R16, respectively.

Ionic taste stimuli directly activate dedicated subsets of TC by passing through ion channels in cell membranes, but the TC types involved are uncertain. In rodents and humans, a Na^+ taste is transduced by influx of Na^+ through an amiloride-sensitive ion channel (ENaC); its structure is drawn in Fig. 10.6. Box 10.4(2) below shows a hamster nerve recording demonstrating the effect of 10-μM amiloride on a response to 100-mM NaCl. The taste of NaCl is not completely accounted for by ENaC sensitivity; a quinine-like taste remains. Sour taste may be generated by influx of H^+ through TRP PKD2L1 + PKD1 channels (structure drawn in Fig. 10.6) in membranes of type III TC. It also has been suggested that

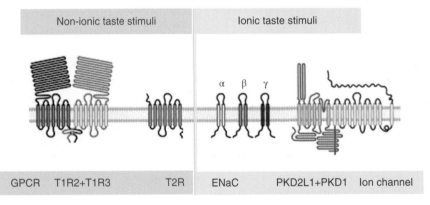

Figure 10.6   Taste bud cells are activated either indirectly by GPCR or directly through ion channels. Sweet sugar acts via heterodimeric GPCR T1R and bitter quinine acts via GPCR T2R; salty NaCl depends on ENaC ion channels, and sour citric acid depends on heterodimeric PKD TRP ion channels. Each eventually initiate neural activity in four independent peripheral taste pathways. (From Yarmolinsky, D.A., Zuker, C.S., & Ryba, N.J. (2009) Common sense about taste: from mammals to insects. Cell, 139, 234–244. Reproduced with permission from Elsevier.)

Box 10.4   Electrophysiological analysis of single neuron & whole nerve responses

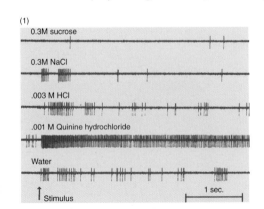

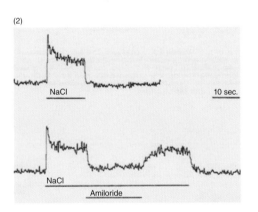

(1) Single gustatory sensory neuron (GSN): five records of action potentials from a single neuron acquired by dividing one rat glossopharyngeal nerve into small fascicles; stimuli were applied to vallate papilla at arrow. Note the strong response (number of action potentials) in response to 1 mM quinine, much stronger than ever seen in the chorda tympani nerve to this stimulus. (See also *Molecular Range* in Glossary) (From Frank, M.E. (1991) Taste responsive neurons of the glossopharyngeal nerve of the rat. *Journal of Neurophysiology*, 65, 1452–1463. Reproduced with permission from the American Physiological Society.)

(2) Whole chorda tympani nerve: two records of rectified, summed action potentials from one hamster chorda tympani nerve. Note 10-μM amiloride inhibits responses to 100-mM NaCl applied to tongue tip. Responses are measured above a cursor aligned with baseline level before stimuli applied. Horizontal lines=application time periods. (From Hettinger, T.P. & Frank, M.E. (1987) Amiloride inhibition of neural taste responses to sodium chloride. In: *Olfaction and Taste*, Vol. IX, (eds. S. Roper & J. Atema), pp. 366–368. NY Academy of Sciences, New York. Reproduced with permission from John Wiley & Sons.)

intracellular acidification has a role in the production of acid taste.

Transduction of nonionic and ionic taste stimuli alike concludes with TC depolarization, which results in activation of **gustatory sensory neurons (GSN)**. Taste nerve responses and behavioral detection of stimuli of all taste qualities depend on adenosine 5'-triphosphate (ATP). Also, within the taste bud, before transmission to the brain, taste stimuli evoke release of serotonin, γ-amino butyric acid (GABA), and norepinephrine, chemicals capable of inhibiting or enhancing independently coded TC messages. The inhibition may provide safety control by reducing effective concentrations of contaminated nutrients.

> Taste receptor (GPCR or ion channel) variants are found in membranes of subsets of taste cells that each detect compounds that elicit distinct taste qualities.

Taste buds occur in several oral receptive fields

Lingual taste buds reside in multiple fungiform papillae, an example shown in Fig. 10.5A, distributed over the dorsal anterior two-thirds of the tongue, in foliate papillae on the lateral edges and circumvallate papillae on the dorsal surface of the posterior one-third of the tongue, as well as on the anterior soft palate and oropharynx, especially the upper laryngeal side of the epiglottis. Locations of the taste bud fields are diagrammed in Fig. 10.7. Frequency distributions of taste buds in mucosa of the lingual and palatal oral cavity and oral pharynx, from which three cranial nerves (CN), VII, IX, and X, in three peripheral ganglia (geniculate, petrosal, nodose) carry taste information to the brain are provided in Table 10.2. Taste buds are more common in foliate papillae and on the palate in hamster (and rat) than in humans. The species difference may relate to the masticatory function of the raised rodent intermolar lingual eminence during feeding. Epiglottal mucosal taste buds, at high proportion in human infants, are much rarer in 80 year olds even though peripheral gustatory function is generally well maintained with aging in humans. This leaves the upper airway less protected from aspiration of food/liquid at advanced age, which may lead to more frequent "choking."

In general, location and chemical sensitivities of each of the three CN taste-bud fields suggest distinct functions. CN VII, confined to the anterior portion of the tongue and palate, specializes in food selection by taste stimulus identification. CN IX, restricted to the posterior third of the tongue, specializes in reflexes of ingestion or rejection, whereas CN X taste buds specialize in airway protection. Studies of rodent behavioral discrimination after cutting individual taste nerves or applying specific inhibitors empirically verify this functional specialization. Thus, stimulus-associated reflex actions rather than taste-quality perceptions may be mapped somatotopically in the oral cavity.

> Taste buds, sensory organs of taste (comparable to retina for vision and cochlea for hearing), are located in distinct oral regions to perform different functions via three cranial nerves, CN VII, IX, and X.

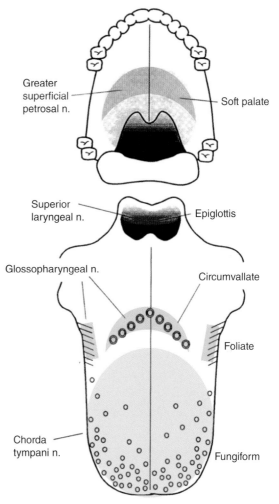

Figure 10.7 Diagram showing human taste bud fields. Fields innervated by CN VII are mostly at the tongue tip but also found on the soft palate. Fields innervated by CN IX are focused at the junction of oral and pharyngeal spaces. CN X innervates taste buds on the laryngeal face of the epiglottis. (See also *Topographic* in the Glossary). (From St John, S.J. & Boughter, J.D., Jr. (2008) The gustatory system. In: *Neuroscience in Medicine* (ed. P.M. Conn), p. 604, Humana Press (Springer), New York. Originally published in Smith, D.V. & Shipley M.T. (1995) The gustatory system. In: *Neuroscience in Medicine* (ed. P.M. Conn) p. 513, JB Lippincott, Philadelphia. Reproduced with kind permission from Springer Science + Business Media.)

Peripheral nerves

GSN are pseudo-unipolar neurons with cell bodies in the three peripheral ganglia listed in Table 10.2. Central and peripheral coursing axonal processes of the neurons are small, either myelinated or unmyelinated. GSN of CN VII travel in the **chorda tympani** (CT), which joins the lingual branch of the mandibular division of the trigeminal nerve (CN V) before reaching the tongue, and the greater superficial petrosal (GSP) nerve, which reaches the soft palate via the vidian nerve as traced in Fig. 10.8. Geniculate central axonal processes travel through the internal auditory meatus to enter the brainstem as the intermediate nerve root, which lies between CN VII and VIII roots. Petrosal central axonal processes of lingual sensory branches of CN IX and nodose central axonal processes of superior laryngeal branches of CN X enter the brain stem within the roots of CN IX and X, respectively.

Table 10.2   The peripheral gustatory pathway

Region	Papillae	% Total TB		CN Branch	Ganglion
		Human	Hamster		
Tongue				VII. Facial	Geniculate
anterior 2/3	Fungiform	20%	18%	Chorda Tympani	
Palate	Islands	6%	14%	Greater Superficial Petrosal	
Tongue				IX. Glossopharyngeal	
posterior 1/3				Lingual	Petrosal
lateral	Foliate	16%	32%		
dorsal	Vallate	31%	23%		
Oropharynx				X. Vagus	Nodose
Epiglottis	Patches	*27%	11%	Superior Laryngeal	

Taste Buds (TB): Region, Cranial Nerve (CN) Branch, and Ganglion (G)

Total taste buds in human = 7902 (*in newborn); hamster = 723 (2% buccal wall/sublingual). (See also *Chorda Tympani* in the Glossary).

(Quantitative data from: Miller, I.J. & Smith, D.V. (1984) Quantitative taste bud distribution in the hamster. *Physiology & Behavior*, 32, 275–285; and Travers, S.P. & Nicklas, K. (1990) Taste bud distribution in the rat pharynx and larynx. *Anatomical Record*, 227, 373–379.)

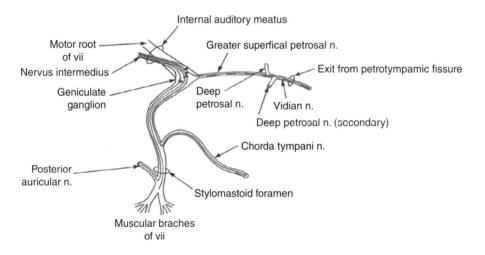

Figure 10.8   Primary afferent taste neurons in the sensory division of CN VII, the facial nerve. The peripheral and central coursing axons of the two sensory branches of CN VII from the rat geniculate ganglion are shown: the chorda tympani to the front of the tongue in orange, and the greater superficial petrosal to the soft palate in green. Centrally, they join to form the intermediate nerve root that enters the brain stem between CN VII and CN VIII (From Gomez, M.M. (1978) The peripheral distribution of the rat geniculate ganglion. PhD Thesis, Wake Forest University, Bowman Gray School of Medicine, Winston-Salem NC. UMI: AAT 7906509.).

Visualization of the CT medial to the mandible coursing from the tympanic bulla to join the lingual nerve is achieved with removal of soft tissue after disarticulation of the temporomandibular joint (anatomy described in detail in Chapter 8, "Temporomandibular Joint"), with removal of its condylar and coronoid processes and the zygomatic arch. This surgical approach and, as important, the ease with which the fungiform taste buds on the tongue tip can be stimulated, has resulted in taste function being defined primarily for a single taste bud field. Box 10.4 contains more information on the techniques used for GSN electrophysiological analysis. Function of individual GSN is measured with single-unit recording (an example is included in Box 10.4(1));

whereas, gustatory sensory nerve function, the combined responses of hundreds of single GSN, is measured by whole-nerve recording (an example is included in Box 10.4(2)).

Gustatory sensory neuron function

Single hamster GSN respond selectively to taste compounds as illustrated for the CT in Fig. 10.9. The neural responses of single neurons in this one taste nerve are compatible with (but less complex than) perceptual "taste worlds" based on all oral sensory nerves (Fig. 10.3). This means more information than received from CT GSN is used by hamsters to make behavioral

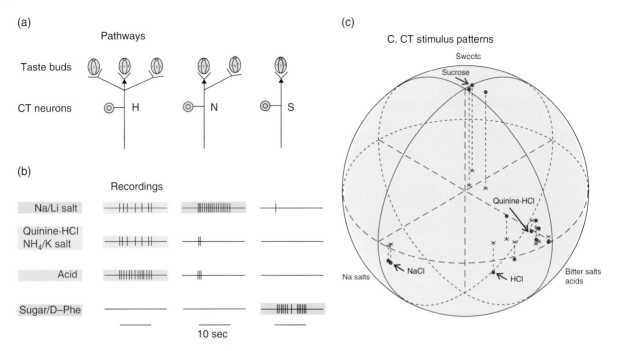

Figure 10.9   Electrophysiological responses of GSN single fibers in the chorda tympani (CT) nerve. Diagrams of (a) taste bud-to-GSN pathways for three physiological types of CT GSN (H, N, S) with (b) decisive single-neuron recordings and (c) a representation of neuronal stimulus patterns for sweets (sucrose, fructose, saccharin), sodium salts (NaCl, NaNO₃), bitter salts (quinine·HCl, KCl, NH₄Cl, MgSO₄), urea, and acids (HCl, citric acid, acetic acid) in MDS three-dimensional space. (See also *Gustatory Sensory Neurons, Sensory Neurons* and *Taste Dimensions* in Glossary). Arrows point to human primary taste stimuli (see Figure 10.1). (From Frank, M.E., Bieber, S.L., & Smith, D.V. (1988) The organization of taste sensibilities in hamster chorda tympani nerve fibers. *Journal of General Physiology*, 91, 861–896.)

discriminations among the tested taste stimuli. The CT contributes sucrose-sensitive (S) and NaCl-sensitive (N) CT GSN that are taste quality **specialists**, the former responding primarily to sweeteners (illustrated in the third column of recordings in Fig. 10.9b) and the latter responding to Na⁺ and Li⁺ halides (illustrated in the second column of recordings in Fig. 10.9b). T1R GPCR and ENaC ion channels (Fig. 10.6), their dedicated TC, and upstream S and N neurons form two peripheral lines to the brain that identify nutrients. In the CT stimulus space in Fig. 10.9c, note tightly clustered sweets and sodium salts falling distant from each other and a looser cluster for other stimuli. Responses to this broader cluster as well as the amiloride-insensitive response to NaCl (illustrated in the first column of recordings shown in Fig. 10.9b), occur in CT H GSN (also known as E GSN because of broad sensitivity to electrolytes). These more variable electrolyte-sensitive CT **generalists** respond to sour HCl and other acids, salty NaCl, bitter quinine and the bitter salts KCl and NH₄Cl. Thus, each cluster in Fig. 10.9c corresponds to activation of the distinct hamster CT neuron types: the highly correlated responses of each of two types of specialists and loosely correlated responses of electrolyte generalists that are possibly composed of several more-specific subtypes.

Individual GSN serve specialist or generalist function. Chorda tympani GSN include specialist detectors of nutrients (sugars and NaCl) as well as nonspecific electrolyte-sensitive generalists that detect stimuli with multiple taste qualities.

Mixing stimuli that activate generalists with stimuli that activate specialists suppresses the specialists' responses. Suppression measured in GSN is asymmetric. There is no reciprocal peripheral specialist stimulus to generalist stimulus suppression. (See also *Generalist* in Glossary). Thus, there is no diminution of generalist signals. Fig. 10.10 illustrates progressively diminished CT S responses to 100-mM sucrose as stronger concentrations of bitter quinine·HCl, which activates CT H GSN, are added. Quinine response increments in generalist GSN quantitatively match response decrements to sucrose specialists, a concurrence suggesting an inhibitory interaction from electrolyte-activated to sucrose-activated TC before neural signals are transmitted to the brain by CN VII. Although the neural, response-size, **intensity** signal for sucrose in S neurons is reduced by adding 1 mM of quinine, consistent with preservation of >75% of CT S neural activity, hamsters' behavioral recognition of 100 mM sucrose is unaffected. Compare "sucrose" and "sucrose + quinine" (S + Q) bars in Box 10.3(2) above. However, sucrose intensity signals when 3 mM and 10 mM of quinine were added were less than 40% of the sucrose-elicited activity on average (Fig. 10.10). One-hundred-mM sucrose elicits a robust 1.43-Hz rhythm that emerges in S GSN tonic responses (Box 10.5(1)). The clarity of this sucrose-induced temporal response is weakened at lower actual sucrose concentration or at the equivalent lower effective concentration in sucrose and quinine mixtures. (See also *Mixture Suppression* in Glossary). Periodic interruption of sweet signals in S GSN may offset adaptation to preserve signal power higher in the gustatory system as do sniffs in the olfactory system (see "Peripheral Activation: Olfactory Mucosa and Olfactory Sensory Neurons" below.).

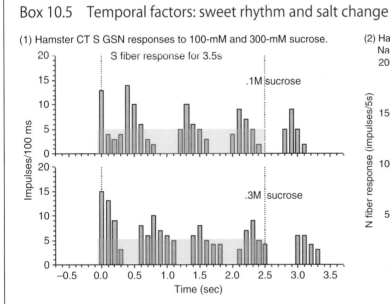

Figure 10.10 CT GSN S-fiber responses to 100-mM sucrose contaminated with increasing concentrations of bitter quinine. The effective concentration of sucrose, as monitored by responses of sweet-specific CT S GSN, descends toward zero as quinine contamination increases from 1 to 10 mM. There is no reciprocal effect of sucrose on quinine responses of CT generalist GSN. (See also *Gustatory Sensory Neurons* in Glossary). The dashed line marks the control mean +2 standard errors, a response level considered to be above background. (From Frank, M.E., Lundy, R.L. Jr., & Contreras, R.J. (2008) Cracking taste codes by tapping into sensory neuron impulse traffic. *Progress in Neurobiology*, 6, 245–263. Reproduced with permission from Elsevier.)

Moreover, ordinarily taste stimuli are perceived transiently above an ambient salinity provided by saliva, a variable formulation described in detail in Chapter 11, "Salivary Glands, Salivary Secretion, and Saliva." For example, the salty quality of NaCl is identifiable as such only when NaCl reaches 10 mM in humans; below this NaCl tastes insipid like water. Peripheral adjustment in effective salt concentrations are experimentally observable in the responses of specific NaCl-detecting N GSN specialist neurons. Box 10.5(2) tracks adaptation of N GSN responses to two, 30-mM sodium salts, the slightly less effective Na-acetate (Ac), and the slightly more effective NaCl before and after exchange of anions (Cl→Ac, Ac→Cl). Switching from Ac to Cl yields dramatic response enhancement while switching from Cl to Ac elicits response diminution. Remarkably, small changes in effective concentrations of stimuli are dynamically exaggerated when imposed on adapted ambient levels in specialist N GSN, an effect that would be hidden in whole-nerve responses to NaCl that also include responses of electrolyte generalists.

> Dynamic sensory self-adaptation and asymmetric response suppression between independent stimuli adjust positive peripheral taste signals for nutrients before transmission to the central nervous system by GSN without altering negative taste signals carried by generalists.

Box 10.5 Temporal factors: sweet rhythm and salt change

(1) Hamster CT S GSN responses to 100-mM and 300-mM sucrose.

(2) Hamster CT N GSN responses to sequential presentation of 30-mM NaCl and Na Acetate (Ac).

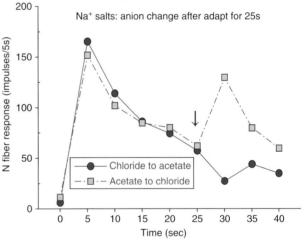

Average 1.43-Hz periodic bursting pattern in CT S GSN responses to two concentrations of sucrose. This powerful rhythm, in spite of reduced effective sucrose concentration with quinine contamination, contributes to coding sweetness until sucrose responses are reduced to <25% by 10-mM quinine. (See also *Quality coding* in Glossary). Vertical dotted lines and shading mark 2.5 sec of a response aligned at zero for the two records. (From Frank, M.E., Formaker, B.K., & Hettinger, T.P. (2005) Peripheral gustatory processing of sweet stimuli by golden hamsters. *Brain Research Bulletin*, 66, 70–84. Reproduced with permission of Elsevier.).

N GSN respond transiently to an anion shift from acetate to chloride or chloride to acetate after 25-sec adaptation (arrow). Slight differences in initial effects of sodium salts (Cl > Ac, seen at time points 5 sec and 10 sec, but lost by the 15-sec time point) are exacerbated after adaptation, demonstrated by shifting anions (Ac→Cl vs. Cl→Ac) at 25-sec time point. (From Frank, M.E. 2008. A perspective on chemosensory quality coding. In: *The Senses: A Comprehensive Reference*, Vol. 4 (sect. eds. D.V. Smith, S. Firestein, & B.K Beauchamp), pp. 339–344. Academic Press, New York. Reproduced with permission from John Wiley & Sons.)

Central neural somatotopic organization

GSN central projections are **somatotopic**. As documented in Table 10.2 above and pictured in Fig. 10.11, oropharyngeal facial, glossopharyngeal, and vagal taste afferents enter the brainstem somatotopically to join the solitary tract and make synaptic contact with the surrounding cells of the nucleus of the solitary tract (nucleus tractus solitarii, NTS) in the medulla oblongata. CN VII from the tongue tip and palate enters the NTS most rostrally, CN IX from the back of tongue follows and CN X from the throat enters most caudally, recapitulating oropharyngeal space. In rodents, terminations of CT taste-responsive neurons are concentrated in a rostro-central (RC) subdivision of the most rostral pole of the NTS. RC NTS neural cell bodies have three general shapes related to their function: the ovoid are intrinsic inhibitory interneurons to process incoming afferent signals, and the multipolar and elongate are projection neurons to access higher regions of the brain.

Primate and rodent gustatory brainstem to thalamocortical projection pathways differ. In primates, including humans, NTS taste neurons project, via the central tegmental tract, to the small-celled medial parvicellular part of the ventral posteromedial nucleus of the thalamus just medial to the somatosensory representation of the tongue. However, in rodents, NTS taste neurons project not directly to the thalamus but to the nearby parabrachial

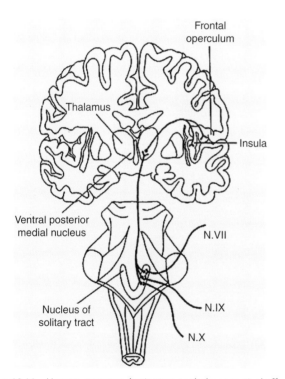

Figure 10.11 Human gustatory brainstem to thalamocortical afferent pathway in the coronal plane. Cranial N VII GSN from the tongue tip enter the rostral tip of the nucleus of the solitary tract (NTS); GSN in cranial N IX from the posterior tongue enter more caudally; and GSN in cranial N X from the throat enter the NTS most caudally. Ipsilateral projections are drawn to the thalamus and primary gustatory cortex (insula and frontal operculum). (See also *Topographic* in Glossary). (From Frank, M.E. & Rabin, M.D. (1989) Chemosensory neuroanatomy and physiology. *Ear, Nose & Throat Journal*, 68, 291–296. Reproduced with permission from Vendome Health Care.)

nucleus (PBN) in the pons to bring regulatory influences into play before signals ascend to the thalamus. Also, NTS neurons, mostly originating from ventral regions, project into medullary oromotor centers to impact secretion of saliva, swallowing, emesis, and other prominent reflexive responses, as noted in chapters 11, "Salivary Glands, Salivary Secretion, and Saliva" and 12, "Orofacial Pain, Touch and Thermosensation, and Sensorimotor Functions."

Thalamic taste neurons project to primary taste cortex, the anterior insula, and adjacent frontal operculum, close to somatosensory cortical representations of the tongue. The bilateral cortical taste regions contain small percentages of neurons responsive to taste stimuli. There is some debate over whether lingual gustatory and somatosensory projections differ in cortical ipsilateral-contralateral hemispheric preference.

> Somatotopy, which is evident in taste receptive fields of CN VII, IX, and X, characterizes the gustatory thalamocortical afferent pathway.

Gustatory central processing

In the hindbrain, NTS brainstem neurons have more complex receptive fields and respond differently across taste qualities than GSN. For example, some NTS neurons respond to sweet and salty stimuli, others are excited by sweet and inhibited by salty stimuli, making average NTS neurons appear less tuned to a single taste quality than GSN. In the NTS, glutamate is an excitatory and GABA is an inhibitory neurotransmitter. The decrease in average quality tuning, without considering the excitatory or inhibitory circuits to and within the NTS, gives the impression that taste quality, rather than being "sharpened" in the brain, is imbedded within spatial and temporal patterns of activity of the central nervous system. Recordings from NTS neurons in unanesthetized awake rats are quite similar to those taken from anesthetized preparations with one exception. More single neurons in awake animals respond to stimuli of a single taste quality; perhaps because tuning circuitry is silenced by anesthesia. Besides spatial features, i.e., differences in rates of response across relevant neurons, temporal response features contain additional information that likely contribute to taste discriminations.

In the forebrain, thalamic taste neurons have more complex response properties than brainstem neurons and project to the primary taste cortex, a pathway likely involved in taste discrimination and perception. **Taste pathways** to the limbic regions (amygdala and hypothalamus) associate motivational and hedonic (preference-aversion) aspects with tastes. While the brainstem is sufficient for facial expressions and motor reflexes of acceptance and rejection, taste aversions, learned when one taste experience is followed by gastrointestinal malaise, require forebrain circuits. Temporal dynamics of brainstem responses to stimuli may contribute to taste-stimulus discrimination but forebrain responses may signify the distinct reactions to taste stimuli. Cortical taste neurons, studied electrophysiologically by positioning micro-electrodes in taste-responsive regions, show higher levels of quality specificity; some cells respond to a "natural" sweet juice containing glucose more than pure glucose, others respond momentarily to preferred stimuli of several taste qualities. In macaque monkeys, a secondary cortical taste area in the orbitofrontal cortex integrates taste, olfactory, and other sensory aspects of foods. Some of its neurons respond less and less as a taste stimulus is repeatedly sampled, showing **habituation**, a "stimulus-specific satiety." Studies on taste-stimulus timing, short response epochs, and mixture interactions are establishing how taste chemicals are identified and acted upon, processing that evolved in a distant past when nutrients were scarce and survival uncertain.

Gustatory brainstem and insular cortex may process tastes differently

The most thoroughly studied taste pathways are from tongue tip and palate to the nucleus of the solitary tract (NTS) in the medulla or from the entire oral cavity through multiple relay centers to the primary **gustatory cortex (GC)** in the insula. Methods and results of two studies follow. One is on the **convergence** of independent GSN signals onto single gustatory NTS neurons; the second is on a gustotopic organization based on taste receptor (TR and ENaC) specificity in isolated GC patches.

GSN converge onto NTS neurons. Fig. 10.12 presents results from NTS single-unit recording (see Box 10.4(1)) with sharp microelectrodes inserted stereotaxically into the dorsal, orosensory tip of the rat NTS. Recording sites were histologically reconstructed from

this region where the majority of small inhibitory and excitatory taste-responsive neurons reside. In this study, Travers, Pfaffmann, and Norgren (1986) show that single NTS neurons have CT lingual NaCl-specific and GSP palatal sucrose-specific fields consistent with the greater tongue tip salt sensitivity and greater palatal sugar sensitivity. NTS neurons also have combined CT–tongue and GSP–palate receptive fields. As illustrated in Fig. 10.12, combined fields may have stimulus-specific or generalist-type function. NTS combined-field specialists respond to NaCl on palate and tongue. NTS combined-field generalists respond to sucrose on the palate and NaCl on the tongue, combining peripheral quality and place domains. Combining signals from distributed active sites dedicated to the same taste quality might serve to increase detection; whereas, combining palatal sucrose with lingual NaCl would augment distributed preferred nutrient compounds.

> CN VII GSN from tongue and palate convey quality and site-specific information to single NTS brainstem neurons, where it is combined in several different ways.

GC preserves taste receptor quality specificity. Computer-analyzed two-photon calcium imaging of taste-evoked activity in GC layers 2 and 3 was studied in mice. A calcium-sensitive fluorescent dye was injected into regions of the insula where

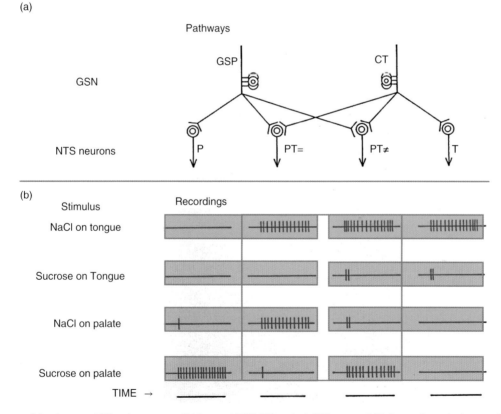

Figure 10.12 Convergence of chorda tympani (CT) and greater superficial petrosal (GSP) GSN on single NTS neurons. (a) Pathways. Rat geniculate ganglion afferents from the palate via the GSP and from the tongue tip via the CT end on neurons in the nucleus of the solitary tract (NTS) to create isolated P (palate) or T (tongue) or combined PT receptive fields (PT= and PT≠). (See also *Convergence* in Glossary). (b) Recordings. NTS responses from single neurons determined a variety of receptive fields. Results reflect greater palatal sensitivity to sucrose and greater tongue-tip sensitivity to salt. Stimulus and application sites (at left) and examples of NTS action potential responses are shown. Responses to NaCl are shaded blue; responses to sucrose are shaded green. (Derived primarily from data in Travers, S.P., Pfaffmann, C., & Norgren, R. (1986) Convergence of lingual and palatal gustatory neural activity in the nucleus of the solitary tract. *Brain Research*, 365, 305–320.)

taste-sensitive VPM thalamic nucleus neurons project. To look for a "gustotopic" organization within the GC, Chen, Gabitto, Peng, Ryba, and Zuker (2011) used rapid bulk stimulus delivery to the whole oral cavity, optical imaging, and verification by genetic or pharmacologic deletion of taste receptor function (refer to "Peripheral Activation" and Fig. 10.6 above.). Activation of independent discrete GC "hot spots" associated with stimulation of taste cell variants (each specific for one taste quality) were revealed (Fig. 10.13). The bitter spot responded to multiple bitters as do the multiple T2R-containing taste cells. With cycloheximide-specific T2R5 knocked out, stimulation with cycloheximide no longer activated the bitter region, but bitters that activate other T2R did. Discrete quality-specific cortical fields were also found for sweet, selectively deleted in T1R2 knockouts, and for umami substances such as K-glutamate + IMP. Of two taste qualities mediated by ion channels, a GC region specific for NaCl stimulation that was pharmacologically removed with amiloride treatment (which blocks ENaC channels required for Na^+-specific taste) was located. A region specific for sour stimulation was not found; sour sensations may be complex, with acids acting as irritants as well as tastes. Thus, with the whole oral cavity simultaneously stimulated and place information obscured, GC gustotopy in the form of four isolated taste quality-specific regions was discovered in the insular cortex. The hot spots, retaining responses indistinguishable from TC, encompass a small fraction of the entire insula, which also contains circuits for performing multisensory processing. Regions of the human insula influenced by gustatory and olfactory inputs have been identified with neuroimaging. The cortical hot spots, identical in stimulus specificity to peripheral TC, may provide quality identity references that mediate central mixture suppression (See also *Mixture Suppression* in Glossary.) and facilitate moving from perception to action.

Smell

Fundamentals and historical perspective

Olfaction (smell) is actually two senses defined by the two paths by which chemical volatiles gain access to the olfactory epithelium. Orthonasal olfaction samples the external environment via the nose, detecting chemicals that inform nutritional, social, reproductive, and habitat options. See Box 10.1(1) above for information on the peripheral patches of olfactory epithelia dedicated to good- and bad-smelling stimuli sampled orthonasally. Retronasal olfaction evaluates oral chemical volatiles settling in the oropharyngeal cavity that contribute to attraction or repulsion. With arrows, Fig. 10.14 depicts the inhaled nasal, in black, and exhaled oral, in red, routes to odor stimulation. People confuse odors that originate in the mouth for tastes, likely because the taste, odor, and touch are happening simultaneously.

Despite the perceptual confusions, tastes and odors are generated by distinct sensory systems in which stimuli that taste are oral aqueous solutions but stimuli that smell are nasal and oral volatiles. By simply closing the nose, many oral stimuli, such as

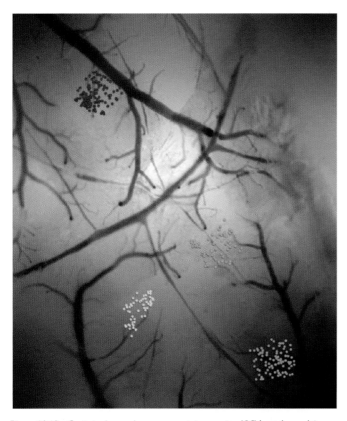

Figure 10.13   Gustotopic map in mouse gustatory cortex (GC) based on calcium imaging. GC regions containing neurons for bitter (■), umami (■), salty (□), and sweet (▤) tastes were located in mice. Increases in intracellular calcium reflected in change in fluorescence ($\Delta F/F = 20–65\%$) were measured in regions receiving input from the taste-responsive thalamus. (See also *Gustatory Cortex* and *Topographic* in Glossary.) A sour-specific region was not found. Stimuli were delivered by rapidly flooding the whole oral cavity. Cycloheximide, quinine, and denatonium; sugars and artificial sweeteners; K-glutamate + IMP; NaCl, NaCl + amiloride; KCl, $MgCl_2$, and citric acid were tested. Optical imaging was combined with genetic (T2R5 & T1R2 knockouts) and pharmacologic (amiloride) functional deletion of taste receptors. (Image courtesy of Jayaram Chandrashekar, Xioake Chen, and Charles Zuker. *Originally published in Science*, 333, 1213 (2011).)

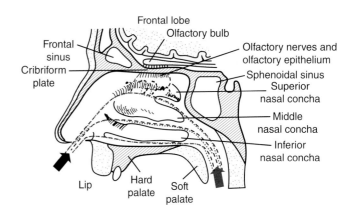

Figure 10.14   A sagittal view through the nasal cavity. Black arrows and dashed lines follow the path of the inhaled air stream, the orthonasal route over the nasal conchae to produce eddies that divert odor molecules in inhaled air toward odor receptors in the olfactory epithelium. Superimposed red arrows and dotted lines follow the exhaled air stream, during which odor molecules in the oropharyngeal space gain access to the olfactory epithelium via a retronasal route from the mouth. (From Shepherd, G.M. (1983) *Neurobiology*, pp. 203–226. Oxford University Press, New York. Reproduced with permission from Oxford University Press.)

Box 10.6   Sensory science: rating bitter intensity and liking or disliking vegetables

(1) Rating scales

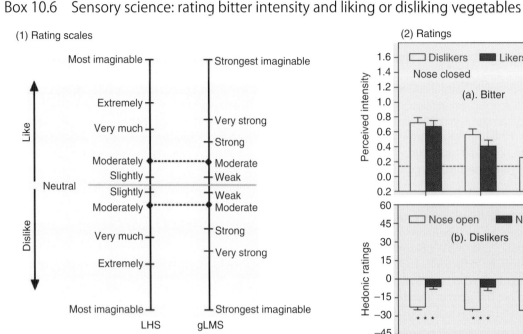

(2) Ratings

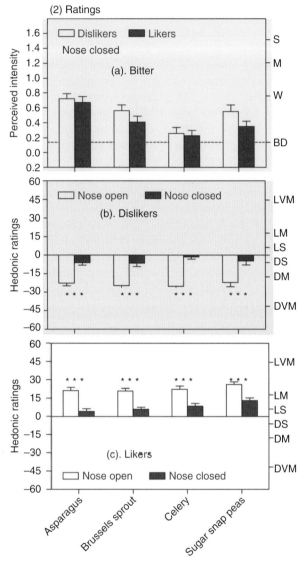

(1) Rating scales accurately reflect people's reactions to items with nutrient status, such as vegetables. A quasi-logarithmic labeled hedonic scale (LHS) for liking (up) and disliking (down) on the left was derived from two general labeled magnitude scales (gLMS) for intensity, one going upward from the neutral position (horizontal line) and one going downward. (From Lim, J., Wood, A., & Green, B.G. (2009) Derivation and evaluation of a labeled hedonic scale. *Chemical Senses*, 34, 739–751. Reproduced with permission from Oxford University Press.) A single upward-going gLMS was used for rating intensity. Bitter intensity (2-a) and strengths of disliking (2-b) or liking (2-c) of four vegetable purees were measured.

For bitter rating: S=strong, M=moderate, W=weak intensity, BD=barely detectable. (See also *Intensity* in Glossary.)

For disliking and liking rating: LVM=like very much, LM=like moderately, LS=like slightly, DS=dislike slightly, DM=dislike moderately, DVM=dislike very much.

*** = statistical significance of increases and decreases.

(2) Ratings of four vegetable purees, liked or disliked, with nose open or closed. Odors (not bitter tastes) were related to disliking or liking.
(From Lim, J. & Padmanabhan, A. (2013) Retronasal olfaction in vegetable liking and disliking. *Chemical Senses*, 38, 45–55. Reproduced with permission from Oxford University Press.)

those recognized as sulfurous or soapy, are discovered to be odors, not tastes. Also, using the rating scales illustrated in Box 10.6(1), vegetables, popularly thought to be disliked because they taste bitter, are found to be primarily disliked for their retronasal odors. Note psychophysical rating data supporting this conclusion in Box 10.6(2). The upper graph (a) shows that weak vegetable bitter taste intensity is rated equally by vegetable dislikers and likers. (See also *Intensity* in Glossary.) The center graph (b) shows that disliking of vegetables and the lower graph (c) shows that liking of vegetables each depend on the nose being open.

There are two odor access pathways. Vapors enter through the nose by the orthonasal route and oral chemical volatiles reach the olfactory mucosa by the retronasal route to contribute much to flavors.

Over the years, attempts to define single physical or frequency-based **dimensions for olfaction or taste** were unsuccessful. Adequate taste and **odor stimuli**, in distinct chemical phases, are detected and identified by discrete receptors with multiple individual chemistries, as schematized in Box 10.7(1)

Box 10.7   Chemical senses have as many qualities as receptors

(1)

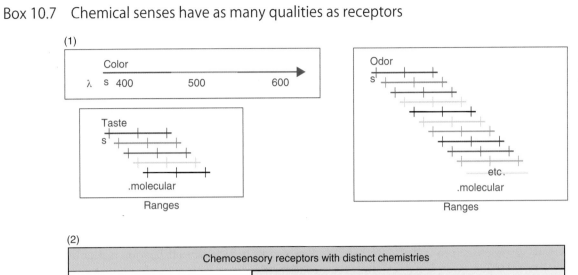

(2)

Chemosensory receptors with distinct chemistries				
		Variants		
		Receptor	Receptor Cell	Sensory Neuron
Olfactory	OR	390	390	
Taste	T1R dimer	2	2	2
	T2R	30	1	1
	ENaC	1	1	1
	PKD dimer	1		1
Total taste		34	5	5
Olfactory & taste		424	395	

(1) Schematics of stimulus dimensions. Colors are based on three pigments with sensitivities peaking at blue, green, and red regions of the visible spectrum of electromagnetic rays. Tastes and odors are based on 34 and 390 receptors tuned to chemicals in aqueous solution and chemical volatiles, respectively. (See also *Sensory Neurons* in Glossary.)

(2) Chemosensory receptors with distinct chemistries. There are 11.5 times as many odor receptors (OR) than there are taste receptors (TR & ion channels); however, because 30 TR2 combine in 1 TC variant, 78 times as many OSN variants than GSN variants send signals the brain, numbers that match with the hundreds of unique odors and handful of unique tastes.

and enumerated in Box 10.7(2). Neither chemical sense is grounded in a single continuous physical dimension, as are the gradually changing vast shades of color created by three cone pigments from a continuum of wavelengths of light.

Chemical stimuli and odor quality

More than 80 years ago, Hans Henning used people's judgments of similarity to create the "smell prism" sketched in Fig. 10.15. His earlier taste tetrahedron represented four abstract gustatory qualities, each the taste of many stimulus compounds (Fig. 10.1). However, the smell prism, a parallel geometric attempt to reduce odors to **primaries**, stipulated six categories of odor objects. Henning labeled the six corners of the prism flowery, foul, fruity, burnt, spicy and resinous; one chemical example is provided for each in Fig. 10.15. Many other objects with distinct odor would

fall under each category. The rose and violet odors are both flowery; the banana and raspberry odors are both fruity; and the odors of decayed meat and decayed fish are both foul. In fact, no model comparable to the three-dimensional "taste world" can be generated for odors because of the high number of independent odor qualities. Henning's six-corner odor prism is still a three-dimensional object, which cannot mathematically represent more than four independent categories. Unlike a tetrahedron, edges and faces of a prism are not all equivalent.

Chemical structures of compounds that give 20 objects their characteristic odors are shown in Box 10.8. The chemicals have short or long carbon chains, have aliphatic, heterocyclic, aromatic, or macrocyclic rings, and contain alcohol, aldehyde, keto, ester, ether, amino, and thiol functional groups. Each chemical itself produces a unique olfactory perception that more or less recapitulates the odor of a particular chemically complex odor

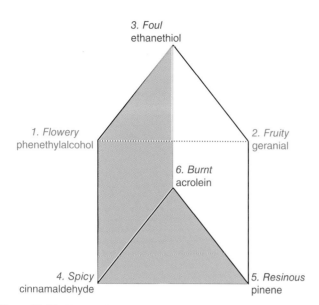

Figure 10.15   Henning's 1924 smell prism represents odor categories (*flowery, fruity, foul, spicy, resinous* and *burnt*) at six corners. The name of a single chemical within each category is positioned nearby. Besides the quality of the ones noted, other distinct odor qualities are perceived in each category. (See also *Quality Primaries* in Glossary.) Examples are *sweaty* isovaleric acid and *fecal* methyl indole under *foul*; or *camphorous* cineole and *sweet* vanillin under *spicy*. Unlike tastes, which readily fall into a few abstract qualia, odors are typically characterized by the names of odor objects, which are first divisible into pleasing or foul and then further sorted under names of objects like spices, flowers, fruits, excrement, carrion, and vomit. (See also *Quality* in Glossary.)

object, whether delivered by oral or nasal route. Natural odor objects often contain a cocktail of odorous chemicals, but one or two key dominant components are responsible for much of the odor character.

> Single volatile chemical compounds are capable of providing characteristic odors to many odor objects.

Given the plethora of distinct odors, it should have been no surprise when Linda Buck and Richard Axel discovered that there are many hundreds of mammalian **odor receptors (OR)**. Buck and Axel were awarded the 2004 Nobel Prize in Physiology and Medicine for their work on rodent olfaction, which is much more complex, with 1000 to 1200 OR, than primate olfaction, with 300 to 400 OR. See Fig. 10.16 for numbers of OR in a sample of mammals. The fewer human OR do not interfere with people tracking the odor of chocolate essential oil across a grassy field, however.

Few component stimuli are detected in odor mixtures

Henning's smell prism, seemingly legitimate decades ago, represents few of the multitude of distinguishable **odor qualities** associated with environmental processes, objects, and events. Unsurprisingly, unlike the few tastes or the many familiar gradually varying colors, people often need assistance with naming odors when presented in a controlled laboratory setting. This "memory" problem likely stems largely from the existence of countless independent odors, many

never before encountered. It happens despite the human capability to recall odors per se more vividly than other sensory experiences and to identify many hundreds of individual odors in natural settings. How components of mixtures are identified, which is not merely based on evoked memories, remains a mystery.

An important clue is found in everyday experience, where odor stimuli are more than likely combined in complex mixtures. Unexpectedly, under these circumstances, identifying single critical odors is made more manageable. This is consistent with David Laing's discoveries that humans identify only the strongest mixture component that endures over time, failing to recognize no more than four equally strong odors concurrently. As for tastes in the less elaborate gustatory system (see "Chemical Stimuli and Taste Quality" above), in the olfactory system mixture suppression reduces identification of many simultaneously appearing odors to few, a coding process epitomized by **dominance** (overshadowing) between independent odors that results in adjustments of effective concentration based on relative odor salience.

A simple laboratory protocol (See Table 10.1, above), which simulates the temporally dynamic natural settings in which odors are usually identified, was used to quantitatively study this odor coding process. Results of an experimental study of the four odor stimuli drawn in Box 10.9(1) show the identification advantage of any one extra stimulus in three-component and four-component mixtures in Box 10.9(2). Selective sensory adaptation quickly, in a matter of seconds, reduced intensities of already-present ambient compounds to promote identification of the later-appearing extra compounds. Multiple odors of the cocktail of compounds generated by most odor objects are likewise soon reduced to a few strong, remembered "characteristic" odors, such as those presented in Box 10.8. In humans, identification of moderately intense odors occurs in the half-second needed to complete a single sniff.

> Individual odor objects are identified in complex mixtures found in natural settings because selective adaptation and mixture suppression together highlight key chemicals, a strategy also used for the less numerous tastes.

Peripheral activation: olfactory mucosa and olfactory sensory neurons

The olfactory sensory neurons (OSN), numbering as many as 5×10^6 within 2- to 5-cm^2 bilateral patches of olfactory mucosa, line parts of superior and middle nasal turbinates (conchae) and the nasal septum, as drawn in Fig. 10.14 above. During normal breathing, the nasal conchae divert airflow upward, deflecting air laden with odor molecules toward OSN apical membranes. Orthonasal "breathing in" samples external odors through the nose. Retronasal "breathing out" samples oropharyngeal odors in the mouth that combine with oral tastes to form *flavor*.

In contrast to taste reception, which engages taste bud receptor cells within a taste-bud cellular network prior to GSN activation, odor reception is accomplished by a single cell type, the bipolar OSN shaded green in Fig. 10.17. As pictured, electro-olfactogram (EOG) slow potentials (surface negative voltages) are recorded electrophysiologically with an electrode placed at the olfactory mucosal surface

Box 10.8   Odor objects captured by one compound

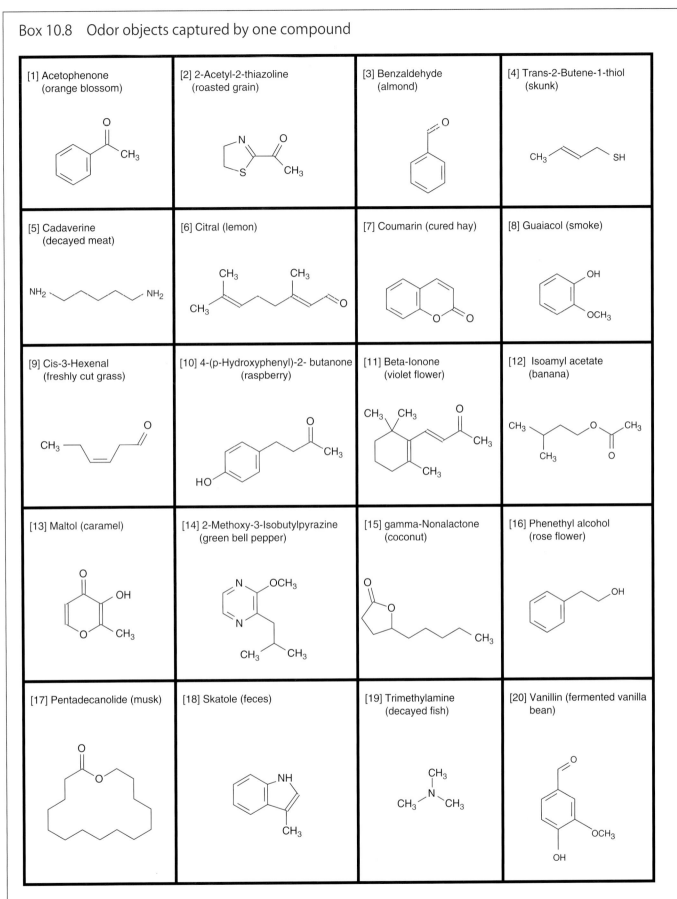

[1] Acetophenone (orange blossom)	[2] 2-Acetyl-2-thiazoline (roasted grain)	[3] Benzaldehyde (almond)	[4] Trans-2-Butene-1-thiol (skunk)
[5] Cadaverine (decayed meat)	[6] Citral (lemon)	[7] Coumarin (cured hay)	[8] Guaiacol (smoke)
[9] Cis-3-Hexenal (freshly cut grass)	[10] 4-(p-Hydroxyphenyl)-2- butanone (raspberry)	[11] Beta-Ionone (violet flower)	[12] Isoamyl acetate (banana)
[13] Maltol (caramel)	[14] 2-Methoxy-3-Isobutylpyrazine (green bell pepper)	[15] gamma-Nonalactone (coconut)	[16] Phenethyl alcohol (rose flower)
[17] Pentadecanolide (musk)	[18] Skatole (feces)	[19] Trimethylamine (decayed fish)	[20] Vanillin (fermented vanilla bean)

The 20 chemicals pictured all occur in nature and have unique odors that together represent a wide range of chemical structure and odor variety. Each chemical itself produces a distinct perception that more or less evokes the complex "odor object" in parentheses. They include pleasant food odors: citral (lemon) and maltol (caramel); flower odors: acetophenone (orange blossom) and beta-ionone (violet flower); and foul odors: trans-2-butene-1-thiol (skunk) and trimethylamine (decayed fish). (See also *Odor Stimuli* in Glossary.)
(From Hettinger, T.P. (2013) Unpublished.)

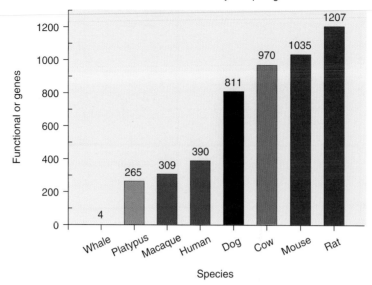

Numbers of olfactory receptor genes

Figure 10.16   Species vary in numbers of functional olfactory receptor genes. Mammals contend with quite diverse olfactory environments that require identification of a few or many distinct odor objects. Rodent ecological niches, for example, encompass many more odorous chemicals than those of humans. On the other hand, sea-living whales recognize few chemical volatiles. All but whales sense more odors than tastes. (Data from the literature: Niimura, Y. & Nei, M. (2007) Extensive gains and losses of olfactory receptor genes in mammalian evolution. *PLoS One*, 2, e708; Kishida, T., Kubota, S., Shirayama, Y., & Fukami, H. (2007) The olfactory receptor gene repertoires in secondary-adapted marine vertebrates: evidence for reduction of the functional proportions in cetaceans. *Biology Letters*, 3, 428–430; Olender, T., Lancet, D., & Nebert, D.W. (2008) Update on the olfactory receptor (OR) gene superfamily. *Human Genomics*, 3, 87–97).

Box 10.9   Prior selective adaptation reduces odors detected in multicomponent mixtures to a few

(1) Four water-soluble chemicals with distinct independent odors.

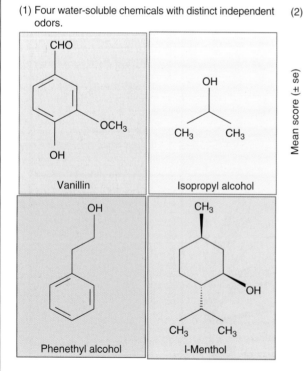

(2) Identification of components in three or four component mixtures is improved by selective adaptation.

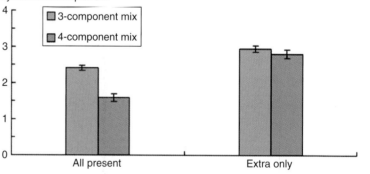

The odor stimuli used to study temporally dynamic odor coding. Subjects were familiarized with the vanilla, rose, alcohol, and mint odors of vanillin, phenethyl alcohol, isopropyl alcohol, and l-menthol.

Comparison of the correct identification of every mixture component that is present ("all present"; veridical identification) with the correct identification of single components that are added after prior presentation of the other components ("extra only"; dynamic odor identification). A simulation of natural smelling was used in which subjects were presented with two-component mixtures quickly followed by three-component mixtures or three-component mixtures quickly followed by four-component mixtures. The subjects identified fewer components in four-component mixtures than three-component mixtures, but had their greatest success in identifying extra odors in mixtures after selective adaptation of the other odors in mixtures of either three or four components (p < .0001). Score = number of correct identifications. (From Goyert, H.F., Frank, M.E., Gent, J.F., & Hettinger, T.P. (2007) Characteristic component odors emerge from mixtures after selective adaptation. Brain Research Bulletin, 72, 1–9. Reproduced with permission from Elsevier.)

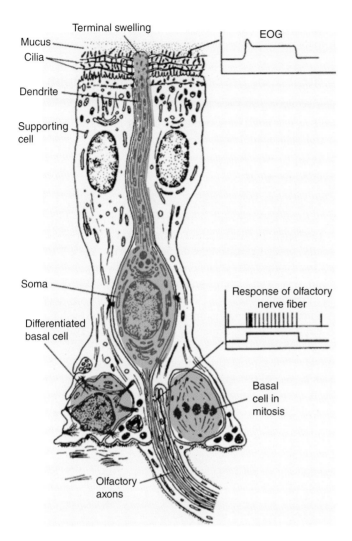

Figure 10.17 Olfactory mucosa: diagram of essential cellular components and electrophysiological responses of an olfactory sensory neuron (OSN). A mature OSN with dendrite and axon and two mature supporting cells, as well as dividing and immature differentiated globose basal stem cells are pictured. OSN EOG slow potentials are obtained with surface recording electrodes and OSN action potentials of nerve fibers obtained with basal electrodes. EOG recorded from awake humans are presented in Box 10.1(1). EOG = electro-olfactogram. (From Banister, L.H. (1976) Sensory terminals of peripheral nerves. In: *The Peripheral Nerve* (ed. D.N. Landon), pp. 396–463. Chapman & Hall, London. Reproduced with permission from John Wiley & Sons.)

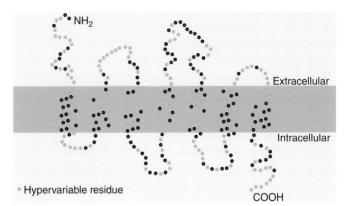

Figure 10.18 Olfactory receptor (OR) located in OSN "cilial" membrane. Olfactory receptors, G-protein-coupled receptors (GPCR) with seven transmembrane domains, code for the tremendous number of odors. The OR genes, 1% of the human and 3% of the mouse genome, form the largest mammalian multigene family. The OR amino acid residues, represented as circles in the diagram, vary within the OR GPCR family. Blue circles denote residues that were quite variable among the handful of receptors originally sequenced. (From Buck, L. B. (2005) Unraveling the sense of smell (Nobel lecture), *Angewante Chemie* (International ed. in English), 44, 6128–6140. Reproduced with permission from John Wiley & Sons.)

epithelium degenerates if OSN axons are injured; but in time it may reappear. Reconstitution, which depends on severity of injury to the epithelial cells, begins with increased mitotic activity of GBC to produce, at successive stages, transit amplifying and neuronal precursors, followed by appearance of immature OSN, which reach maturity with extension of an axon toward the olfactory bulb, a necessity for eventual odor perception.

Olfactory receptor variants are expressed in dedicated subsets of OSN

Olfactory receptors (OR) are GPCR proteins with seven hydrophobic transmembrane segments like opsins in the retina. OR contain multiple "hypervariable" residues (as illustrated in Fig. 10.18), which is consistent with the many OR variants. OR ligands associate with transmembrane GPCR binding sites as retinal (retinaldehyde) binds rhodopsin (the chemical basis for vision) in the retina. A tissue-specific G protein α subunit (G_{olf}) and adenylyl cyclase provide the basis for the second-messenger pathway for olfactory signaling that results in stimulus-evoked release of cyclic adenosine monophosphate, cAMP. With the opening of a specific cyclic-nucleotide-gated Na^+ channel, OSN depolarize and action potentials are generated in the OSN axon. The cation channel involved is homologous to the channel involved in visual transduction. Although comparable biochemical machinery suggests analogies between odor perception and color vision, an important exception is noted in Box 10.7(1). Stimulus domains for chemical odor receptors are multiple and discrete; whereas the single physical visual stimulus domain is continuous.

and OSN action potentials are recorded with a microelectrode inserted at the base of the olfactory epithelium. The EOG assays generator potentials that precede action potentials in OSN axons. Fine-diameter axons, 0.1 to 0.3 μm, comprise the "fila olfactoria" (CN I), in which single Schwann cells surround small bundles of axons that project through the skull to the **olfactory bulb** through the cribriform plate of the ethmoid bone.

Olfactory "cilia" (10 to 20) extend about 0.1 mm into the mucus from the olfactory knob at the top of the dendritic process of a bipolar OSN. The cilial membranes contain the molecular odor receptors (OR). OSN, which turn over in adults, have a 60-day life span. Besides OSN, the olfactory mucosa contains horizontal basal cells, multipotent progenitor globose basal stem cells (GBC), illustrated in Fig. 10.17, and Bowman's glands that secrete mucus. Sustentacular (supporting) cells store secretory granules and extend microvilli into the mucus layer. The olfactory

The peripheral olfactory system uses a single cell type, the olfactory sensory neuron (OSN), for GPCR stimulus reception, cAMP-gated transduction and axonal signal transmission to the brain.

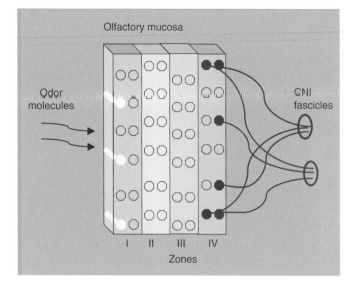

Figure 10.19 Functional organization of olfactory sensory neurons (OSN) in the olfactory mucosa. Four populations of OSN, each individual OSN expressing a single OR variant, are segregated in four mucosal zones (I, II, III, IV). Within a zone OR variants are randomly distributed. Axons of OSN, CN I, form the olfactory nerve layer of the olfactory bulb after passing though the cribriform plate in the skull. In this diagram, odor stimuli course behind a panel of receptors to activate OSN dendrites, represented as white shapes at the left edge of zone I. OSN expressing a single OR variant (red or blue circles) send axons in fascicles *en route* to a few glomeruli of the olfactory bulb. (See also *Olfactory Bulb* and *Topographic* in Glossary.) (Based on a review by Mori, K., Nagao, H. & Yoshihara, Y. (1999) The olfactory bulb: coding and processing of odor molecule information. *Science,* 286, 711–715.)

Regions of the olfactory mucosal surface differ in sensitivity to chemicals. For example, *n*-butanol, an unpleasant odor, is more effective with the EOG recording electrode placed on the anterior, but *d*-limonene, a pleasant odor, is more effective when the electrode is placed on the posterior mucosal surface. This spatial distribution is consistent with discovery of four separate OR sub-families each exclusively expressed in OSN that are randomly dispersed in one of four mucosal zones. This epithelial zonal somatotopy, illustrated in Fig. 10.19, is transformed into an OR-variant odotopy in the olfactory bulb. The many OSN expressing 1 OR variant project CN I axonal fascicles to a few olfactory bulb sites.

Effective OSN stimulus compounds elicit short-latency excitatory responses to chemicals specified by the single expressed OR variant. Many individual OSN are narrowly tuned, that is activated by compounds of similar structure and odor, but some OSN are quite broadly tuned, as must be their expressed OR. Typically, an individual stimulus compound activates a particular set of two or more OSN and likewise also activates a set of two or more corresponding OR. In two studies on central odor processing considered below either aldehydes of varying carbon chain length were used to decipher rabbit olfactory bulb inhibitory circuits or acetophenone was used to determine the capacity of transgenic mice missing a single OR variant to make behavioral discriminations. Single OR may be activated by chemicals having a particular functional group with specified carbon chain lengths; for example the **molecular range** of OSN expressing OR I7 includes heptyl (C7), octyl (C8), nonyl (C9), and decyl (C10) aldehydes. Other OR favor ligands with several functional

groups; for example OSN expressing OR M71, respond to the aromatic ketone acetophenone and the aldehyde benzaldehyde.

Central odor processing in olfactory bulb

OSN expressing one OR converge on a few sites in the olfactory bulb, the five-layer, initial central locus for odor processing at the base of the human brain.

The olfactory bulb processes odor signals specified by OR

OSN axons enter the complex, layered bulb in the superficial olfactory nerve layer to form excitatory synapses with primary dendrites of mitral and tufted cells, output neurons, within spherical neuropil, the olfactory glomeruli, in the deeper glomerular layer. The excitatory neurotransmitter is glutamate. Mitral cells respond selectively to odor quality and intensity. As illustrated in Box 10.10(1) for two OSN variants colored red and blue, one medially positioned and one laterally positioned glomerulus receives exclusive input from the hundreds of OSN expressing each OR variant. Thus, olfactory bulb glomeruli are central functional units that collect the information originating in the stimulus activation of a single OR variant. In rodents, each of the approximately 1000 OSN variants exclusively targets two of the approximately 2000 glomeruli. Based on retrograde OSN tracing from injections of a few glomeruli, specific **topographic** projections from the mucosa to the bulb were suspected well before OR were characterized, but tracing of OR in OSN axons to the bulb with RNA in situ hybridization histochemistry firmly established this remarkable functional topography.

> Single OR variants define individual OSN molecular ranges and their few olfactory bulb projection sites.

Intrinsic periglomerular (PG) cells, which form inhibitory synapses with primary dendrites of mitral cells (M) in multiple glomeruli in the olfactory bulb, are well positioned to generate lateral inhibition between mitral cells, as shown in the circuit diagram: $M_1 \rightarrow PG \rightarrow M_2$, in Box 10.10(2). Furthermore, in the external plexiform layer, secondary dendrites of mitral cells receive inhibitory synapses from granule (GR) cells, also intrinsic to the bulb, providing a circuit for feedback inhibition: circuit GR→M in Box 10.10(2). Periglomerular and granule cells use the inhibitory transmitter GABA.

Periglomerular and granule cells, among the rare self-renewing neurons in adults, are generated in the brain's subventricular zone within walls of the lateral ventricles to join bulbar circuits throughout life. Reciprocal excitatory-inhibitory synapses (indicated in Box 10.10(2) with two arrows going in opposite directions) occur between dendrites of output and intrinsic cells of the olfactory bulb. A human reciprocal synapse between mitral and granule cells is illustrated in Box 10.11(1) with an electron micrograph in which synapses are identified by pre- and postsynaptic morphological features. The mitral and granule cell layers form the deepest layers of the olfactory bulb.

Regions of the bulb are functionally specialized for processing classes of odor chemicals. For example, aromatic hydrocarbons activate mitral cells in the ventral-medial bulb but aldehydes

Box 10.10 Olfactory bulb glomeruli each process OSN input from a single OR variant

(1)

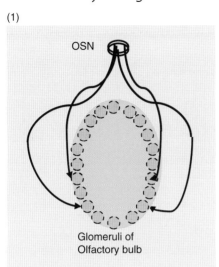

(2)

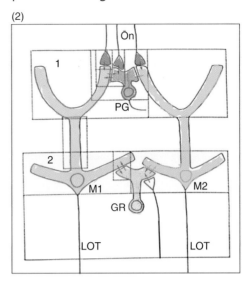

(1) Stereotyped projections of OSN to olfactory bulb, coronal plane. Hundreds of OSN carry signals, generated by stimulus activation of a single OR variant, to one lateral and one medial glomerulus in each bulb. In humans there are 800 glomeruli in the olfactory bulb. Red and blue paths represent input from two OR variants to two glomeruli each. (See also *Olfactory Bulb* in Glossary.)

(2) Inhibitory processing in the olfactory bulb sharpens odor detection. Each glomerulus contains primary dendrites [1] and secondary dendrites [2] of 25 output cells (e.g., mitral cells M1 (orange shading) & M2 (blue shading)) that eventually transmit incoming olfactory nerve (ON) signals downstream via axons in the lateral olfactory tract (LOT). Within the bulb, odor signals are processed by inhibitory interneurons, the (a) periglomerular (PG) and (b) granule (GR) cells, which likely contribute to rapidly adapting sensations and perceptual mixture-component dominance. (From Shepherd, G.M. (1977) The olfactory bulb: a simple system in the mammalian brain. In: Handbook of Physiology, Section 1: The Nervous System. (ed. E.R. Kandel), pp. 945–968. American Physiological Society, Bethesda MD. Reproduced with permission from the American Physiological Society.)

activate mitral cells in the dorsal-medial bulb. Within an aldehyde (CHO)-sensing region, individual mitral cells may be tuned to specific carbon-chain lengths. As Box 10.11(2) suggests, inhibitory inputs from neighboring glomeruli responsive to 5-, 6-, 8-, and 9-CHO may sharpen tuning of a mitral cell with a 7-CHO best stimulus. Similar processing may suppress responses to compounds within stimulus mixtures. Human inability to identify odors of equally intense compounds in mixtures of more than four compounds is, perhaps, in part because of this circuit.

OR-based odotopic neural activity across the olfactory bulb is shaped by OR- specific excitatory input to few sites and complex intrinsic inhibitory networks. Mitral cells show excitatory-inhibitory responses when stimulated. A low stimulus level elicits a simple excitatory response; a higher level elicits a short excitatory response followed by inhibition. This inhibition, lengthening with increasing stimulus strength, may be inhibition of excited mitral cells by granule cells via reciprocal synapses. Resulting rapid self-adaptation may be the key to the olfactory competence of transgenic mice with most glomeruli receiving input from a single OR variant, M71 (Box 10.12(1)). Behavioral data in Box 10.12(2) show that these mice could not tell acetophenone, ligand of the preponderant M71 receptor, from water. This surprising disappearance may involve universal nonspecific interglomerular inhibition evoked by the acetophenone stimulus sufficient to shut down mitral cell output from

the entire olfactory bulb. Although stimulating with acetophenone may have overwhelmed bulbar mutually inhibitory circuitry, the very same transgenic mice could discriminate among stimuli that activated a few remaining OR other than M71. For example, they discriminated between pinene and ethyl acetate, which weakly activated the same few distinct glomeruli in transgenics as in wild-type mice. An intact complex intrinsic bulbar inhibitory circuitry, although sparse, may be sufficient for odor perception.

Thus, the olfactory bulb, with its exquisite multifactor functional topography, layered structure, and inhibitory networks, may extract and refine specific stimulus features as do primary neocortices for other senses.

Inhibitory interneurons, intrinsic to the olfactory bulb, sharpen molecular ranges of output neurons, quicken self-adaptation and initiate mixture-suppression, elements of neural networks resembling primary sensory cortex.

Central odor processing in olfactory cortex

Axons of bulbar relay neurons extend without interruption to the three-layer "primary" olfactory cortex composed of multiple regions, of which the piriform cortex is by far the largest. These

Box10.11   Bidirectional synapses: sharpening OR evoked responses by interneurons in olfactory bulb

(1)

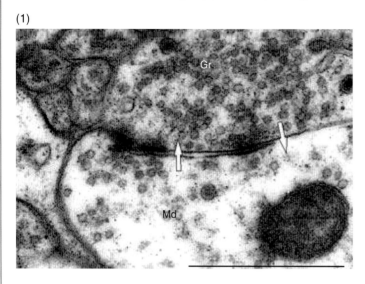

(2)

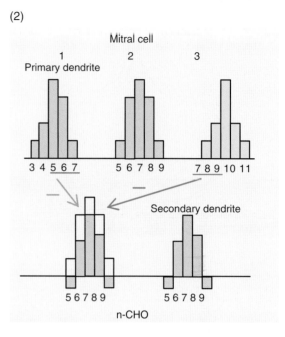

(1) Electron micrograph showing excitatory dendrodendritic synapse between mitral cell secondary dendrite (Md) and granule cell spine (Gr) (upward arrow), and reciprocal inhibitory granule to mitral cell synapse (downward arrow) in human. Small spherical vesicles close to the mitral cell presynaptic membrane and an asymmetric membrane thickening in the granule cell postsynaptic membrane typify excitatory synapses. An elliptical cluster of vesicles in the granule cell spine and symmetric presynaptic and postsynaptic membrane thickenings typify inhibitory synapses. (From Whitman, M.C. & Greer, C.A. (2007) Synaptic integration of adult-generated olfactory bulb granule cells: basal axodendritic centrifugal input precedes apical dendrodendritic local circuits. Journal of Neuroscience, 27, 9951–9961. Reproduced with permission from the Society of Neuroscience.)

(2) Processing of excitatory signals captured by primary dendrites of aldehyde-responsive mitral cells in olfactory bulb. Activation of mitral cell primary dendrites 1 and 3 sharpens the molecular range of mitral cell 2 by inhibiting its secondary dendrites (indicated by gold and green arrows). Inhibitory circuits could help explain "monoclonal nose" results shown in Box 10.12. n-CHO = straight-chain aliphatic aldehyde. (Proposed by Yokoi, M., Mori, K., & Nakanishi, S. (1995) Refinement of odor molecule tuning by dendrodendritic synaptic inhibition in the olfactory bulb. Proceedings of the National Academy of Sciences USA, 92, 3371–3375.) (See also *Molecular Range* in Glossary.)

olfactory regions comprise the rhinencephalon, a **paleocortex**. They receive input that is not first relayed through the thalamus, as are gustatory and other sensory projections en route to neocortex.

Olfactory paleocortex has properties unlike sensory neocortex

Mitral- and tufted-cell axons exit the olfactory bulb in the lateral olfactory tracts (LOT) to make direct connections with the multiple regions of olfactory cortex on the basal surface of the human frontal lobe drawn in Fig. 10.20. The olfactory cortex is three-layer, paleocortex composed of five distinct regions. They are the anterior olfactory nucleus, olfactory tubercle, piriform cortex, anterior cortical amygdaloid nucleus, and lateral entorhinal cortex. Numerous connections among these regions arise mostly from the anterior olfactory nucleus, piriform cortex, and entorhinal cortex. Unlike in six-layer sensory neocortex, strong excitation is sparse but stimulus-elicited inhibition is widespread in the piriform cortex, the most studied of the regions of the olfactory cortex. Piriform cortex, without columnar organization but instead with widely spaced discrete internal connections and many external connections to regions with different functions, is more like an association area

than primary sensory cortex. The piriform cortex and olfactory tubercle, which may influence odor discrimination and perception, connect directly (or via a relay in the medial dorsal thalamus) to orbitofrontal and ventral agranular insular cerebral cortices, two structures also in taste pathways. The amygdala and entorhinal cortex in the ventral forebrain make connections with the hypothalamus or hippocampus, structures involved in homeostasis, emotion, motivation, and learning. Thus, output neurons of the olfactory bulb project directly, or via a few synapses, to the limbic system and diencephalon, **diverse projections** that help explain why odors elicit complex specific situational and emotional memories in addition to odor qualities. Based upon the non-perceptual effects of odors, aromatherapies have been devised to alleviate psychological stress by eliciting memories of pleasant, familiar, and meaningful experiences.

> Processed olfactory information from mitral and tufted relay neurons in the olfactory bulb is directed to the multiple regions of olfactory paleocortex, which directly interact with brain regions specialized for non-sensory functions.

Box10.12   Monoclonal-nose mice cannot discriminate M71 ligand acetophenone from water

(1)

Transgenic, 95% OSN express M71

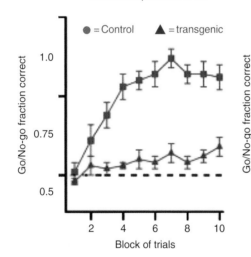

(1) Acetophenone receptor M71 (stained green) found in most OSN of "monoclonal nose" transgenic mice. Endogenous OSN each express one OR variant of those populating one of four zonal regions of the olfactory mucosa, but no such zones are evident for the 95% M71 OSN transgenics (Tg). Control OSN target two glomeruli on opposite sides of each olfactory bulb, but Tg OSN non-specifically contacted most glomeruli, overlapping those specifically associated with OSN expressing other OR. Electro-olfactograms showed Tg olfactory mucosa responds to odors. Fluorescent imaging of Tg olfactory bulb detects presynaptic activity that likely detects intensified inhibition.

(2)

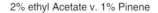

(2) Discrimination of acetophenone from air and ethyl acetate from pinene by transgenic mice (Tg) with M71 "monoclonal noses." Tg mice failed to correctly identify acetophenone, ligand of M71 OR expressed in 95% of OSN. Tg M71 OSN contacted the majority of olfactory bulb glomeruli. Yet Tg mice discriminated ethyl acetate from pinene, ligands for other endogenously expressed receptors in 5% of Tg OSN, which each projected to the specific pair of glomeruli occupied in wild-type mice. Thus interglomerular processing is necessary for odor perception. (From Fleischmann, A., Shykind, B.M., Sosulski, D.L., Franks, K.M., Glinka, M.E., Mei, D.F., Sun, Y., Kirkland, J., Mendelsohn, M., Albers, M.W,. & Axel, R. (2008) Mice with a "monoclonal nose": perturbations in an olfactory map impair odor discrimination. Neuron, 60, 1068–1081. Reproduced with permission from Elsevier.)

Flavor emerges from taste, odor and somatosensations combined when consuming food and drink

Flavor is best defined as a medley of taste, retronasal odor and somatosensations (discussed in more detail in Chapter 9, "Oral Mucosa and Mucosal Sensation") that emerges from food and drink in the mouth. Examples of flavor-elicited, event-related fMRI brain images are shown to the left in Fig. 10.21a. (See also *flavor* in Glossary.) The images were taken from human insular cortex where taste and odors add together in a super-additive fashion (shown in the graphs in Fig. 10.21b on the right), meaning the mixture responses exceed sums of responses to individual component stimuli. Super-additive flavor responses are specific to congruent mixtures, such as sucrose and vanillin (reminiscent of vanilla ice cream, for example); incongruent mixtures, such as NaCl and vanillin may result in the converse, mixture suppression. Mixture suppression occurs when two or more tastes or odors with distinct qualities are presented together, as was shown above in "Chemical Stimuli and Taste Quality" and "Chemical Stimuli and Odor Quality." Retronasal odors and tastes become congruent by learning, from often experiencing them together. Much is still

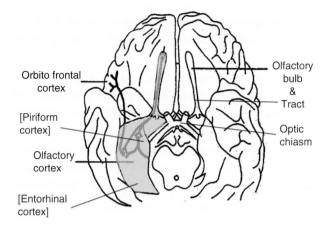

Figure 10.20   Ventral surface of the human brain with the temporal lobe deflected on the right side to expose regions of the three-layer olfactory cortex at the base of the frontal lobe. The piriform cortex is the region that processes signals from the olfactory bulb for conscious perception of odors, whereas, the entorhinal cortex is the region that processes olfactory signals for olfactory memory. (From Frank, M.E. & Rabin, M.D. (1989) Chemosensory neuroanatomy and physiology. *Ear, Nose & Throat Journal*, 68, 291–296. Reproduced with permission from Vendome Health Care.)

unknown about how olfactory paleocortical inputs may combine with gustatory inputs in the insular neocortex.

> Brain regions involving perception, memory, and flavor (the merging of oral odors and tastes) are beyond the olfactory cortex.

Oral chemosensation

The senses of taste and smell resemble each other in many ways. They both respond to chemicals that affect survival, but tastes are oral aqueous solutions whereas odors are either retronasal oral volatiles or orthonasal environmental vapors. The receptor cells of each sense turn over in adults. In each sense, the number of receptor varieties approximates the number of perceived pure stimulus qualities. There are hundreds of odors as there are hundreds of odor receptors; there are five tastes but dozens of taste receptors; yet, a single taste cell functional variant may accumulate all 30 T2R bitter receptors. Tastes and smells are critically processed by sequential peripheral selective self-adaptation and central mixture suppression among stimuli with

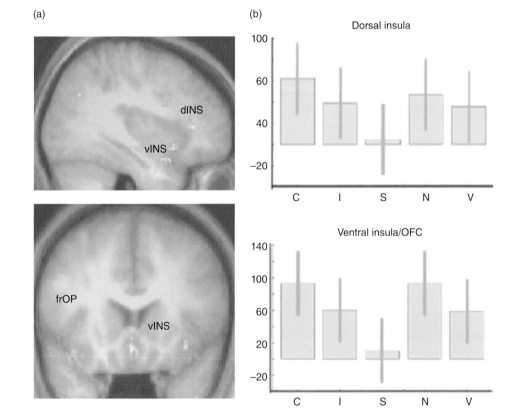

Figure 10.21   Event-related fMRI brain images of a flavor region in the human insular cortex in which taste and odor mixtures elicited enhanced brain responses. (a): Flavor regions of the brain where odors delivered retronasally are more powerful than odors delivered orthonasally. dINS=dorsal insula, vINS/OFC=anterior ventral insula extending into caudal orbitofrontal cortex, frOP=frontal operculum. (b): In flavor regions congruent (C) mixture responses to sucrose (S) plus vanillin (V), greater than incongruent (I) mixture responses to NaCl (N) and vanillin (V), are super-additive (greater than sum of component responses added together). (From Small, D.M. (2012) Flavor is in the brain. *Physiology & Behavior*, 107, 540–552. Reproduced with permission from Elsevier.)

distinct qualities. This dynamic concatenation emphasizes recent and strong odors or tastes present in the complex mixtures encountered in natural situations. The distinct chemosensory qualities perceived rely on dedicated, rather than distributed, elements of neural circuitry in which exact pathways differ but eventually intersect.

The cells that detect taste stimuli are enclosed in multicellular taste buds, which process taste information before transmission to the brain by GSN. However, the cells that detect odor stimuli *are* OSN. They are specialists or generalists carrying specific information from odor receptor to the olfactory bulb in the brain where it is focused by inhibitory networks, which may also contribute to mixture suppression. Although GSN are also either specialists or generalists, as the information proceeds specialists converge with other specialists in the brainstem or are relayed further to appear as patches in the insular gustatory cortex. The olfactory and gustatory pathways combine in the insular cortex where tastes appear to appropriate congruent odors. This process, requiring odors to be present orally, helps explain why people confuse loss of smell (**anosmia**) with a loss of taste (**ageusia**).

Clinical correlations

A general dentist may be the first health care professional to be approached about a loss or distortion of taste. Referral to a specialist in oral medicine for diagnosis is necessary to establish whether the "taste" problem may stem from the common confusion of odor for taste. Seventy percent of patients complaining of taste loss have measurable smell loss; whereas just 10% of them have the taste loss about which they complain. As noted in "Central Odor Processing in Olfactory Bulb," odors of food and drink reaching the olfactory epithelium by the oral route are centrally combined with congruent tastes to form oral flavor. The well-documented association between Parkinson's disease and smell loss, which reliably appears earlier than motor symptoms, is readily detected by testing olfaction via the oral or nasal route. Compared to olfaction, true tastes may be protected from loss by peripheral redundancy. GSN in four cranial nerves have separate receptive fields spaced across the oropharyngeal mucosa. If the presenting problem turns out to be olfactory, referral to an otorhinolaryngologist specializing in nasal-sinus disease is most appropriate. In 40% of olfactory patients, odor stimuli fail to reach the olfactory mucosa due to loss of nasal patency, and in 20% the OSN axonal processes are injured by head trauma. Testing of a single odor stimulus can detect either of these more common chemosensory conditions. Specialized chemosensory clinics are equipped to measure olfactory losses by testing abilities of patients to detect low concentrations (thresholds) and identify odors (identification), but smell distortions, dysosmias, which occur during the reconstitution of injured OSN, are difficult to measure. When the presenting problem turns out not to be olfactory, abnormal oral microbial flora, medications, oral health practices, the possibility of damage to the CT nerve, and depression brought on by the taste problem should be considered. More common than true taste weakness, taste distortions frequently appear as a persistent bad taste in the mouth (phantogeusia), which may be associated with oral burning. Unfortunately, unlike taste losses measured in specialty clinics by applying chemical solutions or minute anodal electrical currents (without the need for cumbersome solutions), there are no techniques available to validate or quantify phantom tastes. Luckily, most dysguesias (tastes with distorted quality) resolve spontaneously in an average of 10 months.

Case study

A 50-year-old woman on visiting her dentist for an annual exam reported, "I've lost my taste. Food and drink are bland and cooking and eating with friends and family are no longer enjoyable." The dentist's mind searched through a list of possible causes for taste loss that he'd learned in dental school. "It might be related to abnormal microbial flora, medications, oral health practices, damage to the chorda tympani nerve, burning mouth, or depression." He recalled. He asked the patient. "Do you experience burning in your mouth?" She responded. "No, but nothing has the familiar tastes I'm used to. Carrots aren't carrots, bananas aren't tasty, and my favorite lamb stew could just as easily be tofu. I noticed this problem about three weeks ago. It has me worried." Then the dentist recalled, "People often confuse taste and smell!"

He asked his patient, "Are you willing to sample a few harmless pure solutions to see if you can identify what they taste like?" She said "Sure." Then the dentist went to his lab to prepare three solutions and type a list of names to choose from. He returned and presented the solutions, one at a time, for her to sip and spit; and water to rinse her mouth with between samples. His test was derived from the easy to apply "Candy Smell Test" that uses "aromatized" sorbitol candies. The patient's responses were "sugar" for two of the solutions and "water" for the third. For complete results on the test see Table 10.3.

After clearing away the cups, the dentist returned and the patient asked, "Did I get them right?" The dentist answered. "Each of your three answers was correct; two of three contained sugar." "You can taste." He continued, "However, you didn't notice that one of the two that contained sugar also contained vanillin; vanilla odor plus sugar taste would taste like vanilla candy."

Given these data, the dentist questioned the patient. "You noticed losing taste about three weeks ago? Did anything unusual happen on that day?" The patient responded, "I was participating in a bike-for-life event and fell. I injured my knee when I hit the road." The dentist asked her, "Did your head hit the pavement?" She replied, "Yes, I bumped my head and had quite a bad headache for the rest of that day."

(Continued)

(Cont'd)

The dentist then felt he could explain her condition and recommended she seek an appointment in a clinic specializing in diagnosing chemosensory **disorders** to verify his simple test and obtain a prognosis for her loss of smell due to head trauma. He said "Food flavors are composed of tastes in solution and volatiles from odors smelled via a 'mouth to nose' route. They are often confused with tastes because they come from the mouth. The olfactory nerve could be damaged by stretching due to a blow to the head and recovery is often possible because the olfactory receptors are capable of reconstituting themselves from stem cells in adults." (See also *Olfactory Receptors in Glossary*.)

Table 10.3   Test of olfactory competence of patient who reports "I can't taste"

Solution	Stimulus	Rinse	Correct Choice	Response
1	sucrose	water	sugar	sugar
2	water	water	water	water
3	sucrose + vanillin	water	sugar + vanilla	sugar

For each stimulus, there are three choices: sugar, water, and sugar + vanilla.

(Test based on "candy test" in Renner, B., Mueller, C.A., Dreier, J., Faulhaber, S., Rascher, W., & Kobal, G. (2009) The candy smell test: a new test for retronasal olfactory performance. *Laryngoscope*, 119, 487–495.)

Acknowledgements

The author thanks Dr. Thomas P. Hettinger for expert contribution to the treatment of the chemistry of taste and smell stimuli in this chapter, which is so important for appreciation of chemical senses.

References

1. Adler, E., Hoon, M.A., Mueller, K.L., Chandrashekar, J., Ryba, N.J., & Zuker, C.S. (2000) A novel family of mammalian taste receptors. *Cell*, 100, 693–702.

2. Axel, R. (2005) Scents and sensibility: a molecular logic of olfactory perception (Nobel lecture). *Angewante Chemie* (International ed. in English), 44, 6110–6127.

3. Bradley, R.M. (1995) *Essentials of Oral Physiology*. Mosby, St. Louis.

4. Buck, L. & Axel, R. (1991) A novel multigene family may encode odorant receptors: a molecular basis for odor recognition. *Cell*, 65, 175–187.

5. Bufe, B., Hofmann, T., Krautwurst, D., Raguse, J.D., & Meyerhof, W. (2002) The human TASR216 receptor mediates bitter taste in response to β-glucopyranosides. *Nature Genetics*, 32, 397–401.

6. Chen, X., Gabitto, M., Peng, Y., Ryba, N.J., & Zuker, C.S. (2011) A gustotopic map of taste qualities in the mammalian brain. *Science*, 333, 1262–1266.

7. Cowart, B.J. (2008) Taste dysfunction: a practical guide for oral medicine. *Oral Diseases*, 17, 2–6.

8. Doty, R.L. (2012) Olfactory dysfunction in Parkinson disease. *Nature Reviews, Neurology*, 8, 329–339.

9. Finger, T.E., Danilova, V., Barrows, J., Bartel, D.L., Vigers, A.J., Stone, L., Hellekant, G., & Kinnamon, S.C. (2005) ATP signaling is crucial for communication from taste buds to gustatory nerves. *Science*, 310, 1495–1499.

10. Hettinger, T.P. & Frank, M.E. (1990) Specificity of amiloride inhibition of hamster taste responses. *Brain Research*, 513, 24–34.

11. Holbrook, E.H., Wu, E., Curry, W.T., Lin, D.T., & Schwob, J.E. (2011) Immunohistochemical characterization of human olfactory tissue. *Laryngoscope*, 121, 1687–1701.

12. Isaacson, J.S. (2010) Odor representations in mammalian cortical circuits. *Current Opinion in Neurobiology*, 20, 328–331.

13. Johnson, D.M., Illig, K.R., Behan, M., & Haberly, L.B. (2000) New features of connectivity in piriform cortex visualized by intracellular injection of pyramidal cells suggest that "primary" olfactory cortex functions like "association" cortex in other sensory systems. *Journal of Neuroscience*, 20, 6974–6982.

14. Livermore, A. & Laing, D.G. (1998) The influence of odor type on the discrimination and identification of odorants in multicomponent odor mixtures. *Physiology & Behavior*, 65, 311–320.

15. Mombaerts, P., Wang, F., Dulac, C., Chao, S.K., Nemes, A., Mendelsohn, M., Edmondson, J., & Axel, R. (1996) Visualizing an olfactory sensory map. *Cell*, 87, 675–686.

16. Nara, K., Saraiva, L.R., Ye, X., & Buck, L.B. (2011) A large-scale analysis of odor coding in the olfactory epithelium. *Journal of Neuroscience*, 31, 9179–9191.

17. Shi, P. & Zhang, J. (2009) Extraordinary diversity of chemosensory receptor gene repertoires among vertebrates. *Results & Problems in Cell Differentiation*, 47, 1–23.

18. Spector, A.C. & Glendinning, J.I. (2009) Linking peripheral taste processes to behavior. 2009. *Current Opinion in Neurobiology*, 19, 370–377.

19. Wong, G.T., Gannon, K.S., & Margolskee, R.F. (1996) Transduction of bitter and sweet taste by gustducin. *Nature*, 381, 796–800.

20. Zhao, H., Ivic, L., Otaki, J.M., Hashimoto, M., Mikoshiba, K., & Firestein, S. (1998) Functional expression of a mammalian odorant receptor. *Science*, 279, 237–242.

Glossary

Adaptation: Self-adaptation is a decrease in response while continuously presenting the same stimulus. Cross-adaptation is a decrease in response to stimulus B presented immediately after stimulus A without rinse; it does not occur when A and B are independent (activating different receptors). If A_1 and A_2 use the same receptor, when weaker A_1 precedes stronger A_2, there is a transient response increment, and vice versa, when A_2 precedes weaker A_1, there is a transient response decrement, as there are when A_1 and A_2 are two concentrations of the same compound.

Chorda tympani: The chorda tympani (CT) is the branch of the facial cranial nerve (CN VII) with cell bodies in the geniculate ganglion, which transmits action potentials to the brain from taste buds in the fungiform papillae on the tip of the tongue.

Coding quality: Coding quality is the means, spatial and temporal, by which neuronal responses distinguish among tastes and odors. Taste and odor representations differ by separately activating gustatory and olfactory systems. This is spatial coding, as is representation of sweet and salty tastes, or vanilla and rose odors, in separate GSN or OSN. Temporal coding involves patterns in timing of neuronal activation regardless of which neurons are activated. The 1.43-Hz temporal rhythm is a redundant temporal code for sweeteners that are also coded for spatially in S GSN.

Convergence: Convergence of inputs from different oral receptive fields (palate, tongue tip) and for different taste qualities (sweet sucrose and salty NaCl) is seen in responses of single NTS neurons.

Disorders: *Anosmia* and hyposmia, or *ageusia* and hypogeusia, respectively refer to complete or partial loss of smell and taste that are objectively measured by threshold or identification. Dysosmia and dysgeusia are distorted smell and taste, respectively, which are subjective impressions not readily measured. Most complaints of taste loss are actually losses in the appreciation of oral odors.

Diverse projection pathways: Taste and odor sensory codes are linked with codes for other functions. Visceral reflexes, as well as secondary and higher order pathways for behavior, emotion, motivation, memory, and cognition (connections to amygdala and hippocampus in the subcortical limbic lobe on the medial face of a brain) are included. The thalamus influences access to the cerebral cortex and the hypothalamus influences feeding and drinking.

Dominance: Stimulus dominance in mixtures is achieved in three ways.

1. Prior selective adaptation of components of mixtures $(A \rightarrow A+E)$ leads to decreased identification of the adapted (ambient) component (A) and increased identification of the added (extra) component (E).

2. Asymmetric suppression of mixture components $(C \rightarrow D\downarrow)$ leads to decreased response intensity of one component (D).

3. Mutual suppression of independent stimuli $(A\downarrow + B\downarrow)$ leads to reduction in response to mixture components compared to response to component stimuli presented alone.

Dynamic selective adaptation and static asymmetric suppression are peripheral; whereas, mutual reciprocal suppression among independent stimuli must rely on central processing. Mixture processing strategies silence signals from contaminated nutrients and perform *a dynamic chemosensory analysis* to highlight strong, recent components in our complex, varying chemosensory environments.

Ethanol: Individual chemosensory stimuli may activate multiple TR and OR. Ethanol tastes sweet and bitter and has an odor. It also irritates via somatosensory nerves. Ethanol has a complex quality.

Flavor: Responses to mixtures of different tastes, orthonasally detected odors, or tastes plus odors are typically suppressed. However, responses to mixtures of congruent tastes with oral odors in the insular flavor cortex are enhanced (super-additive). Odors and tastes become congruent when experienced together often.

Generalist: A generalist is a broadly tuned gustatory or olfactory sensory neuron (GSN or OSN) that responds to stimuli with distinctly different taste qualities. An example is CT E (also known as H) GSN that respond to electrolytes with salty, sour, and bitter tastes.

Gustatory sensory neurons (GSN): Gustatory sensory neurons reside in three cranial nerves (CN): VII, IX, and X.

Gustatory cortex: The gustatory cortex (GC) lies in the anterior insula and adjacent frontal operculum, brain regions sparsely inhabited by taste-sensitive cells.

Habituation: Habituation is a change in response to the same stimulus presented repeatedly, with time and rinse between presentations.

Identification: Chemosensory qualities detected by 424 taste and odor receptors allow us to identify and discriminate among chemicals important for our health and survival.

Intensity: Chemosensory stimuli, which increase in intensity (strength) with increased actual concentration, may be reduced in effective concentration (relative salience) when adapted or suppressed in mixtures. Once above a detection threshold, taste and odor perceptions increase in intensity, as do sensory neural response sizes, until saturation is attained. Increases in intensity are behaviorally measured directly with rating scales or indirectly by identification, which increases in accuracy with increased stimulus intensity.

Mixture suppression: The key rules for perception of mixtures are:

1. Mixture components with greatest intensity dominate;

2. A maximum of four equally intense mixture components are detectable at one time.

Molecular range: Molecular range is the breadth of activation of OSN and GSN by chemicals varying in chemical structure. Chemicals confused with one another comprise response profiles. Ranges and profiles may be narrow, including few chemical structures, or wide, including many structures.

Odor stimuli: Vaporous odor stimuli, delivered by exhaling or inhaling, are chemicals that are not deconstructed into functional groups but themselves produce the unique odors of complex odor objects.

Olfactory bulb: The two olfactory bulbs of rats contain approximately 4000 separate glomeruli that are activated by olfactory sensory neurons (OSN). Each glomerulus, a central functional unit, captures signals from a single OR variant. Glomeruli number is consistently several times OR-variant number across species. Humans and elephants have 52%, rats 29% and mice 17% OR pseudogenes, which evolved by pseudogenization thought to derive from release from positive evolutionary pressure.

Olfactory receptors (OR) and taste receptors (TR): Taste receptors and olfactory receptors are GPCR (G-protein-coupled receptors) that detect chemosensory stimuli. Individual stimuli may activate multiple TR and OR.

Olfactory sensory neurons (OSN): Olfactory sensory neurons coalesce in cranial nerve I.

Other connections: Taste and odor sensory codes are linked with codes for other functions. Visceral reflexes, as well as secondary and higher order pathways for behavior, emotion, motivation, memory, and cognition (connections to amygdala and hippocampus in the subcortical limbic lobe on the medial face of a brain) are included. The thalamus influences access to the cerebral cortex and the hypothalamus influences feeding and drinking.

Paleocortex: Unlike the mammalian six-layer sensory neocortex, responses of the olfactory three-layer, piriform paleocortex are distributed neither somatotopically nor in clusters of cells with specific functions, and responses are more often than not inhibitory.

Quality: The senses of gustation and olfaction detect multiple taste and odor qualities with chemosensory receptors. Chemosensory stimuli also motivate action, provoke hedonic (preference-aversion) responses, and generate the uplifting memories used in aromatherapy.

Quality primaries: Primaries for color vision derive from Helmholtz's demonstration that all colors can be produced by combinations of blue, green, and red light. Taste quality primaries are brought up more frequently than odor quality primaries, likely because they are few in number (four on the tetrahedron). However, primaries in chemical senses are controversial. Color theory has primaries add to produce a new color, unrecognizable in the components, such as the combining of red and green light to produce yellow, but individual mixture components are recognized in taste and odor mixtures.

Sensory neurons: Gustatory sensory neurons (GSN), with peripheral and central axonal processes of cell bodies located in peripheral ganglia, carry information via action potentials from activated taste receptors (TR) on taste cells (TC) in taste buds to the brain. Olfactory sensory neuron (OSN) dendrites are activated to produce slow potentials, monitored by electro-olfactograms (EOGs), with stimulus binding to odor receptors (OR) embedded in OSN cilial membranes. OSN also carry information via action potentials to the brain via their axons.

Specialist: A specialist is a finely tuned sensory neuron (GSN or OSN) that responds to stimuli of the same taste quality, a peripheral labeled line. Examples are CT S GSN that respond to stimuli behaviorally confused with sucrose; and CT N GSN that respond to stimuli behaviorally confused with NaCl.

Taste aversion: Taste aversions may be natural (unlearned) or learned. Unlearned aversive reflexes to bitter and sour stimuli occur in human newborns and in rodents without a forebrain. Conditioned taste aversions (CTA) are established in animal subjects by a single pairing of the taste stimulus (the conditioned stimulus, CS) in drinking water followed by intraperitoneal injection of a toxin (the unconditioned stimulus, US) that results in gastrointestinal malaise. CTA are quantified as suppression of control drinking of naturally preferred, neutral or aversive taste stimuli mistaken for the CS.

Taste confusion: Confusing the tastes of two compounds (such as sucrose and saccharin) indicates they have similar taste quality, whereas distinguishing the tastes of compounds (such as sucrose and quinine) without error indicates they have discriminable tastes. A "taste confusion matrix," derived from numerous identifications of many compounds, defines discriminability (or dissimilarity) for all pairs of the tested compounds. Discriminability of two stimuli can be quantified as T_2 (in bits of information transmitted from stimuli to subjects' responses), which ranges from 0.0 for complete overlap to 1.0 for non-overlapping identifications of a sample of ten stimuli.

Taste dimensions: Multidimensional scaling (MDS), designed originally to help evaluate human judgments on the similarity of a set of items, is a quantitative analysis that provides visualization of a complex data set as distances in a multidimensional space. The distances represent dissimilarities among items as well as possible. Understanding gustatory dimensionality (four qualities represented in three-dimensional space) benefits from MDS of hamster CTA behavior, human taste confusions, and hamster GSN molecular ranges of multiple taste stimuli.

Taste stimuli: Ionic and nonionic water soluble compounds elicit tastes. Ionic electrolytes are detected by ion channels directly to produce salty taste via ENaC and sour taste via PKD2L1-PKD1; whereas nonionic sweet and bitter tastes depend on GPCR.

Topographic: Much topographic mapping of sensory function is *somatotopic*, with a body surface receptive field mapped to the brain. Oral taste regions and olfactory receptors are somatotopically mapped to the nucleus of the solitary tract and olfactory mucosal zones, respectively. Gustotopic mapping in the gustatory cortex and odotopic mapping within the olfactory bulb are topographic representations of TR and OR properties, respectively. Preference-aversion hot spots comprise a hedonic topography in the olfactory mucosa. There is no general chemical topographic representations of taste or smell stimuli in the brain.

PART V
ORAL EFFECTORS

Chapter 11 Salivary Glands, Salivary Secretion, and Saliva

Arthur R. Hand

Department of Craniofacial Sciences and Cell Biology, School of Dental Medicine, University of Connecticut

Salivary glands are exocrine glands located in and around the oral cavity. There are three major paired glands located extraorally, the parotid, submandibular, and sublingual glands. Additionally, numerous small minor glands are present in the submucosal tissues throughout the oral cavity, except in the gingivae and parts of the hard palate. The salivary glands produce saliva, an aqueous fluid containing electrolytes, other small molecules, proteins, glycoproteins, and mucins. Saliva coats and protects the oral tissues, initiates digestion, and facilitates speaking, chewing, and swallowing. The structure of the salivary glands, the mechanisms underlying saliva secretion, and the composition and functions of saliva will be described in this chapter.

Structure

Histological organization

Salivary glands consist of epithelial cells, collectively termed the glandular **parenchyma**, that are specialized for the synthesis of various organic molecules, the secretion of these molecules along with water and electrolytes, and their transport to the oral cavity. The gland cells are organized into **acini** (s. **acinus**) or **secretory endpieces** (the terminology used in this textbook) and **ducts** of different caliber and structure (Fig. 11.1). The secretory endpieces may be spherical or tubular in shape and are the sites of fluid and protein/glycoprotein secretion. The ducts are tubular in shape, and begin as small ducts connected to the endpieces that increase in size as they merge and eventually form a large main duct that empties into the oral cavity. Also present within the gland are connective tissue cells and extracellular matrix, called the **interstitial tissue** or **stroma**, that surrounds and

supports the parenchyma. Fibroblasts and their products (collagen, elastic and reticular fibers, proteoglycans, and glycoproteins), mast cells and other immune system cells (lymphocytes, macrophages, dendritic cells, plasma cells) are regularly found in the stroma. The connective tissue forms a **capsule** around the gland, and partitions or **septa** of connective tissue extend into the gland and organize it into **lobes** and **lobules** (Figs. 11.1 and 11.2). Blood vessels and nerves travel in the connective tissue septa and are distributed throughout the stroma, supplying the gland cells with nutrients and oxygen and removing waste products and stimulating saliva secretion, respectively.

> The epithelial cells of salivary glands are arranged in secretory endpieces connected to the oral mucosa by a system of ducts and supported by connective tissue containing blood vessels and nerves.

Two types of secretory cells are found in the endpieces: **serous cells** and **mucous cells**. The endpieces may be composed of all serous cells, all mucous cells, or may be mixed, with both serous and mucous components.

Serous cells

In a serous endpiece, the cells are roughly pyramidal in shape, with a broad basal surface adjacent to the basal lamina and connective tissue stroma, and a narrow apex that, along with the apices of adjacent serous cells, forms a lumen in the center of a spherical endpiece (Fig. 11.3). The cells are joined by junctional

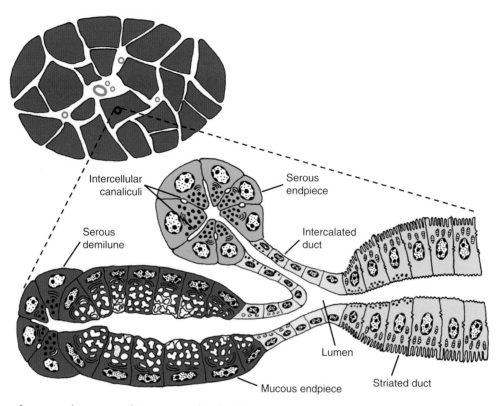

Figure 11.1   Diagram of serous and mucous endpieces, intercalated and striated ducts.

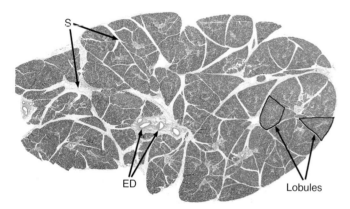

Figure 11.2   Submandibular gland illustrating lobular organization of the gland. Individual lobules (two examples are outlined) are separated by connective tissue septa (S) containing excretory (interlobular) ducts (ED), blood vessels, and nerves.

complexes that include tight and adhering junctions and desmosomes. The luminal surface area is increased by extensions of finger-like **intercellular canaliculi** down the lateral sides of the cells. Serous cells have a spherical, basally located nucleus, abundant basal rough endoplasmic reticulum, a prominent Golgi complex, and numerous secretory granules, about 1 μm in diameter, that are stored in the apical cytoplasm (Figs. 11.4 and 11.5). Serous cells synthesize proteins and glycoproteins, which are transported from the rough endoplasmic reticulum to the Golgi complex, where they are modified, condensed, and packaged into the secretory granules.

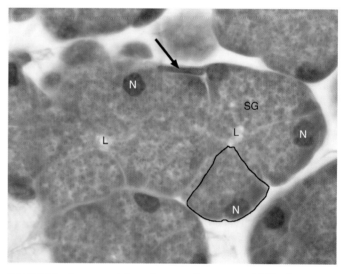

Figure 11.3   Serous endpiece. Serous cells are pyramidal in shape (example outlined), with a broad base adjacent to the connective tissue stroma and a narrow apex abutting a central lumen (L). The nuclei (N) are located in the basal cytoplasm, and the supranuclear cytoplasm is filled with secretory granules (SG). The elongated nucleus of a myoepithelial cell (arrow) is located along the basal surface of the endpiece.

Mucous cells

In a mucous endpiece, the cells may have a pyramidal or cuboidal shape, and the endpieces are typically tubular in shape with a relatively wide lumen (Fig. 11.6). The apical ends of adjacent

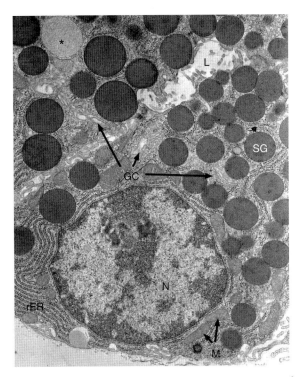

Figure 11.4   Serous cell. Electron micrograph showing portions of three serous cells. A spherical nucleus (N), cisternae of rough endoplasmic reticulum (rER), and several mitochondria (M) are located in the basal cytoplasm. The Golgi complex (GC) is located near the nucleus, and an immature (forming) secretory granule (*) is seen at the upper left. Dense secretory granules (SG) fill the apical cytoplasm adjacent to the lumen (L).

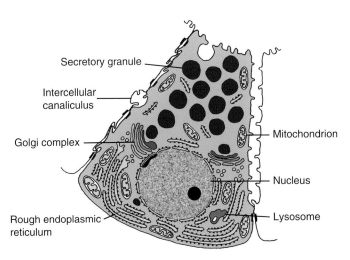

Figure 11.5   Diagram of a serous cell.

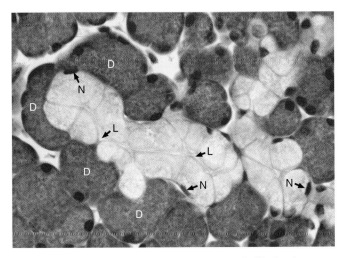

Figure 11.6   Mucous endpiece. Several mucous cells filled with pale-staining mucous granules form a tubular endpiece. Only a few flattened mucous cell nuclei (N) are visible in this section. The lumen (L) extends the length of the tubule. Several serous demilunes (D) surround the mucous tubule.

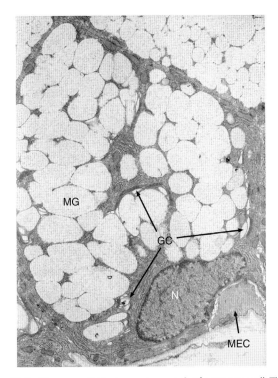

Figure 11.7   Mucous cell. Electron micrograph of a mucous cell. The flattened nucleus (N) is located basally, and rough endoplasmic reticulum is present mainly in the basal cytoplasm. The Golgi complex (GC) is extensive, and the supranuclear cytoplasm is packed with pale mucous secretory granules (MG), many of which are fused with adjacent granules. A myoepithelial cell process (MEC) is present at the base of the mucous cell. (From: Hand, A.R. (1986) In *Oral histology: inheritance and development*, 2nd edn. (eds. D.V. Provenza & W. Seibel). Lea and Febiger, Philadelphia. Reprinted by permission of Lippincott Williams & Wilkins.)

mucous cells are joined by junctional complexes to form a lumen, but mucous endpieces lack intercellular canaliculi. The nuclei of mucous cells usually are somewhat flattened and compressed against the base of the cell, and have denser chromatin than the nuclei of serous cells. The mucous cells have basally located rough endoplasmic reticulum, an extensive Golgi complex, and large, pale, poorly staining secretory granules that fill the apical

cytoplasm (Figs. 11.7 and 11.8). The main products of mucous cells are mucins, which have a polypeptide core that is highly glycosylated during transit through the Golgi complex.

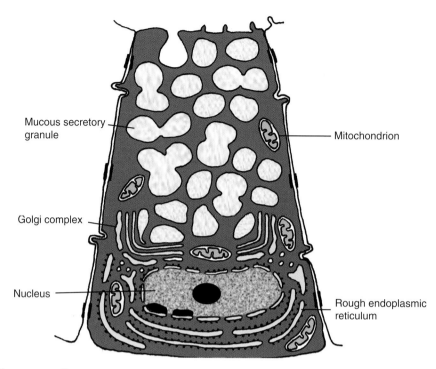

Figure 11.8 Diagram of a mucous cell.

In glands containing mucous endpieces, it is common to find a few serous cells in a characteristic relationship to the mucous cells. In these **mixed endpieces**, mucous cells are arranged in a typical tubular endpiece structure, and serous cells form a crescent at the blind end of the tubule, called a **serous demilune** (Fig. 11.6). The serous cells have a narrow apical extension and intercellular canaliculi that reach the lumen of the mucous tubule.

> Serous cells contain protein rich secretory granules and stain intensely with hematoxylin and eosin; mucous cells contain mucin-filled granules and are poorly stained in routine preparations.

The above description of serous and mucous cells implies a clear distinction between these two cell types. In reality the differences are less distinct. The oligosaccharide component of serous glycoproteins can range from neutral to acidic in nature, with histochemical characteristics similar to those of mucous glycoproteins; hence some authors use the term **seromucous** to describe these cells. Moreover, some serous cells are known to produce some of the same mucins that mucous cells make, and some mucous cells produce non-glycosylated proteins. The histological appearance of fixed mucous cells described above, common to mucous cells throughout the body, is believed to be caused by swelling of the mucous granules during the preservation of the cells by chemical fixatives. When mucous cells are preserved by rapid freezing, which is believed to more closely reflect the native state, their structure is remarkably similar to that of serous cells.

Myoepithelial cells

A third cell type found in secretory endpieces is the **myoepithelial cell**. Although epithelial in origin, myoepithelial cells are similar in structure and function to smooth muscle cells. They are located between the basal membrane of the secretory cells and the basal lamina and have a stellate shape with numerous branching processes that are filled with contractile filaments (actin and myosin) and wrap around the endpieces (Figs. 11.9, 11.10, and 11.11). Contraction of myoepithelial cells squeezes the endpiece and forces the primary saliva in the lumen into and along the duct system. Myoepithelial cells also have an important role in maintaining the integrity of the secretory endpieces. They help the secretory cells maintain their polarity, and they secrete protease inhibitors and antiangiogenesis factors. Myoepithelial cells also are found in some parts of the duct system, where they tend to have a fusiform shape with fewer processes.

> The processes of myoepithelial cells wrap around the endpieces and their contraction forces the primary saliva into the duct system.

> Thus, the three main cell types of the secretory endpieces of salivary glands serve specific functions in the production and secretion of saliva and have distinct histological appearances.

Ducts

The duct system of salivary glands consists of three distinct structural components: **intercalated ducts**, the first duct leading from the secretory endpiece; **striated ducts**, the main intralobular component of the duct system; and **excretory ducts**, located in the interlobular connective tissue.

Intercalated ducts

Intercalated ducts have a small diameter, less than that of the endpieces, and are composed of cuboidal shaped cells with a relatively undifferentiated appearance (Figs. 11.12 and 11.13). The first cells of the duct, adjacent to the endpiece, may have a

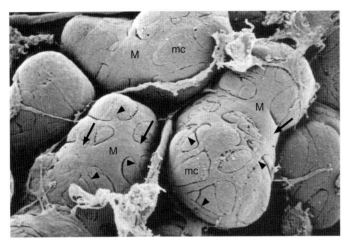

Figure 11.9   Myoepithelial cells. Scanning electron micrograph showing myoepithelial cells (M) covering the basal surface of mucous endpiece cells (mc) in the rat sublingual gland. Broad processes (arrows) extend from the cell bodies, and give rise to smaller processes (arrowheads). (From: Nagato, T. et al. (1980) A scanning electron microscope study of myoepithelial cells in exocrine glands. *Cell and Tissue Research*, 209(1), 1–10. Reprinted by permission of Springer Science + Business Media.)

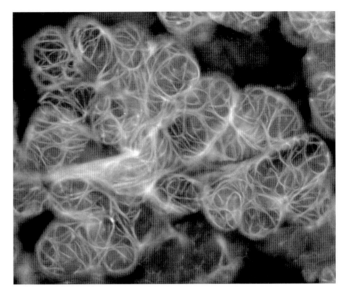

Figure 11.10   Myoepithelial cells. Fluorescence micrograph of myoepithelial cells surrounding the secretory endpieces of the rat sublingual gland. Actin filaments in the processes are labeled with fluorescent phallacidin, an actin-binding compound from the mushroom genus *Amanita*. (From: Murakami, M. et al. (1991) Effect of parasympathectomy on the histochemical maturation of myoepithelial cells of the rat sublingual gland. *Archives of Oral Biology*, 36(7), 511–517. Reprinted by permission of Elsevier.)

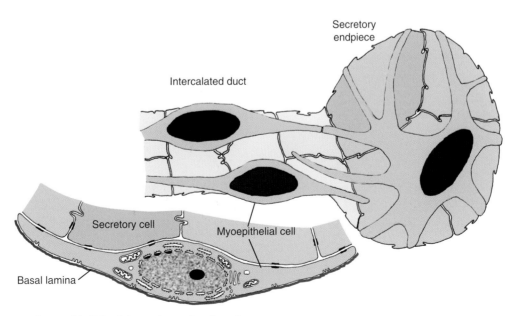

Figure 11.11   Diagram of myoepithelial cells in section and surface views.

few apical secretory granules that contain small amounts of some secretory proteins or mucins. These small ducts merge with the ducts leading from adjacent endpieces to form a larger intercalated duct, and these may again merge prior to emptying into a striated duct. As noted above, fusiform-shaped myoepithelial cells are present in intercalated ducts, oriented longitudinally with respect to the duct.

Striated ducts

Striated ducts are present in abundance in the parotid and submandibular glands, less frequently in the sublingual gland, and rarely in minor salivary glands. They are not found in the pancreas or other exocrine glands, thus they serve to distinguish the major salivary glands histologically from other glands. These ducts have a simple columnar epithelium, a diameter greater than that of the endpieces, and larger lumina than those of the endpieces and intercalated ducts (Fig. 11.14). The nuclei are spherical to oval in shape and located more or less centrally in the columnar duct cells. The cytoplasm contains abundant mitochondria, a few cisternae and tubules of rough and smooth endoplasmic reticulum, lysosomes, and peroxisomes. Some cells have small secretory granules and/or endocytic vesicles in the apical cytoplasm. The basal cell membranes as well as the lateral membranes are highly infolded and interdigitate with similar membrane folds of adjacent cells (Figs. 11.15 and 11.16). The cytoplasm in between these membranous partitions is filled with elongated mitochondria. In the light microscope, the infolded membranes and mitochondria create an impression of lines or "striations" extending from the base of the cell toward the nucleus, thus giving these ducts their name. Numerous capillaries and small venules are present in the connective tissue around the striated ducts. Within the lobule, these ducts merge into larger striated ducts, which may have occasional small basal cells that do not extend to the ductal lumen.

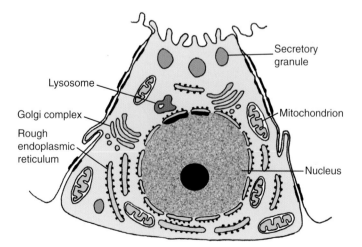

Figure 11.12   Intercalated ducts. Intercalated ducts (ID) are shown in longitudinal (upper panel) and cross section (lower panel). The diameter of the intercalated duct is considerably smaller than that of the endpiece. The duct cells are low cuboidal to cuboidal in shape; nuclei of myoepithelial cells (arrows) are present along the basal surface of the ducts.

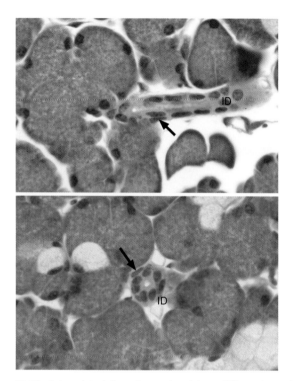

Figure 11.13   Diagram of an intercalated duct cell.

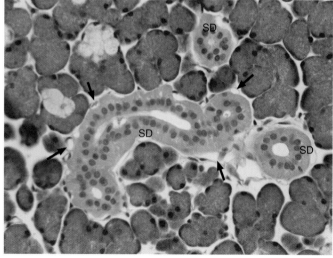

Figure 11.14   Striated ducts. Cross and longitudinal sections of striated ducts (SD). The ducts are lined by a simple columnar epithelium, and their diameter is usually greater than that of the endpieces. Numerous small blood vessels (arrows) are present adjacent to the striated ducts.

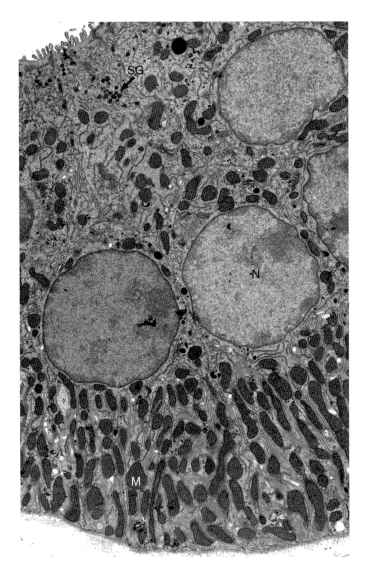

Figure 11.15 Striated duct. Electron micrograph showing portions of several striated duct cells. The basal and lateral cell membranes are highly infolded and interdigitate with similar infolded membranes from adjacent cells. The cells contain numerous mitochondria (M), especially in the cytoplasmic partitions between the infolded basal membranes. Small secretory granules (SG) are present in the apical cytoplasm. (This micrograph was originally published in the *Journal of Biological Chemistry*. Evans, R.L. et al. (2000) Severe impairment of salivation in Na⁺/K⁺/2Cl⁻ cotransporter (NKCC1)-deficient mice. *Journal of Biological Chemistry*, 275(35), 26720–26726. © The American Society for Biochemistry and Molecular Biology.)

Excretory ducts

As the large striated ducts leave the lobule and enter the connective tissue septa, they become excretory (interlobular) ducts. Excretory ducts are larger in diameter and have wider lumina than striated ducts, and are surrounded by relatively dense connective tissue. The epithelium of the ducts is pseudostratified, with columnar cells that extend from the basal lamina to the lumen and basal cells that contact the basal lamina but do not reach the lumen (Fig. 11.17). The columnar cells are somewhat

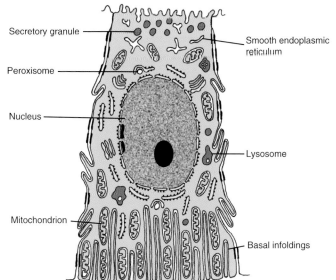

Figure 11.16 Diagram of a striated duct cell.

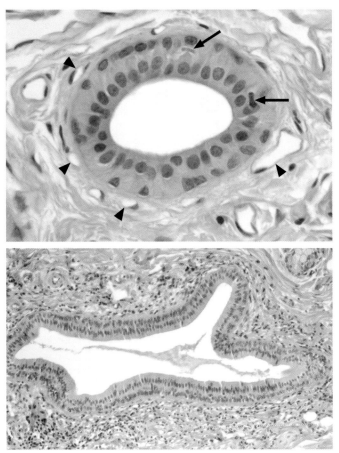

Figure 11.17 Excretory duct. Excretory ducts are located in the interlobular connective tissue septa. Smaller excretory ducts (upper panel) are lined by a pseudostratified epithelium and have a larger lumen than the intralobular striated ducts. Numerous small blood vessels (arrowheads) are located adjacent to the duct. Nuclei of two dendritic cells are indicated by the arrows. Larger excretory ducts may have a stratified cuboidal or stratified columnar epithelium (lower panel) or a stratified squamous epithelium close to the oral opening.

similar in appearance to the striated duct cells, but have fewer basolateral membrane infoldings and fewer mitochondria. The excretory ducts continue to merge, increasing in size until a single main duct emerges from the gland. Occasional goblet cells are present in the larger ducts, and the epithelium may change to stratified columnar or even stratified squamous near the oral opening.

Other cell types occasionally are found in the ducts. Myoepithelial cells may be present in the striated and excretory ducts, and brush (tuft) cells, presumed chemosensory cells with numerous long microvilli and apical microvesicles, are found in excretory ducts. Migratory cells such as lymphocytes and macrophages may be present in the epithelium throughout the duct system, and dendritic cells (antigen-presenting cells) also are commonly found within the ductal epithelium (Fig. 11.17). Finally, stem cells capable of proliferation and differentiation into other gland cell types are thought to reside in the intercalated and excretory ducts.

> The duct system consists of architecturally discrete components, beginning with intercalated ducts that connect the endpieces to the characteristic intralobular ductal component of salivary glands, the striated ducts, which in turn connect to the interlobular excretory ducts that lead to the oral cavity.

Development

Development of the different salivary glands is initiated at different times during embryonic life. The parotid gland begins its development at four to six weeks, the submandibular gland at six weeks, and the sublingual and minor glands at eight to twelve weeks. The glands begin their development as a proliferation of epithelial cells at specific sites in the primitive oral mucosa. Continued proliferation and growth of the epithelial cells into the underlying mesenchyme results in a solid cord of cells that begins to undergo repeated dichotomous branching, eventually producing a "bush-" or "tree-like" structure (Fig. 11.18). The proliferation and branching is regulated by epithelial-mesenchymal interactions, and occurs by the developmental process of **branching morphogenesis** that also forms the pancreas, lungs, kidneys, and other organs. A variety of growth factors and their receptors and specific transcription factors are necessary for proper development of the glands. As development proceeds, lumina are formed in the ducts and then in the terminal buds, and the epithelial cells begin the process of **cytodifferentiation**. The inner layer of cells differentiate into secretory cells, whereas cells of the outer layer become myoepithelial cells. The secretory cells initiate secretory protein synthesis, secretory granules accumulate in the cytoplasm, autonomic innervation is established, and with the development of functional neurotransmitter receptors the cells attain the ability to secrete saliva. Maturation of the secretory cells and ducts occurs

during the last two months of gestation, and the glands continue to increase in size postnatally.

> Salivary glands develop from the embryonic oral epithelium as solid cords of epithelial cells that undergo repeated branching as they grow into the underlying mesenchyme, eventually forming endpieces and ducts with central lumina.

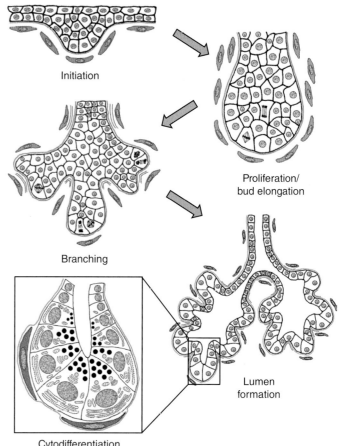

Initiation

Proliferation/
bud elongation

Branching

Lumen
formation

Cytodifferentiation

Figure 11.18   Salivary gland development occurs by the process of branching morphogenesis. The gland is initiated as a proliferation of the oral epithelium, forming a bud that grows into the underlying mesenchyme as a solid cord of epithelial cells. Reciprocal interactions between the epithelium and mesenchyme, involving specific growth factors, receptors, and transcription factors, regulate the developmental process. Continued cell proliferation and branching of the epithelial cord results in terminal buds connected by developing ducts. Deposition of extracellular matrix components stabilizes the clefts formed between adjacent branches. Lumina form in the ducts and terminal buds, and cells of the terminal buds undergo cytodifferentiation to become secretory cells of the endpieces. The basal lamina separating epithelium from mesenchyme is shown as an orange line, mesenchymal cells are green, and differentiated myoepithelial cells are brown. (Modified from Cutler, L.S. (1989) Functional differentiation of salivary glands. In: *Handbook of Physiology: The Gastrointestinal System*, Vol. 3, pp. 93–105. American Physiological Society, Bethesda, MD.)

Major glands

Parotid gland

The parotid is the largest salivary gland. It is located in front of the ear, superficial to the masseter muscle, and the branches of the facial nerve (cranial nerve VII) pass through the gland. Its main duct, **Stensen's duct**, passes forward across the masseter muscle, enters the oral cavity through the buccinator muscle, and opens at the **parotid papilla** on the buccal mucosa opposite the maxillary second molar. Branches of the carotid artery provide the blood supply to the gland. The preganglionic sympathetic nerves innervating the gland originate in the upper thoracic spinal cord and synapse in the superior cervical ganglion, and the postganglionic fibers accompany the blood vessels supplying the gland. The parasympathetic innervation of the parotid gland arises from the inferior salivatory nucleus of the glossopharyngeal nerve (cranial nerve IX) located in the medulla and reaches the otic ganglion via the lesser petrosal nerve. The postganglionic fibers travel to the gland via the auriculotemporal nerve.

The parotid gland is a pure serous gland: all of the secretory endpieces are serous in nature (Fig. 11.19). The serous cells produce a variety of proteins and glycoproteins that have significant roles in protection of the oral tissues and digestion. The intercalated ducts are relatively long, and the striated ducts are prominent. Scattered adipocytes are frequently found in the parenchyma. In older individuals substantial amounts of the parenchyma may be replaced by fat.

> All of the secretory endpieces of the parotid gland consist of serous cells, and the striated ducts are prominent.

Submandibular gland

The submandibular gland is located in the submandibular space, partly inferior to the mylohyoid muscle and extending posterior and superior to the mylohyoid. The main duct of the gland, **Wharton's duct**, runs anteriorly below the mucosa of the floor of the mouth, opening at the **sublingual caruncle** near the base of the **lingual frenum**. The gland receives its blood supply from branches of the lingual artery. As with the parotid, the sympathetic nerves innervating the submandibular gland travel with the blood vessels. The parasympathetic nerves supplying the submandibular gland originate in the superior salivatory nucleus located in the pontine tegmentum, traveling via the facial (cranial nerve VII), chorda tympani, and lingual nerves. The preganglionic fibers synapse in the submandibular ganglion, and postganglionic fibers travel in short nerve roots to the gland.

The submandibular gland is a mixed gland; most secretory endpieces are serous, but a variable number of mucous endpieces with serous demilunes are present (Fig. 11.20). The serous cells are similar to those of the parotid and produce many of the same proteins and glycoproteins, but they also make a number of different proteins, including one of the main salivary mucins, the low molecular weight MUC7. The mucous cells produce both the high molecular weight mucin MUC5B and MUC7. Additionally, they produce a small cysteine-rich protein, trefoil factor 3 (TFF3), which stimulates epithelial repair. Like the parotid, numerous striated ducts are present in the submandibular gland.

> The submandibular gland has both serous and mucous endpieces, with the serous endpieces predominating.

Sublingual gland

The sublingual gland is located just below the mucosa of the floor of the mouth. Its main duct, **Bartholin's duct**, opens with the submandibular duct at the sublingual caruncle. Several smaller ducts, the **ducts of Rivinus**, open along the **sublingual fold** in the floor of the mouth. The blood supply of the sublingual gland is provided by the sublingual artery. Like the submandibular gland, the sublingual receives its postganglionic parasympathetic innervation from the submandibular ganglion.

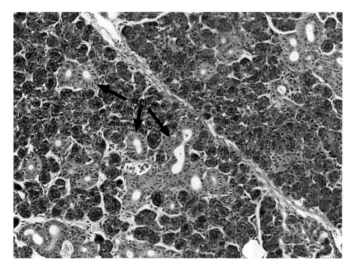

Figure 11.19   Parotid gland. The parotid gland contains serous endpieces and has numerous striated ducts (SD).

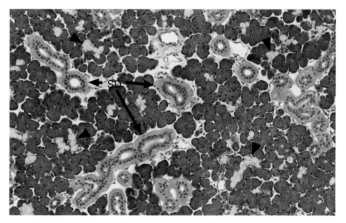

Figure 11.20   Submandibular gland. The submandibular gland is a mixed gland, containing predominantly serous endpieces along with some mucous endpieces (arrowheads) and serous demilunes. Several striated ducts (SD) are present.

The sublingual gland also is a mixed gland; all or most of the secretory endpieces are mucous, with serous demilunes (Fig. 11.21). A few serous endpieces also may be present. The main products of the mucous cells are the mucins MUC5B and MUC7. The serous cells are similar to those of the submandibular gland. The duct system of the sublingual gland is poorly developed; intercalated ducts are short and striated ducts are fewer in number than in the parotid and submandibular glands.

> The sublingual gland consists mainly of mucous endpieces with serous demilunes, and has a poorly developed duct system.

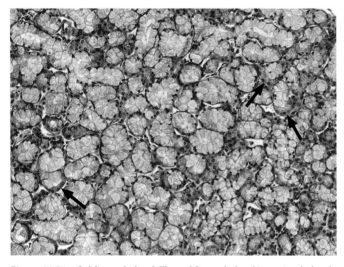

Figure 11.21   Sublingual gland. The sublingual gland is a mixed gland, containing mainly mucous endpieces with serous demilunes (arrows). Fewer striated ducts are present in the sublingual gland than in the parotid and submandibular glands.

The main structural and histological features of the major salivary glands are summarized in Table 11.1.

Minor glands

Minor salivary glands are small aggregates of secretory endpieces and ducts located in the submucosa in most parts of the oral cavity, except for the gingivae, the anterior portion and midline of the hard palate, and the anterior dorsum of the tongue (Table 11.2). The minor glands lack a distinct capsule; their supporting connective tissue is continuous with that of the surrounding submucosa or muscle. The ducts of the minor glands, lined by cuboidal or columnar epithelial cells, open directly onto the mucosal surface. Typical striated ducts generally are lacking, although some of the duct cells may have a few basal membrane infoldings.

Most of the minor glands consist of mucous endpieces that may or may not have serous demilunes (Fig. 11.22). The exception is the lingual serous (von Ebner's) glands located between muscle fibers of the posterior part of the tongue (Fig. 11.23). The ducts of these glands open into the troughs of the circumvallate papillae on the dorsum of the tongue and between the folds of the foliate papillae on the posterolateral surfaces of the tongue. Their association with major concentrations of taste buds suggests that the secretions of the lingual serous glands may have some role in the taste process.

> Most minor salivary glands, except for the lingual serous glands, consist of mucous endpieces with serous demilunes.

Table 11.1   Structural features of the major salivary glands

Component	Parotid	Submandibular	Sublingual
Secretory endpieces	Serous acini	Serous acini, mucous tubules with serous demilunes	Mucous tubules with serous demilunes, occasional serous acini
Intercalated ducts	Long, branching	Moderate length	Short, poorly developed
Striated ducts	Numerous, well developed	Numerous, well developed	Short, poorly developed
Main excretory duct	Stensen's: opens at parotid papilla opposite maxillary 2nd molar	Wharton's: opens at sublingual caruncle	Bartholin's: opens at sublingual caruncle; ducts of Rivinus: open along sublingual fold
Connective tissue capsule	Well defined	Well defined	Poorly developed
Blood supply	Branches of external carotid a.	Lingual a.	Sublingual a.
Nerve supply	Parasympathetic: cranial n. IX via lesser petrosal n., otic ganglion, auriculotemporal n. Sympathetic: superior cervical ganglion, following blood supply	Parasympathetic: cranial n. VII via chorda tympani n., lingual n., submandibular ganglion Sympathetic: superior cervical ganglion, following blood supply	Parasympathetic: cranial n. VII via chorda tympani n., lingual n., submandibular ganglion Sympathetic: superior cervical ganglion, following blood supply
Development begins	4th–6th fetal week	6th fetal week	8th fetal week

Table 11.2 Minor salivary glands

Gland	Location	Histological Structure
Labial	Submucosa of lips	Mucous endpieces, serous demilunes
Buccal	Submucosa of cheeks	Mucous endpieces, serous demilunes
Palatine	Posterior lateral submucosa of hard palate; submucosa of soft palate and uvula	Mucous endpieces, serous demilunes
Glossopalatine	Isthmus of palatoglossal fold	Mucous endpieces
Anterior lingual (glands of Blandin and Nuhn)	Submucosa of ventral surface of tongue	Mucous endpieces, serous demilunes
Posterior lingual (Weber's gland)	Lamina propria and between muscle fibers of posterior tongue	Mucous endpieces, serous demilunes
Posterior lingual serous (von Ebner's gland)	Lamina propria and between muscle fibers of tongue; ducts open into troughs of circumvallate and foliate papillae	Serous endpieces
Minor sublingual	Submucosa of floor of mouth	Mucous endpieces, serous demilunes

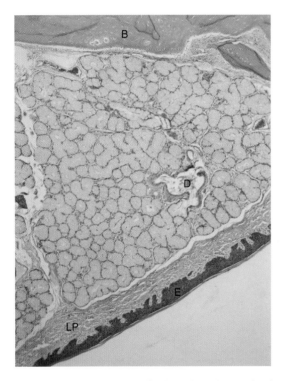

Figure 11.22 Minor salivary gland of palate. The palatine glands consist predominantly of mucous endpieces with serous demilunes. The gland is located in the submucosa of the posterolateral region of the palate; the palatal epithelium (E) and lamina propria (LP) are below, and the bone (B) of the palate is above. Duct (D).

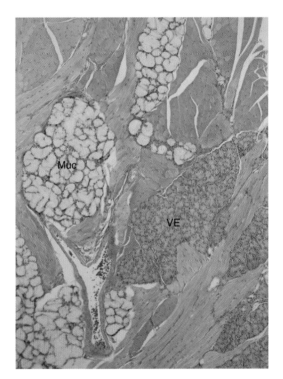

Figure 11.23 Minor salivary glands of tongue. The lingual serous (von Ebner's) glands (VE) are serous glands located between muscle fibers of the tongue. Their ducts open into the troughs of the circumvallate papillae and the folds of the foliate papillae. The posterior mucous (Weber's) glands (Muc) consist of mucous endpieces with serous demilunes. Their ducts open onto the dorsum of the tongue, posterior to the circumvallate papillae.

Salivary secretion

The secretion of saliva is controlled mainly by the autonomic nervous system. The salivary glands are innervated by parasympathetic and sympathetic unmyelinated fibers that are distributed in small bundles to the endpieces and ducts. The nerve fibers may penetrate the basal lamina and make close contact with the epithelial cells (**intraparenchymal innervation**) or remain in the interstitial connective tissue (**extraparenchymal innervation**). Typical synaptic structures are not present at the presumed sites of innervation.

Several reflex mechanisms are involved in stimulating saliva secretion. The taste of food substances and chemicals is the most potent stimulus for saliva secretion. Cranial nerves VII, IX, and X convey taste sensations to the nucleus of the solitary tract (NST) in the medulla oblongata. NST neurons carry taste information centrally to the ventral posterior medial nucleus (VPM) of the thalamus and from there to the gustatory cortex as well as to the hypothalamus. NST neurons also project to the salivatory nuclei, an efferent column adjacent to the NST, to reflexively activate preganglionic parasympathetic neurons of cranial nerves VII and IX. These salivatory neurons synapse with postganglionic neurons in peripheral autonomic ganglia that project to secretory cells of the glands. The salivatory nuclei also receive indirect projections from forebrain taste neurons. Mastication of food, sensed through mechanoreceptors in the periodontal ligament and oral mucosa, also stimulates secretion. The somatosensory sensations travel via the maxillary and mandibular branches of cranial nerve V to the principal trigeminal nucleus in the pons and from there to the VPM and the somatosensory cortex. Principal nucleus neurons also project locally to the salivatory nuclei. Additionally, psychogenic mechanisms, e.g., the sight or thought of food, can stimulate secretion.

Fluid secretion

Fluid secretion is an active process, dependent upon the active transport of electrolytes by the secretory cells. The parasympathetic innervation provides the main stimulus for fluid and electrolyte secretion. This is accomplished by the activation of signal transduction pathways in the secretory cells, and the opening/activation of ion channels and transporters in the luminal and basolateral membranes. Acetylcholine, released from parasympathetic nerve terminals in close proximity to the secretory cells, binds to G-protein coupled muscarinic receptors on the basolateral membrane, activating the enzyme phospholipase C (Fig. 11.24). The subsequent generation of inositol trisphosphate (IP_3) results in release of Ca^{2+} from intracellular stores, predominantly the endoplasmic reticulum. The increase in cytoplasmic Ca^{2+} opens Cl^- channels in the luminal membrane and K^+ channels in the basolateral membrane of the secretory cells. Intracellular Cl^- enters the lumen, drawing extracellular Na^+ ions

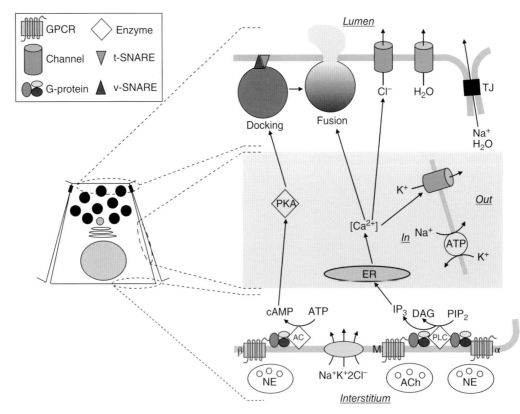

Figure 11.24 Regulation of protein and fluid secretion. Norepinephrine (NE) released from sympathetic nerve terminals binds to the β-adrenergic receptor (G-protein coupled receptor, GPCR) on the basolateral membrane of the secretory cell, resulting in dissociation of the heterotrimeric GTP-binding protein (G protein), G_s. The $G\alpha_s$ subunit increases the activity of adenylyl cyclase (AC), which forms cyclic AMP (cAMP) from ATP. Cyclic AMP activates protein kinase A (PKA), which phosphorylates other proteins, leading to docking of secretory granules to the luminal cell membrane via interaction of v- and t-SNARE proteins on the granule and luminal membranes, respectively. Elevated intracellular Ca^{2+} levels then promote fusion of the granule and luminal membranes, formation of a pore, and release of granule content by exocytosis. Acetylcholine (ACh) released from parasympathetic nerve terminals binds to the muscarinic (M) receptor (GPCR) on the basolateral membrane, resulting in dissociation of the $G_{q/11}$ G protein. The $G\alpha_{q/11}$ subunit activates phospholipase C (PLC), which hydrolyzes phosphoinositol bisphosphate (PIP_2) into inositol trisphosphate (IP_3) and diacyl glycerol (DAG). Inositol trisphosphate binds to the IP_3 receptor on the endoplasmic reticulum, releasing Ca^{2+} into the cytoplasm. The elevated Ca^{2+} levels open K^+ channels on the basolateral membrane and Cl^- channels on the luminal membrane. The accumulation of Cl^- in the lumen draws Na^+ through the tight junctions, and the resulting osmotic gradient causes water to enter the lumen through the tight junction (TJ) and through aquaporin 5 (AQP5) water channels in the luminal membrane. Norepinephrine also elevates Ca^{2+} and stimulates fluid secretion by binding to α-adrenergic receptors (GPCR) and activating phospholipase C.

through the tight junctions to balance the electrochemical gradient. The resulting osmotic gradient pulls water into the lumen, both through the tight junctions and via water channels (aquaporins) in the secretory cell membranes. With strong stimulation that results in high salivary flow rates, HCO_3^- may be formed intracellularly by carbonic anhydrase, enter the lumen via the Cl^- channels, and contribute to the luminal electrochemical and osmotic gradients. During active fluid secretion, intracellular ionic and osmotic balance is maintained by $Na^+/K^+/2Cl^-$ cotransporters, Na^+/H^+ exchangers, and Na^+/K^+-adenosine triphosphatase (Na^+/K^+-ATPase) in the basolateral membrane.

Protein secretion

The secretion of proteins and glycoproteins occurs by the process of exocytosis. Binding of norepinephrine released from sympathetic nerve terminals to G-protein coupled β-adrenergic receptors initiates an intracellular signaling cascade leading to exocytosis in serous cells (Fig. 11.24). Activation of adenylyl cyclase generates cyclic adenosine monophosphate (cyclic AMP), which activates protein kinase A. Protein kinase A phosphorylates other specific proteins, which, along with Ca^{2+}, small GTP-binding proteins and proteins on the secretory granule and luminal membranes, results in docking and fusion of granules with the luminal membrane and release of the granule contents into the lumen. The membranes of the empty granules are removed from the luminal membrane in the form of small endocytic vesicles and either recycled or degraded.

Other neural as well as hormonal mechanisms may stimulate or modulate saliva secretion. Parasympathetic stimulation results in secretion of mucin by mucous cells, and low levels of exocytosis by serous cells. Circulating hormones, particularly those regulating gastrointestinal secretion such as gastrin and cholecystokinin, may stimulate salivary protein secretion. Fluid secretion also may be stimulated by activation of other cell surface receptors. Norepinephrine, binding to α-adrenergic receptors, and substance P, binding to its receptors, can activate the phospholipid-Ca^{2+} pathway described above. The P2X and P2Y purinergic receptors, activated by extracellular ATP, open cell surface Ca^{2+} channels and stimulate Ca^{2+} release from intracellular stores, respectively. Parasympathetic nerves, endothelial cells, and secretory cells produce nitric oxide, which can stimulate secretion through elevation of intracellular Ca^{2+}. Finally, vasoactive intestinal polypeptide, neuropeptide Y, substance P, and calcitonin gene-related peptide may be released from autonomic nerves and locally modulate blood flow, thus controlling the availability of fluid and electrolytes for secretion into saliva, and metabolic substrates necessary for sustaining secretory activity.

> Saliva secretion is stimulated reflexly by afferent taste and oral somatosensory nerves. Fluid secretion is regulated mainly by parasympathetic nerves that activate intracellular phospholipid-Ca^{2+} signaling, whereas protein secretion is regulated mainly by sympathetic nerves via the cyclic AMP-protein kinase A pathway.

The primary saliva produced by the endpieces is modified as it passes through the duct system. The striated ducts function to reabsorb Na^+ and Cl^- ions from the primary saliva, and they secrete K^+ and HCO_3^-. Electrolyte transporters and Na^+/K^+-ATPase are located in the basolateral membrane, which is greatly amplified by numerous infoldings. Mitochondria in the cytoplasm between infoldings provide the energy to drive the Na^+/K^+-ATPase. Due to well-developed tight junctions and a lack of aquaporin water channels, the striated ducts are relatively impermeable to water, so the net result is a decrease in the osmolality of the saliva as it passes through the duct system. The excretory ducts are believed to function similarly.

> Striated ducts modify the primary saliva by reabsorbing Na^+ and Cl^- and secreting K^+ and HCO_3^-.

Myoepithelial cells and duct cells also are innervated by autonomic nerves. In most glands, contraction of myoepithelial cells results from sympathetic nerve stimulation; in some glands, parasympathetic stimulation also may cause myoepithelial cell contraction. Both sympathetic and parasympathetic nerve fibers are found adjacent to striated ducts. Experimental studies have shown that neurotransmitters that increase intracellular Ca^{2+} levels (e.g. acetylcholine) stimulate ductal electrolyte transport, and neurotransmitters that increase intracellular cyclic AMP levels (e.g. norepinephrine, vasoactive intestinal polypeptide) have the opposite effect. Exocytosis of the contents of striated duct cell secretory granules occurs in response to sympathetic nerve stimulation.

Saliva composition and function
Whole saliva

Saliva consists predominantly of water (~99%), however, the inorganic and organic components present in saliva (Table 11.3) have significant roles in oral protection and function. The electrolytes, proteins, glycoproteins, and mucins present in saliva are secreted mainly by the endpieces and ducts of the glands. Whereas the composition of the saliva produced by each of the paired major glands differs, reflecting their cellular makeup, the composition of **whole saliva**, i.e., the fluid in the mouth, is the critical factor in regulation of the oral environment. Whole saliva consists of the secretions of the three major glands, the minor glands, and plasma and cellular constituents contributed by the gingival crevicular fluid. Additionally, whole saliva contains desquamated oral epithelial cells, microorganisms and their products, and food debris.

The volume of saliva produced per day varies from about 600 mL to over 1 L. The amount produced at any given time depends on several factors, including autonomic nervous system activity, body hydration, the time of day, and drug use. As described above, taste and mastication stimulate saliva secretion from the major glands, whereas an increase in sympathetic tone causing vasoconstriction can inhibit secretion. Dehydration, e.g., due to excessive sweating, can reduce saliva output. Secretion

Table 11.3   Composition of whole saliva

Parameter	Characteristics
Volume	600–1,000 mL/day
Flow rate (resting)	0.2–0.5 mL/minute
pH	6.7–7.4
Osmolality	~50–75 mOsm/kg
Electrolytes	Na^+, K^+, Cl^-, HCO_3^-, Ca^{2+}, Mg^{2+}, HPO_4^{2-}, SCN^-, F^-
Protein concentration	~0.5–1.5 mg/mL
Major proteins	Amylase, proline-rich proteins, mucins, histatins, cystatins, peroxidase, lysozyme, lactoferrin, immunoglobulin A, defensins, cathelicidin-LL37
Small molecules	Glucose, amino acids, urea, uric acid, lipids
Other components	Growth factors, insulin, cyclic AMP-binding proteins, serum albumin

from the major glands also follows a circadian pattern, with the greatest (unstimulated) output between noon and 6 p.m., and the least output between midnight and 6 a.m. Although producing only a small volume, the minor glands secrete almost continuously, and therefore have an important role in moistening, lubricating, and protecting the oral mucosa and teeth during sleep. A side effect of many commonly prescribed medications is dry mouth, caused by central or peripheral inhibition of saliva secretion (see "Clinical Correlations").

The flow rate of unstimulated whole saliva varies between 0.2 and 0.5 mL/minute. With maximal stimulation, the whole saliva flow rate can exceed 7 mL/minute. The volume of saliva in the mouth at any given time varies between about 0.6 and 1.2 mL, following and just prior to swallowing. This volume is spread over the entire oral cavity, creating a salivary film 0.07 to 0.1 mm thick coating the mucosa and teeth.

> Whole saliva, the fluid in the mouth, produced at the rate of about 1 L/day, is composed of the secretions of the major and minor glands and fluid from the gingival crevice, and forms a thin film coating all of the oral surfaces.

Clearance

Saliva performs many important functions (Table 11.4). Protection of the oral tissues is one of saliva's most important roles. This includes clearance, buffering, maintenance of tooth integrity, and antimicrobial activity. The dilution and clearance of food debris, microbial acids, and other products is facilitated by the constant flow of the salivary film across the teeth and mucosa. The salivary film moves at different rates, depending on the location and whether secretion has been stimulated or not. Under resting conditions the salivary film moves at about 0.8 mm per minute along the facial surfaces of the maxillary incisors, whereas under stimulated conditions (e.g., food consumption) the film can move at greater than 300 mm per minute along the lingual surfaces of the mandibular incisors. Thus clearance varies in

different parts of the oral cavity, and the rate of clearance is inversely related to the prevalence of dental caries in these regions.

Pellicle

The negatively charged mucins and glycoproteins, with abundant bound water, help to lubricate the mucosa and teeth and allow tissues to slide past one another during chewing, swallowing, and speaking. Additionally, a coating of mucins on the oral surfaces helps to protect against thermal, chemical, and mechanical insults. Many salivary constituents, including mucins, acidic proline-rich proteins (PRPs), statherin, histatins, and cystatins, bind to the enamel surface, forming a **salivary pellicle**. These bound constituents create a reservoir of calcium and phosphate at the tooth surface that opposes demineralization and promotes remineralization of initial caries lesions, especially in the presence of F^- ions.

Buffering

Salivary HCO_3^- and carbonic anhydrase play important roles in counteracting the effects of microbial acids generated from sugars on the hydroxyapatite crystals of enamel and dentin. Salivary HCO_3^- levels increase as salivary flow increases, and in the presence of H^+ carbonic anhydrase in saliva or bound to teeth in the salivary pellicle forms H_2O and CO_2, and the CO_2 escapes into the air. Some buffering also is achieved by HPO_4^{2-} and $H_2PO_4^-$ in saliva, as well as by cationic, histidine-rich proteins. Additionally, urea and ammonia formed by microbial metabolism help to neutralize acids.

Antimicrobial activity

Saliva contains a number of proteins that function in regulating the oral microbial flora. Some of the proteins, such as lysozyme and peroxidase, are enzymes that attack microbial cell walls or generate products that inhibit microbial metabolism. Other proteins, such as mucins, salivary agglutinin (gp340), and the major salivary immunoglobulin, secretory immunoglobulin A (sIgA), bind to and aggregate microorganisms, preventing them from

Table 11.4 Functions of saliva

Function	Effect	Active Constituents
Protection	Clearance, moistening	Water
	Lubrication	Mucins, glycoproteins
	Thermal/chemical insulation	Mucins
	Pellicle formation	Proteins, glycoproteins, mucins
	Tannin binding	Basic proline-rich proteins, histatins
Buffering	pH maintenance	Carbonic anhydrase VI, bicarbonate, phosphate, basic proteins
	Neutralization of acids	Urea, ammonia
Tooth integrity	Enamel maturation, repair	Calcium, phosphate, fluoride, statherin, acidic proline-rich proteins, cystatins
Antimicrobial activity	Innate defense	Lysozyme, lactoferrin, peroxidase, histatins, mucins, agglutinins, defensins, cathelicidin LL-37, SPLUNC family proteins, secretory leukocyte protease inhibitor
	Adaptive immune defense	Secretory immunoglobulin A
	Barrier	Mucins
Tissue repair	Wound healing, tissue regeneration	Growth factors, trefoil factor family peptides
Digestion	Bolus formation	Water, mucins
	Starch digestion	Amylase
	Triglyceride digestion	Lipase
	Nucleic acid digestion	Ribonuclease, deoxyribonuclease
Taste	Solution of molecules	Water
	Taste bud maintenance	Epidermal growth factor, carbonic anhydrase VI

binding to oral tissues. SPLUNC (short palate lung nasal epithelium clone) family proteins, in addition to binding and inhibiting growth of certain bacteria, bind lipopolysaccharide (LPS) and prevent release of inflammatory mediators from macrophages. Some small peptides, such as defensins, cathelicidin LL-37, and the histatins, insert into and disrupt microbial cellular membranes, resulting in osmotic lysis or depletion of various metabolites. Lactoferrin binds iron, reducing its availability to microorganisms, and also disrupts cellular membranes. Secretory leukocyte protease inhibitor (SLPI) binds to and inhibits certain bacteria, and along with several other salivary proteins (e.g. lysozyme, peroxidase, lactoferrin, mucins, defensins, sIgA, and salivary agglutinin) exhibits anti-viral activity.

Wound healing

Growth factors present in saliva, such as epidermal growth factor, and other salivary proteins (e.g., trefoil factor family peptides, histatins) are believed to facilitate wound healing and tissue repair. These factors may induce cell proliferation and migration during wound healing and re-epithelialization in the oral cavity and the digestive tract. Trefoil proteins are thought to promote healing of ulcers in the oral cavity and digestive tract; they are produced by salivary mucous cells and also by keratinocytes of the oral epithelium.

Digestion

Saliva has an important role in eating and digestion. Saliva serves to facilitate mastication and swallowing of food and solubilizes many food constituents. During mastication, the water and mucins in saliva protect the oral tissues and help to create a food bolus suitable for swallowing. Saliva also contains several enzymes that initiate digestion of various dietary constituents. These include amylase, which hydrolyzes starches to maltose and limit dextrins, ribonuclease (RNAse) and deoxyribonuclease (DNAse). Lingual lipase, produced by the lingual serous glands and pharyngeal glands, initiates digestion of dietary triglycerides. Although digestion of these substances is achieved mainly by pancreatic and gastric enzymes, the salivary enzymes may play a significant role in cases of pancreatic insufficiency.

Toxin binding

In addition to digestion of various dietary substances, some salivary proteins function to protect against certain harmful dietary constituents. The basic PRPs and histatins bind tannins, common constituents of many plant-derived foods that may inhibit growth and have various toxic effects, and prevent their uptake by intestinal epithelial cells. Experimental studies have shown that dietary tannins increase the synthesis of basic PRPs by the salivary glands. Cystatins are cysteine peptidase inhibitors and may function to protect against the deleterious effects of plant-derived papain-like enzymes in the diet. Similar to the effect of tannins on basic PRPs, dietary papain increases the expression of cystatins in the salivary glands. Although not considered a harmful substance, consumption of xylitol, a sugar alcohol used as a sugar substitute, increases the activity of peroxidase in saliva.

Taste

The solubilization of food makes possible the detection of taste substances by taste receptors in taste buds of the tongue. Clearance of taste substances by saliva permits detection of new taste stimuli. The taste receptors are adapted to the concentration of Na^+ in saliva; the threshold for the salty taste of NaCl is greater and the supra-threshold intensity is less in the presence of saliva than distilled water. Some components of saliva may interact with taste substances and modify their effect. For example, HCO_3^- in saliva reacts with acid (H^+), reducing its taste intensity, and basic PRPs bind to tannins, diminishing or altering their bitter taste or interfering with taste reception. It has long been thought that the secretions of the lingual serous glands, which bathe the taste buds of the circumvallate and foliate papillae, have a significant role in the taste process. The glands produce some digestive enzymes, antimicrobial proteins, as well as a lipocalin, which has proteinase inhibitory and lipid-binding activity. Saliva from these glands probably serves to refresh the taste buds after a stimulus, as well as to control the microbial flora in the troughs of the papillae. The lingual serous glands, like the parotid and submandibular, secrete carbonic anhydrase VI, which may be a trophic factor for taste buds. Epidermal growth factor in saliva helps to maintain taste buds on fungiform papillae of the tongue.

> Saliva functions to protect the oral tissues through several mechanisms, including lubrication and moistening, clearance of microbes and their products, buffering of acids, prevention of demineralization and promotion of remineralization, antimicrobial activity, wound healing, and binding of toxic substances. Saliva also initiates digestion of food and solubilizes taste substances.

Diagnostic and forensic uses of saliva

Diagnostics

Although only a few organic constituents of saliva are mentioned in this chapter, recent efforts to catalog the entire salivary proteome have revealed the presence of around 2000 unique protein components. Many of these are secretory proteins synthesized and released by the salivary gland cells; others are membrane or intracellular proteins shed from the cells or released from dying cells; still others originate from other tissues and organs, are carried to the glands in blood plasma, and transported across the glandular epithelium or oral mucosa. Because saliva can be collected easily and noninvasively, it has potential as a diagnostic fluid. It is

anticipated that knowledge of all of the proteins present in saliva and determination of the changes in their levels in various disease states will lead to the identification of specific "biomarkers" that can be used to diagnose various diseases. The development, already in progress, of small, tabletop instruments using microfluidics and nanotechnology approaches to perform immunoassays and molecular tests on saliva samples will facilitate point-of-care diagnostics and personalized medicine and dentistry.

Saliva currently is used to test for the presence of various hormones and drugs, including steroids, nicotine metabolites, and other drugs of abuse (e.g., cocaine, marijuana, barbiturates, amphetamines). Several commercial testing products are available. The transfer of these compounds from plasma into saliva is related to their lipid solubility, molecular size, dissociation constant, and protein-binding characteristics. The concentration of cortisol in saliva is widely used as measure of psychological stress, and increases in estrogen levels in saliva are used to predict ovulation times.

Forensics

Saliva also has important forensic uses. Blood types of about 80% of individuals can be determined from a saliva sample, as the oligosaccharide structure on salivary mucins is the same as that on red blood cells that determines blood type. The epithelial cells shed from the oral mucosa are a source of DNA that can be used to determine an individual's genotype and to specifically identify an individual.

> Saliva can be collected easily and non-invasively; complete characterization of its protein components and identification of specific disease biomarkers will advance its use as a diagnostic fluid.

Clinical correlations

Salivary hypofunction

The feeling of a dry mouth, or **xerostomia**, is a relatively frequent clinical complaint. There are several conditions that may lead to the reduced output of saliva, or **salivary hypofunction**. The most common causes of salivary hypofunction are the side effects of many prescribed or over-the-counter medications. Other conditions causing reduced saliva output include autoimmune diseases and head and neck radiation. Decreased saliva and a dry mouth often occur in older individuals. With age, a significant amount of the parenchyma of salivary glands may be replaced by adipose tissue. However, in healthy, nonmedicated older individuals, clinical studies show that unstimulated (resting) as well as stimulated whole saliva output does not differ from that of younger individuals.

In autoimmune diseases, an individual's immune system attacks otherwise normal tissues and organs. In primary **Sjögren's syndrome**, the salivary and lacrimal glands are severely damaged by cells of the immune system, resulting in reduced output of saliva and tears. Sjögren's syndrome may accompany other autoimmune diseases, such as rheumatoid arthritis or systemic lupus erythematosus. The salivary hypofunction causes xerostomia and difficulty in speaking and swallowing. The loss of the protective effects of salivary proteins, mucins, and buffers usually results in an increase in dental caries, mucosal infections, and ulcers. Sjögren's syndrome predominantly affects middle-aged women; it is estimated that as many as four million people in the United States may be affected by Sjögren's syndrome. Measurement of whole saliva flow rate along with biopsy of the minor glands of the lip and histopathological examination are important diagnostic aids in Sjögren's syndrome. Although there is no effective treatment for Sjögren's syndrome, frequent sipping of water or the use of saliva substitutes may help to alleviate some of the symptoms. When some functional gland tissue remains, prescribing oral parasympathomimetic drugs may increase saliva output.

Approximately 40,000 cases of head and neck cancer are diagnosed each year in the United States. Most of these cancers are treated by radiation therapy, and the radiation field generally includes the salivary glands. The glands are extremely sensitive to the effects of radiation, which causes degeneration of the secretory cells and severe loss of secretory function. The effects on the teeth and oral mucosa are similar to those seen in Sjögren's syndrome. At present, there is no effective way to prevent radiation damage to the salivary glands. Some experimental drugs that act as radical scavengers have shown some protective effects in clinical trials. Gene therapy has been proposed as a possible approach to either prevention of radiation damage or restoration of gland function after radiation or autoimmune damage. Experimental animal studies using viral vectors containing different genes administered by retrograde infusion via the oral openings of the gland ducts have shown positive effects. A Phase 1 clinical trial in which the gene for the water channel aquaporin-1 was administered in an adenovirus vector has shown some temporary increases in saliva production.

> Salivary hypofunction may be caused by autoimmune diseases, radiation to the head and neck, and most commonly, by numerous drugs; lack of the protective effects of saliva leads to increased dental caries, mucosal lesions and infections, and a decreased quality of life.

Other conditions

Obstruction of the main excretory duct of a salivary gland may occur through trauma, blockage of an excretory duct, or infection. Biting or trauma to the lip, a common injury, may sever the duct of a minor salivary gland, with the result that mucus pools in the connective tissue. The resulting swelling is called a **mucocele**. A stricture, mucous plug, or calcified body (stone or **sialolith**) may obstruct the duct of a major or minor salivary gland. Symptoms include swelling and pain at mealtimes, which subside within a few hours. Sialoliths form as calcium and phosphate precipitate on membranous or cellular debris in a duct lumen. They occur most frequently in the submandibular gland as calcium concentrations are greater in the serous secretory granules, and consequently in this saliva. Inflammation of the glands, **sialadenitis**, and stagnation of saliva are likely

predisposing factors. Sialadenitis may be caused by bacterial infections ascending the ducts from the oral cavity, or viral infections, especially caused by the mumps virus. Dehydration, leading to decreased output of saliva, predisposes to bacterial infection.

Although rare, a number of benign and malignant tumors affect the salivary glands. They tend to be morphologically and clinically diverse and thus may present difficulties for accurate diagnosis and management. About 80% of salivary gland tumors are benign, and approximately 70% of all tumors are found in the parotid gland. These present a challenge to the surgeon because of the intimate relationship of the parotid gland to the facial nerve. Tumors also may arise in the submandibular and sublingual glands, as well as the minor salivary glands.

Developmental abnormalities may affect the salivary glands. Fibroblast growth factors and their receptors, especially FGF10, play critical roles in the process of branching morphogenesis that occurs during development. Mutations in the FGF10 gene, or the gene for its receptor, FGFR2, can result in the absence (**aplasia**) or underdevelopment (**hypoplasia**) of salivary glands and other organs.

References

1. Baum, B.J., Yates, J.R. III, Srivastava, S., Wong, D.T.W., & Melvin, J.E. (2011) Scientific frontiers: emerging technologies for salivary diagnostics. *Advances in Dental Research,* 23(4), 360–368.
2. Dodds, M.W., Johnson, D.A., & Yeh, C.K. (2005) Health benefits of saliva: a review. *Journal of Dentistry,* 33(3), 223–233.
3. Eveson, J.W. (2011) Salivary tumours. *Periodontology 2000,* 57(1), 150–159.
4. Garrett, J.R., Ekstrom, J., & Anderson, L.C. (eds.) (1998) Glandular mechanisms of salivary secretion. *Frontiers of Oral Biology,* 10, 1–226.
5. Garrett, J.R., Ekstrom, J., & Anderson, L.C. (eds.) (1999) Neural mechanisms of salivary gland secretion. *Frontiers of Oral Biology,* 11, 1–236.
6. Hand, A.R. (1990) The secretory process of salivary glands and pancreas. In: *Ultrastructure of the Extraparietal Glands of the Digestive Tract* (eds. A. Riva & P.M. Motta). Kluwer Academic, Boston.
7. Harunaga, J., Hsu, J.C., & Yamada, K.M. (2011) Dynamics of salivary gland morphogenesis. *Journal of Dental Research,* 90(9), 1070–1077.
8. Lee, M.G., Ohana, E., Park, H.W., Yang, D., & Muallem, S. (2012) Molecular mechanism of pancreatic and salivary gland fluid and HCO_3^- secretion. *Physiological Reviews,* 92(1), 39–74.
9. Malamud, D. (2011) Saliva as a diagnostic fluid. *Dental Clinics of North America,* 55(1), 159–178.
10. Matthews, S.A., Kurien, B.T., & Scofield, R.H. (2008) Oral manifestations of Sjögren's syndrome. *Journal of Dental Research,* 87(4), 308–318.
11. Patel, V.N., Rebustini, I.T., & Hoffman, M.P. (2006) Salivary gland branching morphogenesis. *Differentiation,* 74(7), 349–364.
12. Tabak, L.A. (2006) In defense of the oral cavity: the protective role of the salivary secretions. *Pediatric Dentistry,* 28(2), 110–117.
13. Tandler, B. (guest ed.) (1993) Microstructure of the salivary glands: part I. *Microscopy Research and Technique,* 26(1), 1–91.

Glossary

Acini: Spherical or tubular configuration of secretory endpiece cells arranged around a lumen. (Singular: acinus.)

Aplasia: Defective development or congenital absence of an organ or tissue.

Bartholin's duct: The main duct of the sublingual gland, opening with the submandibular duct at the sublingual caruncle.

Branching morphogenesis: Developmental process in which reciprocal interactions between epithelium and mesenchyme involving growth factors and their receptors leads to repeated splitting or branching of the epithelial buds to create a gland with multiple secretory endpieces connected to a duct system.

Capsule: Connective tissue enclosing an organ.

Cytodifferentiation: The process of development of specialized cells from undifferentiated cells. For example, in salivary glands this involves an increase of endoplasmic reticulum and Golgi complex and the accumulation of secretory granules in acinar cells.

Ducts: Tubular epithelium-lined structures that convey the secretions from the endpiece cells to the oral cavity.

Ducts of Rivinus: The minor ducts of the sublingual gland, opening along the sublingual fold in the floor of the mouth.

Excretory ducts: Larger caliber ducts located in the interlobular connective tissue, eventually forming the main duct of the gland.

Extraparenchymal innervation: Autonomic nerve terminals that remain with the nerve bundle and Schwann cell in the interstitial connective tissue.

Hypoplasia: Underdevelopment or incomplete development of an organ or tissue.

Intercalated duct: The initial segment of the duct system, connecting the secretory endpieces with the striated ducts.

Intercellular canaliculi: Finger-like extensions of the endpiece lumen along the lateral membranes of serous cells.

Interstitial tissue: The connective tissue cells and extracellular matrix components that support the gland parenchyma.

Intraparenchymal innervation: Autonomic nerve terminals that leave the nerve bundle and penetrate the basal lamina to make close contact with the secretory and/or duct cells.

Lingual frenum: The thin band of oral mucosa between the midline of the ventral surface of the tongue and the floor of the mouth.

Lobes: Major subdivisions of an organ visible grossly.

Lobules: Histological subdivisions of a lobe of an organ, separated by connective tissue partitions.

Mixed endpiece: A secretory endpiece containing both mucous and serous cells.

Mucocele: A swelling on the lip mucosa due to the accumulation or pooling of mucin in the connective tissue, caused by the rupture of the duct of a minor salivary gland.

Mucous cell: A secretory cell producing a mucin or mucins, whose cytoplasm typically is filled with pale-staining secretory granules.

Myoepithelial cell: A stellate- or fusiform-shaped contractile cell associated with the secretory endpieces and/or ducts of many exocrine glands.

Parenchyma: The functional components of an organ.

Parotid papilla: A swelling of the oral mucosa on the inside of the cheek, opposite the second maxillary molar, at which the duct of parotid gland opens.

Salivary hypofunction: The objective finding of reduced salivation, usually defined as a resting flow rate of whole saliva of less than 0.1 mL per minute.

Salivary pellicle: The coating of salivary proteins, glycoproteins and mucins on the exposed surfaces of the teeth and the oral mucosa.

Secretory endpiece (acinus): Spherical or tubular configuration of exocrine secretory cells arranged around a lumen and connected to a duct.

Septa: Connective tissue partitions separating the lobes and lobules of an organ.

Seromucous: A descriptive term originally applied to secretory cells with staining properties intermediate between serous and mucous cells, but often used to refer to glycoprotein producing serous cells.

Serous cell: A secretory cell that produces proteins or glycoproteins with various functional activities, that are stored in dense secretory granules that fill the apical cytoplasm.

Serous demilune: The crescent shaped cluster of serous secretory cells at the end of a mucous endpiece.

Sialadenitis: Inflammation of a salivary gland.

Sialolith: A calicified plug or stone obstructing the duct of a salivary gland.

Sjögren's syndrome: An autoimmune disease that affects the salivary and lacrimal glands, resulting in destruction of the secretory cells and reduced output of saliva and tears.

Stensen's duct: The main duct of the parotid gland, opening at the parotid papilla.

Striated duct: The characteristic intralobular component of the duct system of salivary glands, whose principal function is to reabsorb sodium and chloride from the primary saliva produced by the endpiece cells, resulting in a hypotonic final saliva.

Stroma: The supporting connective tissue (interstitial tissue) of an organ.

Sublingual caruncle: The site on either side of the lingual frenum at which the main ducts of the submandibular and sublingual glands open into the oral cavity.

Sublingual fold: A fold in the mucosa of the floor of the mouth formed by the superior border of the sublingual gland and the submandibular duct; the minor ducts (Rivinus) of the sublingual gland open along the sublingual fold.

Wharton's duct: The main duct of the submandibular gland, opening at the sublingual caruncle.

Whole saliva: The saliva present in the mouth (oral fluid), composed of secretions of the major and minor salivary glands, gingival crevicular fluid, white blood cells, oral epithelial cells, oral microbes and their products, and food remnants.

Xerostomia: The subjective sensation of a dry mouth.

Chapter 12 Orofacial Pain, Touch and Thermosensation, and Sensorimotor Functions

Barry J. Sessle

Faculty of Dentistry, University of Toronto

This chapter reviews the neural processes that are involved in the somatosensory and motor functions of the face and mouth. It focuses first on the neural basis of orofacial touch, temperature, and especially pain common in the orofacial region. In addition, attention is given to the neural mechanisms that underlie the numerous reflex and other sensorimotor functions expressed in the orofacial region, particularly those related to mastication (chewing), swallowing, and other associated neuromuscular functions.

The orofacial region is remarkable in its high level of sensory discriminability and sensitivity, reflecting in part its great innervation density and the large amount of brain tissue devoted to the representation of the oral cavity and surrounding facial areas. Furthermore, there are specialized receptor systems associated with the periodontal tissues that support the teeth and with the facial whiskers (vibrissae) that are especially well developed in several subprimates (e.g., rodents). These receptor systems provide an added dimension of sensory experience, and together with the tongue and lips are very important for an individual's ability to explore the environment and control movement and other behaviors. Also noteworthy are that some of the most common pains occur in the orofacial region (e.g., toothaches, headaches, **temporomandibular disorder (TMD)** pain) and can cause considerable long-term suffering. Furthermore, some sensory functions are unique to this region (e.g., taste). The orofacial region also is remarkable in the vast array of sensorimotor

behaviors that it manifests, ranging from relatively simple reflexes (e.g., the jaw-opening reflex) to the very complex sensorimotor activities that are associated with speech, mastication, and swallowing that provide for social communication and the ingestion of food and fluid vital for life. These simple or complex sensorimotor activities utilize sensory inputs into the brain from the receptors in the face and mouth to initiate or guide them, and involve the integrated neuronal activity of many parts of the brain.

Sensory functions

Touch

General characteristics

The ability to sense touch (i.e., tactile sensibility) is extremely well developed in the orofacial region of humans and other animals. In fact some species depend on parts of this region for exploring their environment and even for their very survival. For example, the facial whiskers and perioral tissues are crucial for rodents, especially in infancy, to sense their environment and find nutrients (e.g., from their mother's nipples). In humans, tests to measure touch include **tactile threshold, two-point discrimination**, and **stereognosis** (a term referring to the ability to recognize the form of objects), and these tests have shown that some orofacial areas such as the

Fundamentals of Oral Histology and Physiology, First Edition. Arthur R. Hand and Marion E. Frank.
© 2014 John Wiley & Sons, Inc. Published 2014 by John Wiley & Sons, Inc.

lips and tongue tip have a tactile sensitivity that is better than any other part of the body.

Peripheral processes

As noted in Chapter 9, the orofacial tissues are densely innervated by primary afferent (i.e., sensory) nerve fibers, each of which terminates peripherally at sensory organs termed receptors. These receptors "sense" stimuli applied to the face and mouth as well as changes in the environment, and transduce this sensory information into electrochemical energy, which is then conducted as action potentials along the afferent fibers into the brainstem (i.e., "nerve conduction"). The receptors can be broadly categorized into two types: free nerve endings, and specialized or corpuscular receptors, of which several anatomically distinct examples exist. Many of the receptors primarily associated with myelinated, large-diameter, fast-conducting afferent nerve fibers (A-β afferents, some A-δ afferents) function as **mechanoreceptors** since they respond either transiently to (as velocity detectors) or throughout (as static-position detectors) a mechanical stimulus applied to a localized orofacial area that is termed the receptive field of the afferent. Figure 12.1 shows examples from recordings of afferents supplying periodontal tissues. Since many types of mechanoreceptors are exclusively activated by tactile stimuli and have an anatomically recognized receptor structure and many neurons in the central relay stations (see below) respond exclusively to tactile stimulation, these features support the concept of the specificity theory of sensation (Fig. 12.2). According to this theory, a specific set of receptors and afferent nerve fibers and neurons and relay stations in the central nervous system (CNS) respond exclusively to tactile stimuli, for example, and provide the higher levels of the brain (e.g., cerebral cortex) only

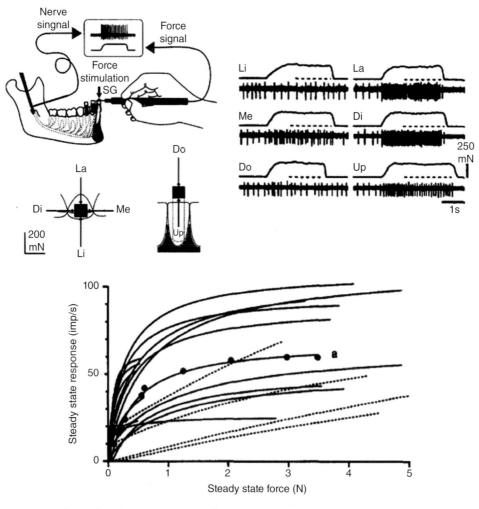

Figure 12.1 Response properties of periodontal mechanosensory afferents recorded in the inferior alveolar nerve in humans during application of forces applied to the central incisor in labial (La), lingual (Li), mesial (Me), distal (Di), downward (Do), and upward (Up) directions. Note the different responses of a single periodontal afferent supplying the tooth when the same magnitude of force is applied in the six different directions; the greatest slowly adapting discharge of the afferent is to the Di force. Also note from their stimulus-response functions that some periodontal afferents show a progressive increase in their response as the force is progressively increased (dotted lines) whereas others show a more rapid increase at low forces but then quickly saturate (adapt). (From Trulsson and Johansson (1996) *Progress in Neurobiology*, 49, 267–284).

with neural information related to touch and not, for example, to pain or temperature. As noted below, this theory has not held up well in accounting for pain.

The mechanoreceptors in the facial skin, oral mucosa, periodontal tissues, and jaw joint (the temporomandibular joint, TMJ) thus provide the sensory inputs into the brain that reflect detailed information of the quality, location, intensity, duration, and rate of movement of an orofacial mechanical stimulus. Some analogous receptor mechanisms account for our ability to detect and discriminate the size of small objects placed between the teeth, their hardness and texture, and bite force. These receptors are located in the periodontal tissues around the root of each tooth, but also receptors in the TMJ and even in jaw muscles make an important contribution. Receptors in the TMJ and the jaw muscles also largely account for our conscious perception of jaw position (mandibular **kinesthesia**).

Central pathways and processes

The major nerve carrying the primary afferent neural signals from the orofacial mechanoreceptors is the trigeminal nerve (the fifth cranial nerve). The low-threshold mechanosensory afferent nerve fibers in the trigeminal nerve pass via the **trigeminal ganglion** (where their primary afferent cell bodies are located) and the trigeminal sensory nerve root into the trigeminal brainstem sensory nuclear complex (Fig. 12.3). The neural signals are transferred (via synaptic transmission) to mechanosensitive neurons at all levels of the trigeminal brainstem sensory nuclear complex, which can be subdivided into a main sensory nucleus and a spinal tract nucleus; the latter is subdivided further into the subnuclei oralis, interpolaris, and caudalis. These second-order neurons conduct the signals onwards through their projections to higher sensorimotor centers but also many of the neurons project to local brainstem regions, including those responsible for activating muscles, and thereby serve as

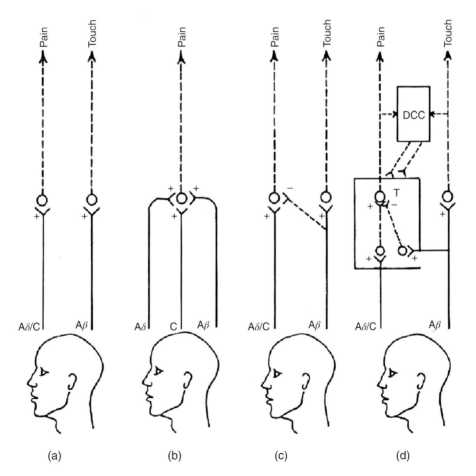

Figure 12.2   The main theories of pain. (a) Specificity theory emphasizes a separate and exclusive peripheral and central pathway for pain compared with, for example, touch. (b) Intensive or summation theory draws attention to the convergence of different afferent fiber types that are activated by different types of stimuli (e.g., noxious, tactile, warm, cool) and that excite (+) central neurons. Pain is coded by a distinctive pattern of activity of central neurons that is evoked by each of the four different stimulus modalities. (c) Sensory interaction theory emphasizes the ability of some afferent fiber inputs (e.g., mechanosensitive) to suppress (−) activity in central neurons relaying nociceptive information. (d) Gate control theory also stresses central interaction of inputs from different afferent fiber types. The interaction of inputs from large-diameter (e.g., A-β mechanosensitive) afferents versus small-diameter (e.g., A-δ and C nociceptive) afferents to central transmission (T) nociceptive neurons is emphasized. This theory also notes the capability of this "gating" mechanism to be modulated (+, −) by descending central controls (DCC). (Modified from Sessle, 1981a.)

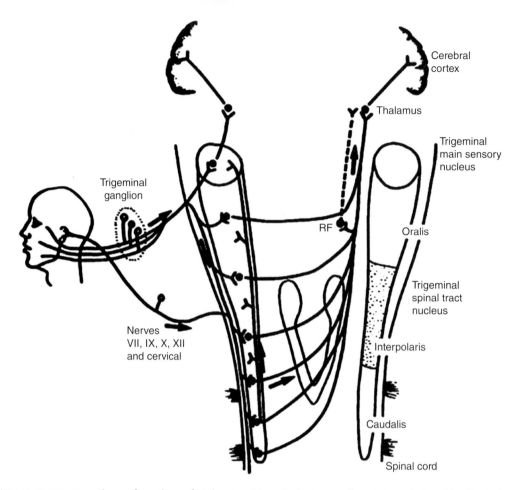

Figure 12.3   Major somatosensory pathways from the orofacial region. Trigeminal primary afferents have their cell bodies in the trigeminal ganglion and project to second-order neurons in the trigeminal brainstem sensory nuclear complex. These second-order neurons may project to neurons in higher levels of the brain (e.g., in the thalamus) or in brainstem regions such as cranial nerve motor nuclei or the reticular formation (RF). The sensory inputs also include orofacial afferents supplying the cornea and sinuses (e.g., maxillary sinus). Not shown in detail are the projections of some cervical nerve afferents and cranial nerve VII, IX, X, and XII afferents to the trigeminal brainstem complex and the projection of many cranial nerve V, VII, IX, and X afferents to the solitary tract nucleus. (Modified from Sessle, 1981b.)

interneurons involved in reflexes or more complex sensorimotor behaviors (see "Sensorimotor Functions and Motor Control" below). Nonetheless, a major projection from trigeminal brainstem neurons is concerned with touch perception, and this pathway projects from the trigeminal spinal tract nucleus and especially the main sensory nucleus to the ventroposterior thalamus (termed the ventrobasal thalamus in subprimates). This projection is principally to the contralateral side of the brain, but an ipsilateral projection also exists (Fig. 12.3). In the thalamus the signals are relayed to third-order mechanosensitive neurons, many of which project to parts of the overlying cerebral cortex. One part is the **somatosensory cortex**, where the cerebral cortical neural processing begins that eventually leads to the perception of an orofacial touch stimulus. An extensive and disproportionate part of this somatosensory cortex is devoted to the representation of the face and mouth, reflecting the importance of sensory information from orofacial tissues compared to other body regions.

The trigeminal brainstem sensory nuclear complex can be subdivided into a main sensory nucleus and a spinal tract nucleus; the latter is subdivided further into the subnuclei oralis, interpolaris, and caudalis.

An extensive and disproportionate part of the somatosensory cortex is devoted to the representation of the face and mouth, reflecting the importance of sensory information from orofacial tissues compared to other body regions.

The second-, third-, and fourth-order neurons in this ascending pathway to the cerebral cortex show many functional properties comparable with those of the mechanoreceptive primary afferent fibers, with a localized mechanoreceptive field and coding of the intensity of the stimulus that results in their activation (e.g., see Fig. 12.4a). They also retain much of the "specificity" of the mechanoreceptors and their mechanosensory primary afferents, thus providing further support

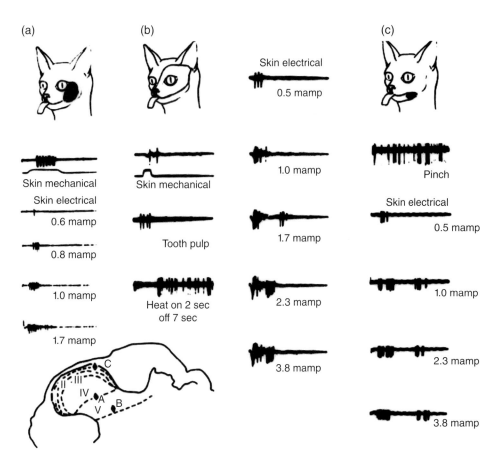

Figure 12.4 Examples of the three major classes of neurons in the trigeminal subnucleus caudalis. Data were derived from electrophysiological recordings in the subnucleus caudalis of a cat. Records in (a) were obtained from a single low-threshold mechanosensitive neuron that could only be activated by light mechanical (tactile) stimulation of the area of facial skin outlined (i.e., the receptive field of the neuron). Note its progressively increasing discharge to mechanical stimulation of the receptive field to increasing intensity levels of electric stimulation of the receptive field; even at high intensities, only a single burst of impulses can be produced. This neuron in (a) was located in layer IV of the subnucleus caudalis, as illustrated below in the cross-section of the medulla. The wide-dynamic-range neuron shown in (b) could be activated by tactile stimulation of its receptive field (outlined) as well as by electric stimulation of the canine tooth pulp, pinch (not shown), and noxious levels of radiant heat applied to the receptive field. Note that with increasing intensity levels of electric stimulation of the receptive field, late as well as early bursts of impulses could be evoked; the late discharge probably reflects inputs from nociceptive afferent fibers (e.g., A-δ and C), and the early burst reflects inputs from faster-conducting mechanosensory afferent fibers (e.g., A-β). This neuron was located in layer V of the subnucleus caudalis. The nociceptive-specific neuron shown in (c) was located in layer I of the subnucleus caudalis and could only be excited by noxious stimulation (e.g., pinch) of the receptive field. The first burst of impulses produced by high-intensity electric stimulation probably reflects inputs from small myelinated (A-δ) nociceptive afferent fibers, and the later burst reflects inputs from the slower-conducting unmyelinated (C) nociceptive afferent fibers. Time duration of records: (a), 50 msec; (b), 100 msec (except heat record: 10 sec); (c), 200 msec (except pinch record: 10 sec). Record to pinch in (c) is at twice the amplification for skin electrical records. (Modified from Sessle, 1981a.)

for the specificity theory of touch. Nonetheless, by means of the complex ultrastructure and regulatory processes that exist at each of the relay sites, considerable modification of the synaptic transmission of the tactile-related signals can occur, as a result of other incoming sensory signals and descending influences from higher brain centers exerted on touch-transmission neurons in the relay sites (Fig. 12.5). Such modulatory processes may explain, for example, how distraction or focusing one's attention on a particular task at hand can depress our awareness of a touch stimulus, e.g., being unaware of all the tactile stimulation of the mechanoreceptors on our forearm and other parts of our body when we are writing a letter or examination or reading a book.

> Considerable modification of the synaptic transmission of the tactile-related signals can occur, as a result of other incoming sensory signals and descending influences from higher brain centers exerted on touch-transmission neurons in the relay sites.

Thermosensation

General features

The ability to sense the temperature of an object or substance is particularly well developed in the orofacial region. Thermal changes of less than 1 °C can be readily detected and discriminated,

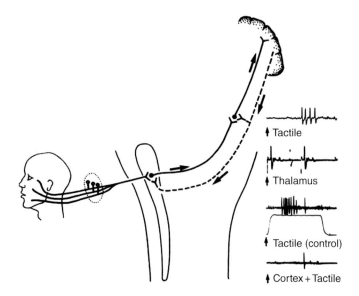

Figure 12.5 Influences from somatosensory cerebral cortex on sensory transmission in the trigeminal system. Tactile information from the face and mouth is relayed to the cerebral cortex via the trigeminal brainstem nuclei and thalamus. Many cortical neurons receiving and processing this information project directly down to the thalamus and brainstem and may modulate sensory transmission in the brainstem and thalamic neurons. Records on the right show such an example of a neuron recorded in the trigeminal brainstem sensory nuclear complex of a cat. The neuron could be activated by mechanical (tactile) stimulation of a localized receptive field on the face. It projected directly to the contralateral ventrobasal thalamus since it could be antidromically excited (viz., backfired) by an electric stimulus delivered to the thalamus, as shown. Note that if the facial tactile stimulus (the electronic analog of which is shown below the third trace) was delivered around the same time as an electric stimulus to the somatosensory cerebral cortex, the neuron's responses to a series of tactile stimuli were markedly depressed. This is evidence of a rapidly conducting feedback loop from the cortex that may depress or limit trigeminal sensory transmission. (Modified from Sessle, 1981b.)

although temperature detection and discrimination can vary depending on the area of thermal stimulation, the magnitude and rate of the thermal changes, whether or not the area has undergone previous thermal changes, and the adapting temperature of the skin or oral mucosa being stimulated.

Peripheral processes

The receptors for temperature change are called **thermoreceptors**, which are activated by a small thermal change in either a cooling (cold receptors) or warming (warm receptors) direction; the former are more common than the latter. They are associated with some of the small-diameter, slow-conducting afferent fibers that are either myelinated (e.g., A-δ afferents) or unmyelinated (C-fiber afferents) and that provide the brain with accurate information on the location, magnitude, and rate of the temperature change.

Central pathways and processes

The main relay site in the brainstem of the afferent signals carried in the orofacial thermoreceptive primary afferent fibers is the trigeminal subnucleus caudalis. Some caudalis neurons are exclusively activated by thermal stimulation of localized parts of

the face and mouth, and this thermal-related information is relayed from these caudalis neurons to the contralateral thalamus and then to the somatosensory cerebral cortex. The properties of peripheral and central neural elements underlying our thermal sensibility fit well with the specificity theory.

Taste

Only three aspects of taste are briefly mentioned here since taste is comprehensively covered in Chapter 10. First, like pain (see below), taste has cognitive, affective, and motivational dimensions as well as a sensory-discriminative dimension. For example, some tastes are pleasurable and we are motivated to seek them out, whereas other tastes have the opposite effect. In fact, humans have innate as well as acquired taste preferences, and the food industry is well aware of our inborn preference for sweetness (our "sweet tooth"). Second, taste sensibility is now known not to be confined to specific areas of the tongue; extralingual (e.g., palatal) taste buds may also make an important contribution to our taste. Third, several factors may modify taste, e.g., decreased saliva, poor oral hygiene, wearing of dentures, local anesthetics, plant extracts, other sensory experiences (such as smell). In addition, genetic, metabolic, and endocrine factors and the age of the individual may also influence taste sensibility.

Pain

General characteristics

Pain can cause great human suffering and represents a major economic burden on society through healthcare costs, time lost from work, etc. Moreover, in the case of orofacial pain conditions, they are very common (e.g., toothaches, headaches, TMD) and are often chronic and disabling.

Pain is now conceptualized as a multidimensional experience that includes a sensory-discriminative component that allows us to discriminate the quality, location, intensity, and duration of a noxious stimulus (i.e., a tissue-damaging stimulus). However, pain also encompasses cognitive, motivational, and affective (emotional) dimensions that can vary from individual to individual and can modify a person's response to the stimulus. Thus, the pain a person experiences can depend not only on the magnitude of the noxious stimulus but also on factors such as the meaning to the person of the situation in which the pain occurs, the person's emotional state and motivation to rid themselves of the pain, and even racial and cultural background and gender. A clinical consequence of this multifactorial nature of pain is that it can complicate diagnosis and treatment of pain for the clinician. It also makes the experimental study of pain exceedingly difficult.

> Pain is a multidimensional experience that includes sensory discriminative, cognitive, affective, and motivational dimensions. The pain a person experiences can depend not only on the magnitude of the noxious stimulus but also on factors such as the meaning to the person of the situation in which the pain occurs, the person's emotional state and motivation to rid themselves of the pain, and even racial and cultural background and gender.

Concepts of pain

The neural basis of pain is still only partly understood, but considerable advances have been made in the last few years. These insights into pain and especially its mechanisms have to a large extent come from studies of animals. The classic concept for explaining pain and the other somatic sensations is the specificity theory (Fig. 12.2). While it seems to explain other sensations such as touch (see above), specificity theory has been shown to have a number of limitations in trying to explain pain on the basis of a specific peripheral and central system. Consequently other theories have been proposed to account for the complexity and multidimensionality of pain, including the **gate control theory of pain**, which has attracted the most interest and research in the past 50 years (Fig. 12.2). Although it has its own limitations, it nonetheless provides a good conceptual framework for considering the multifactorial nature of pain. A major tenet of the gate control theory is its emphasis on the sensory interaction that occurs within the brain between the tactile-related neural signals carried into the brain by the large-diameter, low-threshold primary afferent fibers (principally A-β afferents, see above), and those signals conveyed by the small-diameter, high-threshold afferent fibers (some A-δ and C fiber afferents). The peripheral terminals of many of the latter fibers have a high threshold and are activated only by noxious stimuli. If, as a result of this interaction, the activity in these nociceptive afferent fibers prevails, central "pain-transmission" neurons are excited (the "gate" opens) and bring into action the central processes related to the perception of and reactions to noxious stimulation. The theory also emphasizes descending central neural controls (i.e., emanating from higher brain centers) related to the cognitive, affective, and motivational dimensions of pain that through their influences on the central transmission neurons can modulate the gate for pain.

Peripheral processes

Some nociceptive primary afferent fibers are specifically sensitive to noxious stimuli, whereas others respond to innocuous stimuli as well. The nociceptive afferents are small in diameter and slow conducting (A-δ and C fiber afferents), and they terminate in the peripheral tissues as free nerve endings, termed nociceptors. Injury or inflammation of orofacial tissues not only activates some of the numerous nociceptive afferent endings in the tissues, for example, tooth pulp afferents (Fig. 12.6), but may also induce an increased excitability of these endings and adjacent nociceptive endings. This **peripheral sensitization** is important in the increased pain sensitivity that can be detected clinically at a peripheral injury or inflammation site (e.g., as in arthritis, myositis, and pulpitis). The increased pain sensitivity may be reflected as an exaggerated perceptual response to noxious stimuli (**hyperalgesia**) or as a pain response to a stimulus (e.g., tactile) that is normally innocuous (**allodynia**), and the involvement of adjacent afferent endings beyond the initial injury site is a peripheral process contributing to the spread of pain in these tissues (Table 12.1). Several chemical mediators, including some normally associated with

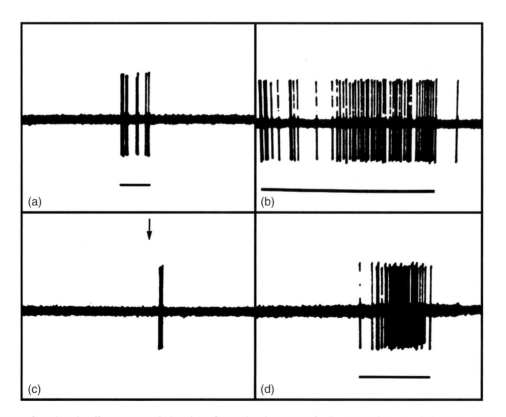

Figure 12.6   Responses of tooth pulp afferents recorded in the inferior alveolar nerve of a dog. Note that stimuli that cause pain when applied to human teeth could excite the pulp afferent(s), as shown by its response to (a) mechanical probing of dentin of the tooth supplied by the afferent as well as to (b) an air blast, (c) hypertonic calcium chloride (arrow), and (d) drilling applied to the dentin. Time calibration: 1 sec. (From Narhi et al. (1982) *Archives of Oral Biology*, 27, 1053–1058).

actions within the central nervous system (CNS) (e.g., excitatory amino acids such as glutamate; opioids), are involved in activating the nociceptive afferent endings or in producing or modifying peripheral sensitization by interacting with ion channels or membrane receptors on the nociceptive afferent endings (Fig. 12.7). Some of these ion channels and membrane receptors are activated by noxious mechanical and thermal stimuli (e.g., the

TRP channels described in Chapter 9). In addition, non-neural processes, such as satellite glial cells in the trigeminal ganglion and immune cells in peripheral tissues such as the tooth pulp, may modulate the nociceptive afferent excitability in these tissues. Also noteworthy is the documentation of sex differences in some of these peripheral processes that may account at least in part for the sex differences in the prevalence of a number of orofacial pain states. Moreover, some drugs that are commonly used to relieve orofacial pain (e.g., aspirin) may exert their analgesic action by interfering with some of these peripheral mechanisms.

Table 12.1   Relationship of parameters of peripheral sensitization of a nociceptive afferent to sensory perceptual correlates of pain.

Peripheral Sensitization	Sensory Perception
Decreased activation threshold	Allodynia
Increased responsiveness to noxious stimuli	Hyperalgesia
Involvement of adjacent nociceptive afferent endings	Pain spread

Several chemical mediators are involved in activating the nociceptive afferent endings or in producing or modifying peripheral sensitization.

Several drugs that are commonly used to relieve orofacial pain (e.g., aspirin) may exert their analgesic action by interfering with some of these peripheral mechanisms.

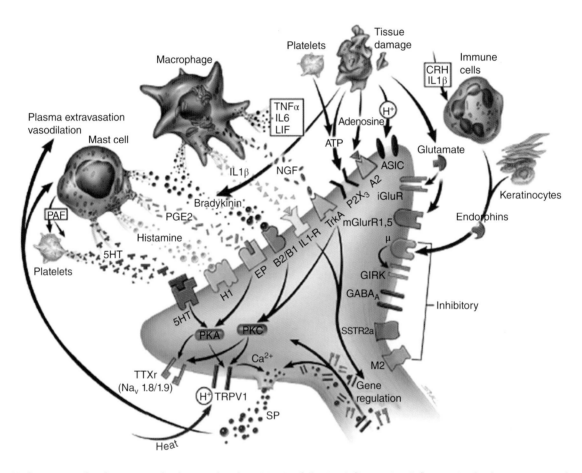

Figure 12.7   Mediators in orofacial tissues involved in peripheral sensitization following inflammation. Inflammation leads to numerous chemicals being released from macrophages, mast cells, immune cells, and injured cells that act on ion channels or membrane receptors on peripheral nociceptive afferent nerve endings and thereby may alter the sensitivity of the endings. Some of these mediators can increase the excitability of the nociceptive afferent endings (i.e., peripheral sensitization); others may exert inhibitory effects. Several of these mediators are shown. ASIC, acid-sensing ion channel; CRH, corticotrophin-releasing hormone; GIRK, G protein coupled inward rectifying potassium channel; 5-HT, serotonin; iGluR, ionotropic glutamate receptor; IL-1β, interleukin-1-beta; IL-6, interleukin-6; LIF, leukemia inhibitory factor; μ, mu-opioid receptor; M_2, muscarinic receptor; mGluR, metabotropic glutamate receptor; NGF, nerve growth factor; PAF, platelet-activating factor; PGE_2, prostaglandin E_2; PKA, protein kinase A; PKC, protein kinase C; SSTR2A, somatostatin receptor 2A; TNF-α, tumor necrosis factor alpha; TrkA, tyrosine kinase receptor A; TRPV1, transient receptor potential vanilloid 1; TTXr, tetrodotoxin-resistant sodium channel. (From Meyer et al., 2006.)

Central pathways and processes

The nociceptive primary afferent fibers supplying the face and mouth project via the trigeminal ganglion to the trigeminal brainstem sensory nuclear complex, especially to the subnucleus caudalis (see Fig. 12.3). Here they release chemical mediators that are synthesized in the primary afferent trigeminal ganglion cell bodies and transported to their peripheral (in orofacial tissues) and central (in the brainstem) endings; these include glutamate and the neuropeptide substance P, which activate the neurons by acting, respectively, on glutamatergic and neurokinin receptors on the neurons. Many caudalis neurons receive the signals from orofacial nociceptive primary afferents and, thus, can respond to noxious stimulation of the face and mouth (including the teeth), TMJ, or jaw and tongue muscles. There are two types of these neurons: **nociceptive-specific neurons** that respond exclusively to noxious stimuli, and **wide-dynamic-range neurons** that respond to innocuous as well as noxious stimuli (e.g., Fig. 12.4b, 12.4c). These two types of neurons relay nociceptive information to neurons in the contralateral thalamus, from where it is relayed from analogous nociceptive-specific and wide-dynamic-range neurons to the overlying cerebral cortex or other thalamic regions. While parts of the thalamus or cortex are involved in the various components of pain behavior (perception, motivation, etc.), the precise function of each region is still not fully understood. Also unclear is the function of the rostral components of the trigeminal brainstem complex. While they are especially concerned with the relay of tactile information (see above), they also may play a role in orofacial pain mechanisms. For example, afferent fibers from the tooth pulp, generally assumed to represent a nociceptive input, synapse with neurons present not only in the subnucleus caudalis but also in the more rostral components of the complex.

Control of pain

The procedures available for the control of pain are numerous (Table 12.2), ranging from pharmacologic approaches such as local and general anesthetics and analgesic drugs (e.g., aspirin, morphine) to therapeutic procedures such as acupuncture, transcutaneous electric stimulation (TENS), cognitive behavioral therapy, hypnosis, and psychiatric counseling; neurosurgical procedures are also are available for severe pain conditions unrelieved by the other approaches. These various procedures are aimed at blocking pain signals either in peripheral tissues (e.g., aspirin), before nerve impulses enter the brain (e.g., local anesthetics), or within the brain (e.g., general anesthetics and many analgesic drugs).

As mentioned above, the trigeminal brainstem sensory nuclei have a complex structural organization by which their neurons can interact in complex ways with many other parts of the CNS. These interactions involve inhibitory processes that modulate nociceptive transmission and that are widespread in the brain. Some of these processes also are involved, as noted above, in modifying touch as well as reflex activity and more complex behavioral functions (see "Sensorimotor Functions and Motor Control"). Inhibitory modulation of nociceptive transmission in the trigeminal and spinal systems can occur through (1) sensory interaction and (2) descending central control mechanisms, as postulated by the gate theory of pain (see above). For example, the activity of trigeminal nociceptive neurons can be markedly suppressed by large fiber afferent inputs activated by tactile stimulation of orofacial tissues (i.e., sensory interaction); in some situations, even small-fiber nociceptive afferent stimulation may also suppress their activity. In addition, there are descending central controls, e.g., stimulation of brain sites such as the midbrain periaqueductal gray matter and the nucleus raphe magnus in the lower brainstem (Fig. 12.8) that descend in the CNS and produce inhibition of the nociceptive neurons and can have marked analgesic effects in humans and experimental animals.

> Inhibitory modulation of nociceptive transmission in the trigeminal and spinal systems can occur through (1) sensory interaction and (2) descending central control mechanisms.

The discovery of these modulatory effects on nociceptive transmission has enhanced our understanding of pain mechanisms and helped develop better pain control procedures. The

Table 12.2 Various methods used for management of orofacial pain

Pharmacological methods	Psychological methods	Physical methods
Local anesthetics	Information	Jaw exercises
Nonopioid analgesics	Education	Stretch therapy
Salicylates	Counseling	Massage
Acetaminophen	Biofeedback	Heat/cold
Nonsteroidal anti-	Stress Management	Ultrasound
inflammatories	Relaxation	Soft laser
Steroids	Hypnosis	Acupuncture
Opioids	Cognitive-behavioral therapy	TENS
Anxiolytics and sedatives	Psychotherapy	Oral splints
Antiepileptics, anticonvulsants		
Antidepressants		
Muscle relaxants		
Serotonin agonists		
NMDA receptor antagonists		

(a)

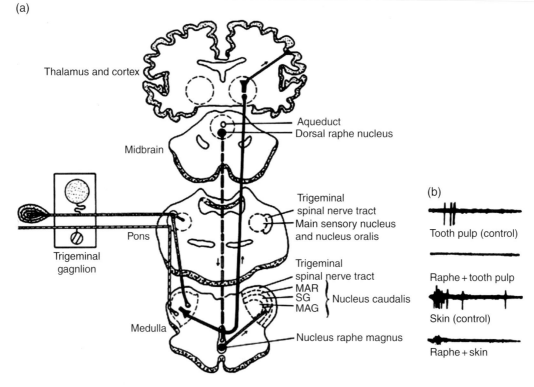

Figure 12.8   Diagram of a descending modulatory pathway in the brain that may suppress activity of neurons in the trigeminal nociceptive pathway. (a) shows that some nociceptive neurons (i.e., nociceptive-specific neurons) in trigeminal subnucleus caudalis receive and relay information only from small-diameter primary afferent fibers (cross-hatched pathway, see lower small cell body in Trigeminal ganglion), whereas other nociceptive neurons (i.e., wide-dynamic-range neurons) relay information from small-diameter afferent fibers and from large-diameter primary afferent fibers (stippled pathway, see upper large cell body in Trigeminal ganglion). These nociceptive neurons predominate in layers I [marginalis, MAR] and V of the subnucleus caudalis. Substantia gelatinosa (SG) and magnocellularls (MAG) are other layers of the subnucleus caudalis. Responses of both types of neurons to noxious orofacial stimuli can be suppressed by descending influences from the dorsal raphe nucleus in the periaqueductal gray and in nucleus raphe magnus (dashed pathway), as shown for the nociceptive neuron illustrated in (b). This neuron was recorded in an animal's subnucleus caudalis and responded with a brief burst of two action potentials when a light mechanical (tactile) stimulus was applied to its receptive field on the face, and the neuron could also be activated when an electrical stimulus was applied to the canine tooth pulp and when noxious radiant heat was applied to the receptive field; it was thus classified as a wide-dynamic-range neuron. These responses could be markedly suppressed when an electrical stimulus was also delivered to one of the raphe nuclei. Time duration of records: 100 msec (except heat record: 10 sec). (From Dubner et al., 1978.)

inhibitory effects involve the release of endogenous (i.e., naturally occurring) chemicals that either may activate the descending control systems and cause them to release neurochemicals (e.g., norepinephrine and 5-hydroxytryptamine, or serotonin) which act on the nociceptive-transmission neurons or are released from interneurons in the vicinity of the nociceptive-transmission neurons (Fig. 12.9). A well-known example of these endogenous substances is the opioid chemical enkephalin, which is a peptide that is pharmacologically similar to the opiate drugs such as morphine. When this endogenous opiate-like chemical is injected into certain parts of the brain, it produces analgesic effects, and if applied locally in the vicinity of nociceptive neurons such as those in the trigeminal subnucleus caudalis (or analogous neurons in the spinal cord), the activity of these neurons to noxious stimuli can be suppressed. Other neurochemicals in the CNS such as γ-amino butyric acid (GABA) and glycine also are involved. Thus, pain-suppressing systems occur naturally within the brain, and a number of important therapeutic procedures exert their analgesic effects, at least in part, by utilizing such systems. For example,

procedures involving skin, muscle, or nerve stimulation (TENS and acupuncture) may exert their reported analgesic effect in part by exciting afferent pathways to the brain that ultimately lead to activation of endogenous opioid-related analgesic systems. And the action of narcotic analgesics such as morphine has been linked to such systems. Placebo analgesia, which contributes to the effect of most pain-relieving procedures, also involves some of these systems.

> Pain-suppressing systems occur naturally within the brain, and a number of important therapeutic procedures exert their analgesic effects, at least in part, by utilizing such systems.

Some segmental and descending pathways have the opposite effect, namely they can facilitate nociceptive transmission, and thereby contribute to the enhancement of pain, as might occur for example in the development and persistence of a chronic pain state. Descending facilitatory influences are also involved in the enhanced pain levels associated with fear or

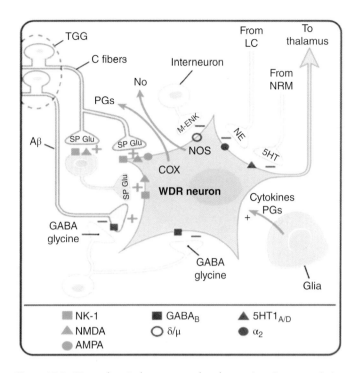

Figure 12.9 Neurochemical processes related to nociceptive transmission in the trigeminal subnucleus caudalis. In this example, activation of nociceptive fibers leads to the release of glutamate (Glu) and substance P (SP) which diffuse across a synapse to a wide-dynamic-range (WDR) neuron which projects to the thalamus. Glutamate binds and activates either NMDA or AMPA glutamatergic receptors, whereas SP binds and activates neurokinin (NK-1) receptors. The afferent fibers can activate (+) the WDR neuron directly, or indirectly via contacts onto excitatory interneurons. Several intracellular signal transduction pathways have been implicated in modulating the responsiveness of the nociceptive neurons, including the protein kinase A (PKA) and protein kinase (PKC) pathways. The neurons can themselves modulate nearby cells by synthesis and release of prostaglandins (PGs) via cyclooxygenase (COX) and of nitric oxide (NO) that involves nitric oxide synthase (NOS). Glia also can modulate nociceptive processing by release of substances such as cytokines and prostaglandins (PGs). Descending terminals of fibers originating in CNS regions such as the nucleus raphe magnus (NRM) or locus coeruleus (LC) can release serotonin (5-HT) or norepinephrine (NE), the effect of which is principally inhibition (-) of the neuron. In addition, the neuron has receptors for substances released from other neurons (interneurons) within the subnucleus caudalis: met-enkephalin (M-ENK), glycine, and γ-aminobutyric acid (GABA). Drugs that alter these receptors or neurotransmitters have potential as analgesics. TGG=trigeminal ganglion. (From Hargreaves and Goodis, 2002.)

anxiety. Facilitatory interactions also occur between various convergent afferent inputs to trigeminal nociceptive neurons in the CNS and contribute to the **referral of pain**, where pain may be felt at the site of injury or pathology and also, or instead, at other distant sites. Several orofacial pain states (e.g., TMDs, some toothaches) not uncommonly manifest pain referral, and this complicates diagnosis of the pain condition.

Another related and especially noteworthy facilitatory effect is that which may be initiated by injury or inflammation of peripheral tissues and which can result in a prolonged increase in excitability of nociceptive neurons in the CNS; an outline of the process and examples of the neuronal change are shown in Figure 12.10. This **central sensitization** appears to be an important process contributing to the hyperalgesia, allodynia, and pain referral (see above) that characterize pain resulting from an orofacial injury or inflammation. Moreover, the development and maintenance of a central sensitization state is thought to underlie most chronic pain conditions. Central sensitization reflects a neuroplasticity of the nociceptive pathways in the CNS, and emphasizes that the nociceptive system is not hardwired (like a telephone system) but is dynamic and plastic, and its excitability can change from one moment to another depending on the messages its nociceptive-specific and wide-dynamic-range neurons receive from peripheral tissues, and on the CNS state of the individual. A number of brain chemicals such as those operating through glutamatergic, neurokinin, opioid, GABA, and 5-hydroxytryptamine receptor mechanisms contribute to or modulate these central neuroplastic changes induced by peripheral injury or inflammation. Other factors that influence these changes include genetic and environmental factors as well as non-neural (e.g., glial) cells.

> Central sensitization appears to be an important process contributing to the hyperalgesia, allodynia, and pain referral that characterize pain resulting from an orofacial injury or inflammation. It is also thought to underlie most chronic pain conditions.
> The nociceptive system is not hardwired but is dynamic and plastic.

Sensorimotor functions and motor control

Muscle

There is a vast array of both simple and highly complex motor activities in the orofacial region. Some of these, such as chewing, drinking, and swallowing, are fundamental behaviors required for survival. Movements of the jaw and the surrounding muscles are integrally involved in behaviors as diverse as mastication (chewing), drinking and suckling, manipulation of objects with the tongue, lips, and cheeks, and communication through facial expressions and speech.

Peripheral processes

The peripheral motor elements of these activities are the muscles of the jaw, tongue, face, pharynx, larynx, and palate and the motor axons (the α-efferents) that supply them. Each of the skeletal muscles of the face, jaws, and tongue is under the control of the brain through its motor innervation, which is derived from the α-motoneurons in the brainstem. A single α-motoneuron and the several muscle fibers that it supplies by its α-efferent are known collectively as the **motor unit**. Impulses from the motoneuron are conducted along its α-efferent to the muscle fibers and bring

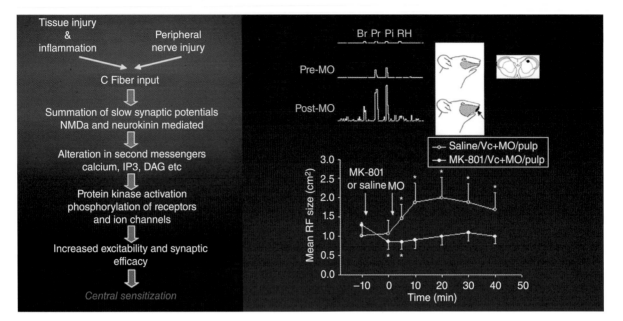

Figure 12.10   Trigeminal central sensitization. As noted on the left, injury or inflammation of orofacial tissues or nerve fibers results in a barrage of action potentials conducted into the brainstem by nociceptive afferents (e.g., C fibers). The glutamate and neuropeptides (e.g., substance P) released from the afferents' brainstem endings (e.g., trigeminal subnucleus caudalis) act respectively on glutamatergic (e.g., NMDA) and neurokinin (e.g., NK-1) receptor subtypes on nociceptive neurons to influence intraneuronal second messenger and phosphorylation processes that result in a hyperexcitability of the neurons, i.e., central sensitization. Illustrated on the right is an example of central sensitization in the rat trigeminal subnucleus caudalis (Vc). The nociceptive-specific neuron shown underwent changes in its response and mechanoreceptive field (MF) properties after application of the inflammatory irritant mustard oil (MO) to the right maxillary molar pulp of the rat. The top series of traces show the neuronal responses to brush (Br), pressure (Pr), pinch (Pi), and radiant heat (RH) applied to the MF in control conditions prior to MO application (i.e., Pre-MO). Bottom traces show the neuronal responses to the same stimuli 20 minutes after MO application (i.e., Post-MO). Note that after MO application to the molar pulp, this neuron developed a lowered activation threshold such that it became responsive to Br and RH of the MF; it also became more strongly responsive to Pi stimuli. The right side of the figure shows that the neuron's MF also expanded, 10 minutes after MO application. These neuroplastic changes in the MF and response properties of the neuron reflect a central sensitization. The neuronal recording site of the neuron in subnucleus caudalis is shown on the far right. The graph at the bottom shows the time course of the MF expansion after MO application as well as the ability of the NMDA receptor antagonist MK-801 (but not its vehicle isotonic saline) applied to caudalis to prevent this MF expansion, pointing to the involvement of NMDA receptor mechanisms in the production of the central sensitization in the caudalis neuron. (Adapted from Chiang et al. (1998) *Journal of Neurophysiology,* 80, 2621–2631.)

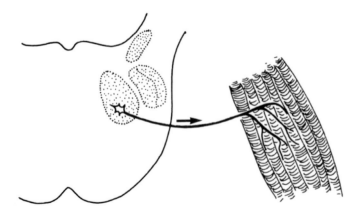

Figure 12.11   Single motor unit innervating a jaw muscle. Diagram shows an α-motoneuron in the trigeminal motor nucleus with its α-efferent (i.e., motor axon) that supplies a number of the muscle fibers within the muscle. (Modified from Sessle, 1981.)

about muscle contraction through the process of neuromuscular transmission (Fig. 12.11).

Like those elsewhere in the body, these muscles of the face, jaws, and tongue consist basically of a **passive viscoelastic com-**

ponent (e.g., tendons, ligaments, fascia) and an **active contractile component** comprising numerous individual striated (contractile) muscle fibers, also known as extrafusal muscle fibers. Both components may contribute to the tension or tone that these muscles exhibit at rest or during contraction. Also like other muscles, the relative contribution of each component of these muscles appears to be a function of muscle length, with the viscoelastic component especially contributing to tension in the muscle when it is stretched. The contraction of the muscle can result in shortening or development of tension or both. For example, the masseter muscle may shorten and produce a jaw-closing movement against a constant load (isotonic contraction), or the muscle may show no appreciable change in length but instead produce contractile tension (isometric contraction), such as when an individual bites together on the maxillary and mandibular teeth. In the jaw-closing muscles, the maximal muscle twitch tension (which may reflect the involvement of both active and passive components of muscle) actually occurs with the jaws separated several millimeters and not with the teeth in occlusion (as was frequently thought to be the case in the past).

In general, muscles are made up of extrafusal muscle fibers that show rapid and/or slow twitch contraction properties.

Physiologic and histochemical analyses have shown that one type, sometimes referred to as fast (or white) muscle, is rapidly contracting yet quickly fatigable, whereas the second type (slow, or red, muscle) is slowly contracting and fatigue resistant and thus more suited for movements requiring sustained contraction, as in the case of a certain posture of a limb or the mandible. Other types also exist and have intermediary properties. All types have been identified in the muscles of the face, mouth, and jaws. The fast fibers predominate, although the relative proportions may vary between species and between different parts of the same muscle. Some of these muscles, such as those of the jaw, have contraction times that are almost as fast as the fastest muscles in the body, yet the muscles show great fatigue resistance.

The **electromyogram (EMG) of a muscle** can be recorded using electrodes that are placed within a muscle or on the skin or mucosa overlying the muscle and detect the muscle's electrical impulses associated with motor unit activity. Examples are shown in Figure 12.12. The recorded EMG provides information on the start, duration, and termination of a muscle's activity. When a muscle's contraction is isometric (i.e., no change in length, such as when the teeth are clenched in the case of the masseter muscle), the amplitude of the muscle's EMG activity is a good measure of the force developed by the muscle. Even more information can be gained if EMG monitoring is done in conjunction with another system that records position or movement so that, for example, a particular position or movement of the mandible can be related to the activity of the muscle or muscles involved in the position or movement. The EMG technique has been used in numerous experimental studies (e.g., relating muscle activities to jaw movements during chewing), and as an aid in diagnostic (e.g., for suspected neuromuscular pathologic conditions) or therapeutic (e.g., biofeedback) approaches.

The peripheral sensory elements of muscle are receptors and their associated afferent nerve fibers. They include free nerve endings and their small-diameter afferents that conduct signals to the CNS about noxious stimuli and possibly stretch of muscle. There are also specialized receptors, such as the stretch-sensitive **muscle spindle** which provides the brain with sensory information about muscle length, and the **Golgi tendon organ** which is particularly sensitive to muscle tension. The muscle spindle is a complex receptor since it has a dual afferent supply from large-diameter (Group Ia, II) afferent nerve fibers, and also receives a motor innervation from the gamma (fusimotor) efferent fibers of small gamma motoneurons. The gamma efferent input to the muscle spindle can modify the sensitivity of the spindle afferent fibers to stretch, thereby indirectly assisting or maintaining muscle contraction. In contrast to muscles in most other places of the body, these specialized receptors have a limited distribution in the orofacial region, e.g., they are sparse or absent in jaw-opening muscles (e.g., anterior digastric) and facial muscles.

Central processes

Only limited details are available of the primary muscle afferent pathways and central connections of most of the orofacial musculature, except for the trigeminal mesencephalic nucleus which contains the cell bodies of muscle spindle primary afferent fibers supplying the jaw-closing muscles (e.g., masseter and some of the mechanosensitive primary afferent fibers supplying periodontal tissues). The trigeminal mesencephalic nucleus is the only site in the body where primary sensory cell bodies are located within the CNS. There are several other significant distinguishing features of the orofacial motor systems, compared to the spinal motor system controlling muscles of the neck, limbs, and trunk. (1) Many orofacial muscles lack muscle spindles (as noted above) and also Golgi tendon organs. (2) A gamma-efferent control system is thus absent due to the lack of muscle spindles in many muscles. (3) Reciprocal innervation, where muscle afferent fibers in the spinal system have reciprocally opposite effects on spinal motoneurons supplying agonist and antagonist muscles in a movement, is limited given the sparsity of muscle spindle and tendon organ afferent fibers in the orofacial region; nonetheless, the lack may be compensated for by the powerful regulatory influences provided by afferent inputs from facial skin, mucosa, TMJ, and teeth (see below). (4) Integrative pathways and processes exist to allow for the bilateral activity of muscles; although activity of a particular limb, neck, or trunk muscle can occur on both the left and right sides of the body in some movements, the bilateral activation (or depression) of muscles is particularly prominent in orofacial movements (e.g., chewing, swallowing, coughing, speech).

> There are several significant distinguishing features of the orofacial motor systems compared to the spinal motor system controlling muscles of the neck, limbs, and trunk.

The muscle afferent fibers, as well as cutaneous, intraoral, and TMJ afferent fibers, make excitatory reflex connections in the brainstem with motoneurons located within one or more of the cranial nerve motor nuclei that contain the motoneurons supplying the various orofacial muscles (Fig. 12.13). These brainstem connections are usually indirect and involve interneurons in the trigeminal spinal tract nucleus or the solitary tract nucleus or the brainstem reticular formation. Some of these reflex circuits are rather limited or "simple," involving only one cranial nerve motor nucleus and as few as one synapse (e.g., the monosynaptic jaw-closing reflex) or only a small number of synapses, as reflected in the jaw-opening and horizontal jaw reflexes, facial muscle reflexes, tongue reflexes, and laryngeal, pharyngeal, and palatal reflexes. In addition to these excitatory effects of various orofacial stimuli on the motoneurons reflected in reflexly induced activation of the muscles, inhibitory effects can also be evoked by sensory stimuli (Fig. 12.12). Descending regulatory influences arising from higher brain centers such as the cerebral cortex also can exert facilitatory or inhibitory influences on the motoneurons (see below). The excitatory and inhibitory influences are especially involved in protecting the masticatory apparatus e.g., from biting the tongue during chewing.

The neural circuits underlying these "simple" reflexes and their modulation also provide much of the neural organization

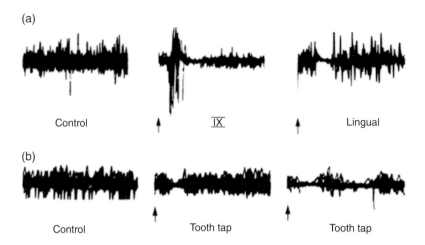

(a)

Control   IX   Lingual

(b)

Control   Tooth tap   Tooth tap

Figure 12.12   Reflex effects evoked in monkey genioglossus (a) and masseter (b) muscles by various orofacial stimuli (arrows). As shown in (a), a genioglossus excitatory reflex could be elicited by glossopharyngeal nerve (IX) stimuli, and this was followed by an inhibitory ("silent") period. Lingual nerve stimulation evoked only a silent period. (b), Similarly, for masseter, reflex effects could be evoked by tactile stimuli applied to the canine tooth. Note that with increasing intensity (from middle to right records), a single silent period was evoked, but that a second silent period is apparent in the third record. Duration of each record was 100 msec. (Adapted from Dubner et al., 1978.)

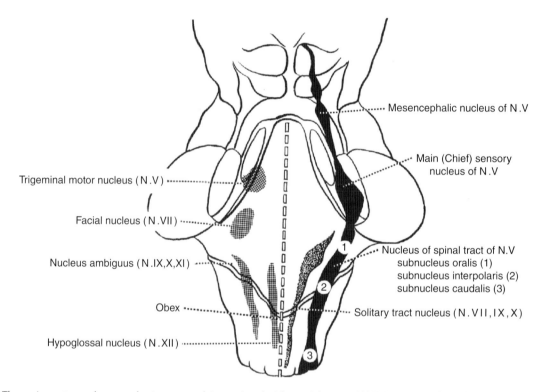

Figure 12.13   The main motor and sensory brainstem nuclei associated with cranial nerves V, VII, IX, X, XI, and XII. The cranial nerve V motor nucleus contains α-motoneurons supplying jaw-closing (e.g., masseter) and jaw-opening (e.g., anterior digastric) muscles, while cranial nerve VII nucleus has α-motoneurons supplying the muscles of facial expression (e.g., orbicularis oris). The nucleus ambiguus contains α-motoneurons supplying muscles of the palate, pharynx, and larynx, and the cranial nerve XII nucleus has α-motoneurons supplying the intrinsic and extrinsic muscles (e.g., genioglossus) of the tongue. For clarity, motor nuclei are presented on the left and sensory nuclei on the right, but each nucleus occurs bilaterally, so sensory and motor nuclei are in close proximity to each other.

upon which are based more complicated motor activities such as the protective reflex synergies of coughing and gagging that involve bilateral activity of interneurons in the solitary tract nucleus or trigeminal brainstem complex and bilateral activation or suppression of motoneurons in several of these cranial nerve motor nuclei. The circuits also contribute to the even more complex rhythmic, automated activities of mastication, suckling, and swallowing; speech is another complex sensorimotor behavior utilizing some of this neural organization (Fig. 12.14).

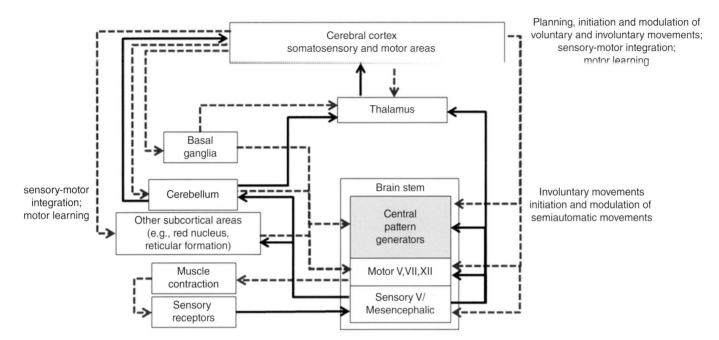

Figure 12.14   Diagram showing the main connections of the orofacial sensorimotor system. There are extensive excitatory and inhibitory interconnections between the different cortical and subcortical regions. The central pattern generators provide the programmed output to cranial nerve motoneurons supplying the muscles active in chewing (the "chewing center") and swallowing (the "swallowing center"). (From Avivi-Arber et al., 2011.)

> The neural circuits underlying these reflexes and their modulation also provide much of the neural organization upon which are based more complicated motor activities such as the protective reflex synergies of coughing and gagging, and the even more complex rhythmic, automated activities of mastication, suckling, and swallowing.

The reflex responsiveness and the tonic activity of muscles can vary depending on a number of factors, including the state of consciousness or sleep, the maturity of the brain, the amount of voluntary control exerted by the subject, and the particular phase of respiration when the reflex is initiated. For example, the anterior digastric, genioglossus, and laryngeal muscles can show a rhythmic, respiratory-linked activity.

Descending regulatory influences were briefly mentioned above. Indeed, there are several direct and indirect inputs to the cranial nerve sensory and motor nuclei in the brainstem from higher brain centers (e.g., cerebral cortex, hypothalamus, basal ganglia, and limbic system) or other parts of the brainstem (e.g., reticular formation and cerebellum). Most of our knowledge of this topic is about cerebral cortical control. Just as there is a cortical region devoted to the sensory representation of the orofacial area, there is another adjacent cortical region that is involved in the voluntary initiation and control of movements in and around the mouth. Although often referred to as the motor cortex, this region is not entirely motor since some of its cortical neurons receive sensory input from muscle, teeth, and other oral structures, to provide, for example, feedback on how an ongoing movement is progressing. Likewise, some of the neurons in the somatosensory cortex also are concerned with motor control.

Studies involving stimulation or removal of this face sensorimotor cortex, as well as recordings in this region of neuron activity in awake animals as they perform jaw or tongue movements, indicate that a particular orofacial movement may be controlled by one or more separate and discrete intracortical loci, the neurons of which project to cranial nerve motoneurons supplying the muscle(s) involved in that movement. In some of these loci, stimulation may evoke tongue and jaw movements resembling lapping, chewing, or swallowing; a separate area also occurs for speech.

Humans and experimental animals in which the face sensorimotor cortex has been removed or injured by surgery or accident may still be able to produce reasonable orofacial movements and can masticate and swallow their food. Although subtle changes in motor control may occur following cortical damage, the cerebral cortex does not appear to be essential for swallowing and mastication to occur. This emphasizes the importance of subcortical centers in the control of movements in and around the mouth. Subcortical regions such as the basal ganglia, hypothalamus, and brainstem reticular formation have important regulatory influences over the motoneurons involved in these movements. Some of these subcortical regions play important roles in the state of consciousness, as well as in stress, emotion, and other psychologic factors implicated in disorders such as TMDs (see below).

Some of the higher brain centers, including the face sensorimotor cortex, are also involved in the learning of orofacial sensorimotor skills, such as learning to chew or play a musical wind instrument. Learning is dependent on the ability of the CNS to undergo neuroplastic changes, and the neuroplastic capability of the face sensorimotor cortex and other higher brain centers allows for such learning. The neuroplasticity has also recently been reported to underlie our ability to adapt our sensorimotor functions to a changing external environment, such as intraoral changes to the dental occlusion, loss of teeth, and pain.

> The ability of the face sensorimotor cortex and other higher brain centers to undergo neuroplastic changes allows for learning and our ability to adapt our sensorimotor functions to a changing external environment, such as intraoral changes to the dental occlusion, loss of teeth, and pain.

Mastication, swallowing, and related neuromuscular functions

Mastication

The primary role of dental practice is to maintain both the structural and the functional integrity of the masticatory system, and the primary role of chewing (also termed mastication) is to break down foodstuffs for subsequent digestion by means of the masticatory forces generated between the teeth. In many animal species, including humans, most of the structural requirements for mastication are present at birth, and yet the sophisticated neuromuscular function that we know of as mastication does not immediately manifest itself in toto at birth. Rather, the feeding requirements of the animal are addressed by the neuromuscular system for suckling that is present at birth, and there is a considerable and variable postnatal learning period before mastication is fully manifested.

Individuals may vary in the effectiveness or efficiency with which they accomplish masticatory function. Subjects with a good dentition usually have better masticatory efficiency than those with a poor dentition (viz., missing teeth or dentures). However, those with low efficiency do not, on the whole, compensate by increasing the number of chews. There is little difference in the number of chewing strokes between individuals irrespective of the dentitional state, and subjects with low efficiency tend to swallow larger food particles.

> The primary role of chewing is to break down foodstuffs for subsequent digestion by means of the masticatory forces generated between the teeth.

Mastication is characterized by three-dimensional cyclic jaw movements (vertical, lateral, and anteroposterior) and facial and tongue movement patterns that are produced by the integrated bilateral contraction of jaw, facial, and tongue muscles (Fig. 12.15). The pattern of masticatory jaw movements differs between individuals and between animal species. In addition to these inherent differences, a number of factors have been shown to influence various components of the masticatory cycle or series of cycles, and these include dentitional state, consistency of the food bolus, and masticatory habits of the individual.

While the forces on the teeth during mastication are usually in the 5- to 10-kg range, they can vary depending on such factors as the teeth concerned (molars exert the greatest force, incisors the

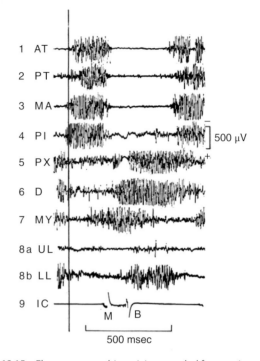

Figure 12.15 Electromyographic activity recorded from various muscles during a natural chewing cycle in a human subject; the recordings were made from jaw (1-6); tongue (7); and facial (8) muscles. The vertical line indicates onset of activity in the right anterior temporalis muscle. Letters M and B indicate, respectively, onset and offset of contact of the opposing incisor teeth. AT, anterior temporalis; PT, posterior temporalis; MA, masseter; PI, medial (internal) pterygoid; PX, lateral (external) pterygoid; D, digastric; MY, mylohyoid; UL, upper lip, LL, lower lip; IC, incisor contact. (From E. Moller (1966) *Acta Physiologica Scandinavica*, 69, 1 (suppl. 280).)

least), tooth-cusp configuration, consistency or toughness of the diet, practice, the wearing of dentures, the presence of pain or periodontal disease, and the distance that the jaws are separated when the forces are applied. Even greater forces are developed during biting: maximal biting forces on a tooth usually range from approximately 20 to 200 kg.

Mastication was long thought to be based on alternating simple jaw reflexes of jaw opening and jaw closing, but the current concept is that the cyclic, patterned nature of chewing depends on a brainstem center comprising a **central neural pattern generator**, the "chewing center" that may involve several groups of neurons in the brainstem. This center is sensitive to descending regulatory influences from higher brain centers and to sensory inputs originating from orofacial receptors. The sensory inputs may be especially important as a young infant learns how to masticate and acquire masticatory skills. They may be involved in actively (i.e., reflexly) guiding masticatory movements and the position of the jaw when the teeth come into occlusion (e.g., through activation of periodontal mechanoreceptors) and when the jaw is slightly open at "rest," (i.e., in postural position) (e.g., through activation of muscle and TMJ receptors).

> Both mastication and swallowing are dependent on central neural pattern generators in the brainstem.

Swallowing

Swallowing typically is triggered by stimulation of mechanoreceptors and chemoreceptors in the posterior pharyngeal wall or the epiglottic part of the larynx. Swallowing can be induced voluntarily, but food or liquid must be present for the volitional swallow to occur readily, e.g., volitional swallowing is markedly impaired by local anesthesia of the pharyngeal or laryngeal mucosa. This implies that central descending influences (e.g., via neural signals from the cerebral cortex to the brainstem "swallow center"; see below) related to a command for swallowing to occur require peripheral support (viz., sensory inputs to the brainstem from the larynx or pharynx) before the voluntary desire to swallow can be effected. The marked decrease that occurs in nocturnal salivary flow and the resultant decrease in peripheral stimulation may explain the low incidence of swallowing during sleep (about 50) compared with its incidence during waking hours (more than 500); alternatively, a relatively direct effect of the CNS processes underlying the sleep state on the activity of the central neural mechanisms underlying swallowing could account for or contribute to the low nocturnal incidence of swallowing.

As well as its obvious alimentary (ingestive) function, swallowing also can function as a protective reflex of the upper airway, since the act of swallowing prevents the intake of food or fluid into the airway. Swallowing also is associated with a cessation of breathing, i.e., normally swallowing and respiration are mutually exclusive. Unlike mastication which is sensorimotor behavior learned after birth and which is sensitive to CNS influences and sensory inputs, swallowing is innate and manifested as early as fetal life; it is a reflexly triggered, all-or-nothing motor activity, and it is relatively insensitive to sensory or central control. But, like mastication, swallowing is dependent on a central neural pattern generator in the brainstem. Swallowing involves oral, pharyngeal, and esophageal phases reflected in a rigid, temporal sequence of integrated muscle activities driven by the cranial nerve motoneurons; the integration is provided by the output to the motoneurons from the brainstem central neural pattern generator, the "swallow center". The sequential activities of many muscles of the tongue, jaw, face, palate, pharynx, larynx, and esophagus provide the means by which a food or liquid bolus is propelled from the oral cavity to the stomach (Fig. 12.16). Other key features of the swallowing process are protection of the airway and prevention of reflux (regurgitation) (see Table 12.3).

> Unlike mastication which is sensorimotor behavior learned after birth and which is sensitive to CNS influences and sensory inputs, swallowing is an innate, reflexly triggered, all-or-nothing motor activity that is relatively insensitive to sensory or central control.

Some of the various muscles involved in swallowing are "**obligate**" **swallow muscles**, meaning they are always active in swallowing; examples are some of the tongue muscles as well as the palatal, pharyngeal, laryngeal, and esophageal muscles. Others are

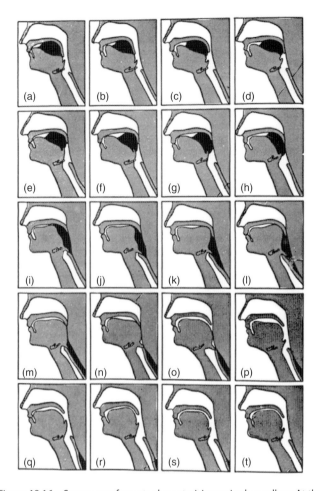

Figure 12.16   Sequence of events characterizing a single swallow. At the start of the swallow, breathing stops (apnea), the soft palate acts as a partition up to the base of the tongue (a, b) and elevates so as to engage the posterior pharyngeal wall and thereby close off the nasopharynx as the food bolus (black) moves backward over the tongue surface (c–e) by the tongue acting as a piston to squeeze the bolus into the pharynx. The bolus is then conveyed down the pharynx by pharyngeal muscle contractions (f j). Note that the epiglottis is tilted backward to help protect the entrance into the laryngeal airway (white); the glottis (not shown) also serves to close off the entrance into the airway. When the bolus arrives at the upper esophageal sphincter (k), the sphincter relaxes to allow the bolus into the upper esophagus (l, m) before it closes again to prevent reflux (regurgitation). Reflux also is minimized by an analogous closing of the lower esophageal sphincter once the bolus enters the stomach. As the bolus moves down the esophagus (n–t), the soft palate relaxes, the epiglottis resumes its position, and the airway is reopened. (Reproduced with permission from Bradley, R.M. (1984) *Basic Oral Physiology*. Year Book Medical, Chicago; adapted from Rushner, R.F. & Hendron, J.A. (1951) *Journal of Applied Physiology*, 3, 622–630.)

"**facultative**" **swallow muscles** in that they show a variable participation in swallowing. The facultative muscles are the facial and jaw muscles, and they may be especially sensitive to alterations in the oral environment and to maturational changes. Therefore, their participation can vary depending, for example, on the consistency or volume of a foodstuff being swallowed, or whether the subject is an infant or adult since there can be age-related differences in the involvement during swallowing of facial muscles (particularly

Table 12.3   Requirements of alimentary swallow

Feature	Factors Involved
Pressure gradient	Tongue muscles Pharyngeal constrictor muscles Esophageal musculature
Prevention of reflux	Tongue/palate apposition Tongue/pharyngeal wall apposition Upper esophageal sphincter closure Lower esophageal sphincter closure
Protection of airway	Palate/pharyngeal wall apposition Elevation of larynx and tilting backward of epiglottis Adduction of glottic folds Apnea

noticeable in the infant) versus jaw muscles (noticeable in the adult). The infantile (visceral or "tooth-apart") pattern of swallowing, as opposed to the adult (somatic or "tooth-together") pattern, is often characterized by a pronounced tongue thrust, and retention of this pattern is thought by some clinicians to be of etiologic significance in certain malocclusions such as anterior open bite. However, tooth-apart swallows are quite normal in adults when a liquid or soft food bolus is being ingested, viz., the teeth may or may not come into occlusion during a normal adult swallow; a major determining factor is the consistency of the bolus.

Other related sensorimotor functions

Suckling is another example of a complex orofacial sensorimotor behavior that is crucial for the neonate. Suckling, mastication, and swallowing are themselves components of even more complex behaviors. They are associated with feeding and drinking which are dependent in particular on the function of higher brain centers such as the hypothalamus. Nonetheless, sensory feedback also is utilized for the initiation, maintenance, and cessation of these ingestive behaviors; for example a "full stomach" stretches gastrointestinal receptors which, through their afferent inputs and connections in the CNS, can inhibit feeding. Many of these higher brain centers also are concerned with other complex functions involving the oral cavity, including oral aggression (e.g., biting), facial expression, and speech.

> Feeding and drinking are dependent in particular on the function of higher brain centers such as the hypothalamus.

Clinical correlations

Orofacial pain conditions

The orofacial region is a common site of pain, and the following provides a brief description and possible mechanisms of several of the most common or interesting orofacial pain conditions. The first is toothache, the most common of orofacial

pains. Toothache usually results from trauma or dental caries affecting the "nerve" of the tooth (the pulp) or the overlying hard tissue, the dentin. Many of the afferent fibers in the tooth pulp terminate in close proximity to odontoblasts (the dentin-forming cells), but some enter the tubules in the dentin, occasionally in close association with the process of the odontoblast (see Chapter 5). The role of these intradental fibers in the sensitivity of dentin to applied stimuli is still unclear. While it is conceivable that intradental neural processes may contribute, most evidence favors a hydrodynamic mechanism that results in the activation of pulpal afferent nerve fibers. The hydrodynamic theory suggests that enamel or dentinal stimuli can cause a displacement of dentinal tubule contents; this, in turn, is thought to bring about a mechanically induced excitation of the nerve fibers. There also is some evidence that the odontoblasts may be involved, through the stimuli causing them to release chemical mediators that activate the pulpal (or intradental) afferent endings.

Most of the nerves in the tooth pulp are small-diameter afferent fibers associated with pulpal sensation, but some are autonomic efferent fibers that are primarily involved in the control of the blood supply of the pulp. The pulpal afferent fibers can be activated by various types of stimuli (e.g., sugar, cold or hot drinks), and, while it is generally assumed that their activation is exclusively related to pain, some research findings suggest that some pulpal afferent fibers and their pathways in the brain may be involved in sensory functions other than pain. For example, pulpal afferents project not only to the trigeminal subnucleus caudalis but also to other parts of the trigeminal brainstem sensory nuclear complex principally involved in processing of tactile information.

> While it is generally assumed that their activation is exclusively related to pain, some research findings suggest that some pulpal afferent fibers and their pathways in the brain may be involved in sensory functions other than pain.

Another group of pain conditions common in the orofacial region are temporomandibular disorders (TMDs). These are more common in women, and present a variety of signs and symptoms, the most frequent of which is pain in the region of the TMJ or jaw muscles or both, limitation of jaw movement, and clicking or crackling (crepitus) in the TMJ. The pain can sometimes be referred to other structures such as the teeth and jaw muscles or even to the neck, and TMDs often are comorbid with other pain conditions such as headaches and fibromyalgia. Salivation and lacrimation, likely reflecting the involvement of the autonomic nervous system, also are frequently manifested in TMDs. The etiology, diagnosis, and treatment of TMDs represent some of the most controversial aspects of dentistry. Occlusal factors associated with, for example, the faulty interdigitation of the upper and lower teeth were long considered to be most important, and as a consequence dentists focused on a dental cause for TMDs in their diagnostic and treatment approaches. But there is now overwhelming evidence of the etiological importance of central factors (e.g., stress related) and of psychosocial influences in most TMD patients. The sensitivity of the TMJ or jaw muscles (reflected in allodynia and hyperalgesia) that is a clinical feature of most TMDs can be explained by peripheral and/or central sensitization phenomena. Because of the uncertainty about the etiology of TMDs, treatment procedures are varied and numerous, and range from ones focused on occlusal factors (e.g., occlusal equilibration) that nowadays have little scientific evidence to support their use, to the administration of anxiety-reducing drugs or muscle relaxants, to counseling and cognitive behavioral therapy.

> The sensitivity of the TMJ or jaw muscles (reflected in allodynia and hyperalgesia) that is a clinical feature of most TMDs can be explained by peripheral and/or central sensitization phenomena.

A much less common orofacial pain condition is **trigeminal neuralgia** (or tic douloureux). It is said to be the most excruciating pain a human can suffer from, and it manifests as paroxysms or bursts of excruciating pain that typically is felt in facial regions supplied by the maxillary and mandibular divisions of the trigeminal nerve, and that usually lasts for a few seconds or minutes, with long periods of remission between the pain attacks. A very interesting but puzzling feature is that the neuralgic attack is usually triggered not by a noxious stimulus but by a light, non-noxious stimulus (e.g., puff of air, wisp of cotton) to localized trigger site(s) in the mouth or perioral region. The etiology of trigeminal neuralgia is, like TMDs, also unclear, and theories relate to either peripheral or central (CNS) etiological factors. It is considered a neuropathic pain state and there is some evidence suggesting that peripheral neural pathological changes, such as those caused by compression of the trigeminal sensory nerve root near the trigeminal ganglion by aberrant vessels or bony outgrowths, are of etiologic importance in triggering the painful attacks. The signs and symptoms of trigeminal neuralgia also are suggestive of changes in the CNS, with dysfunction of the neurons in the trigeminal brainstem sensory nuclear complex. This view is consistent with the effectiveness of certain anticonvulsant or antiepileptic drugs in depressing the activity of trigeminal brainstem neurons. These drugs are now widely used clinically in the management of the condition.

Another orofacial neuralgic condition is postherpetic neuralgia (shingles). It differs from trigeminal neuralgia in that the etiology is more clear, involving the herpes zoster virus that has gained access to the trigeminal ganglion. The pain, when expressed in the orofacial region, usually involves the skin of the ophthalmic division of the trigeminal nerve (i.e., above and around the eye), and there is a selective loss of large myelinated fibers. Within the context of the gate control theory of pain, this loss could conceivably lead to an imbalance of the sensory inputs into the brainstem with an ensuing "opening of the gate" (see above). However, the actual processes underlying the pain are still unclear. A vaccine has recently been developed to manage the condition.

Burning mouth syndrome (BMS), also known as glossodynia or stomatodynia, is a quite common intraoral pain condition particularly found in postmenopausal middle-aged and elderly women. BMS is a constant burning pain that usually is not associated with any clinical evidence of damage or inflammation of the intraoral tissues (e.g., tongue, lips, palate) where the pain is perceived. Its etiology is unclear, although there is emerging evidence that it may reflect a neuropathic pain state. Unfortunately, there is as yet no well-documented effective treatment for BMS.

Yet another poorly understood orofacial pain condition is atypical facial pain; atypical odontalgia or chronic continuous dentoalveolar pain are orofacial pain states now thought to reflect the same or related condition. Unlike trigeminal neuralgia and postherpetic neuralgia, this pain is diffuse, deep, and dull or throbbing in nature. Also, unlike trigeminal neuralgia, trigger zones are typically not associated with the disorder and the pain can be constant for many days. The etiology also is uncertain, although a previous dental procedure (e.g., tooth extraction, root canal therapy) is often the precipitating factor, and its clinical features suggest that central sensitization may be involved.

There are several types of headaches, and some of the most common or well-known primary headaches, are briefly outlined here. Headaches also may be secondary to head or neck injury or vascular disorders, infections, substance abuse, and psychiatric conditions.

The two main types of migraine headaches are migraine with aura (classical migraine), which is accompanied with visual, sensory, or speech problems, and migraine without aura (common migraine). The pain of migraine is usually unilateral, moderate to severe in intensity, pulsating, and aggravated by physical activity, and it may be just a few hours in duration but can last up to three days. Patients also often complain of nausea, vomiting, and increased sensitivity to light and sound. The etiology and pathogenesis of migraines are not fully understood, but both peripheral sensitization and central sensitization and neurogenic-related inflammation of the meninges appear to be involved. In addition to avoidance of triggers that some patients experience (e.g., certain foods, alcohol, odors, hormonal factors, stress) and having rest and quiet in the case of an attack, patients usually benefit from pharmacological therapy based on the use of drugs such as the triptans to help abort an impending attack, and other drugs (e.g., beta-blockers, calcium channel blockers) to manage frequent migraines.

Tension-type headaches are experienced by most persons at least once in their lifetime. These headaches may be infrequent (<12 days/year), frequent (>12 < 180 days/year), or chronic (>180 days/year). Unlike migraine headaches, the pain is a bilateral pressing or tightening pain of mild to moderate intensity and is not aggravated by physical exertion. But like migraine headaches, peripheral sensitization and central sensitization, involving especially muscle afferent inputs into the brainstem, have been proposed as underlying mechanisms. Treatment is to counsel the patient to avoid triggers or precipitating factors such as certain foods and stress, and mild analgesics (e.g., aspirin) also may be needed.

Cluster headache refers to a series of extremely painful attacks (i.e., clusters) that are associated with autonomic nervous system reactions reflected as tears in the eyes, stuffy nose, swelling of the eyelids, and facial sweating. Its exact cause is unknown and, unlike migraine and tension-type headaches, cluster headache generally is not associated with triggers. There is no well-documented cure, but there are various treatment options depending on its severity and other features; these include triptans, ergotamines, and calcium channel blockers. It sometimes can be confused with an acute pulpitis or periapical periodontitis, with unnecessary dental treatment carried out as a result, so it is important for dentists to be aware of its distinctive features.

Temporal arteritis is a severe throbbing or stabbing headache in the temporal region that is usually unilateral and involves inflammation of temporal vessels that are tender to palpation. Its cause is unknown, and most patients benefit from careful use of corticosteroids.

Sensorimotor disorders

Several disorders occur in the neuromuscular system, some affecting peripheral elements of muscle and others affecting CNS regions. Some of the common or well known of these disorders are briefly outlined here, especially those manifested in the orofacial region.

Muscular dystrophy is a group of muscle diseases that are characterized by progressive skeletal muscle weakness due to defects in muscle proteins and death of muscle cells and tissue. Patients show progressive muscular wasting manifested in poor balance, difficulty walking, and also some orofacial motor dysfunction reflected in drooping eyelids and speech impairment. There is no known cure, although physical therapy, occupational therapy, speech therapy, and orthopedic equipment may help.

Myasthenia gravis is another disorder affecting muscle itself, in this case the neuromuscular junction. It is an autoimmune disease involving inhibition of the excitatory effects of the neurotransmitter acetylcholine at the neuromuscular junction. Patients show muscle weakness and fatigability, and muscles in the orofacial region may be involved. Most cases of myasthenia gravis are treated by acetylcholinesterase inhibitors or immunosuppressants.

Two disorders that affect CNS sites, especially motoneurons, are amyotrophic lateral sclerosis (ALS) and poliomyelitis. ALS is often called Lou Gehrig's disease and affects motoneuron function. It is characterized by rapidly progressive muscle weakness, muscle atrophy, and muscle spasticity. Its manifestations include difficulties in speaking, swallowing, and chewing which make eating very difficult and also increase the risk of choking or aspirating food into the respiratory system. The cause of ALS is unclear, although mutations in some genes have been linked to some types of ALS, and there is a familial type of ALS. Polio, in contrast, does have a known cause, since it is a viral, infectious disease producing inflammation in the spinal cord and even the brainstem or higher CNS sites (e.g., motor cortex). As a result, paralysis of muscles can occur, including the orofacial musculature supplied by cranial nerve motoneurons in the brainstem. Fortunately, polio largely has been eradicated in most countries through vaccination programs.

Dystonia refers to motor disorders involving sustained muscle contractions manifested as twisting and repeated movements or abnormal posture. Although the causes of dystonia are not well understood, primary dystonia is thought to reflect pathological changes in CNS areas involved in motor functions, such as the basal ganglia and cerebellum. In the case of other forms of dystonia, the causes range from damage to certain CNS regions, trauma, or the use of certain drugs with actions in the CNS. Dystonia often is manifested in the orofacial region, with oromandibular dystonia affecting the jaw and tongue muscles and thereby producing distorted jaw and tongue movements, and spasmodic dystonia affecting the tongue and laryngeal muscles and thereby causing speech difficulties. There is no cure at present for dystonia, and therapy is limited to minimizing the symptoms.

Tardive dyskinesia is another motor disorder reflected in involuntary, repetitive body movements. It typically is caused by long-term or high-dose use of antipsychotic drugs that act on higher levels of the CNS. Orofacial manifestations are common, such as facial grimacing, lip smacking and pursing, tongue protrusion, and rapid eye blinks. Treatment usually involves reassessment of the antipsychotic drug regime, or using a dopamine-depleting drug.

Parkinson's disease or parkinsonism is a CNS degenerative disorder resulting from the death of dopamine-generating cells in the substantia nigra, although the actual cause of this cell death is still unclear. Motor disturbances are common, especially in the early phase of the disease, with shaking, rigidity, slowness in movements, and locomotor difficulty. Sometimes orofacial motor disturbances may appear. The use of levodopa and dopamine agonists has become the standard pharmacological approach, especially for the early motor symptoms, but the effects of these drugs can gradually lessen as the disease progresses and in some patients the drugs can themselves cause dyskinesia. In severe cases, neurosurgery and deep brain stimulation may be used to reduce the motor symptoms.

Cerebral palsy refers to a group of nonprogressive motor disorders caused by damage especially to motor control centers of the developing brain. It may occur during pregnancy, childbirth or during the first two to three postnatal years. Patients show motor control problems such as balance difficulties and muscle spasticity or spasm. Other symptoms are involuntary facial gestures, and some may have problems with masticatory and swallowing functions and their integration with respiration. There is no known cure, and therapy usually is limited to the treatment and prevention of complications arising from the effects of the disorder.

Bruxism is an abnormal oral activity associated with tooth grinding and clenching. It may occur during waking hours (daytime bruxism) or sleep (sleep bruxism). It can be associated with grinding noises due to tooth contact and can produce wear facets on the teeth. Orofacial pain (e.g., TMDs), headaches, and sleep disturbances also may occur. Bruxism represents one of the most controversial areas in dentistry because its etiology is unclear and a variety of therapeutic approaches have been advocated but with limited scientific underpinning. For many years, it had been thought that occlusal factors were especially involved and much emphasis was placed on "correcting the bite." But there is little evidence to support the view that changes in the dental occlusion are of etiological significance, although it is possible that they may play a role as a risk factor in some individuals. Currently, bruxism is generally considered a parafunctional activity, with most scientific evidence favoring CNS mechanisms in its etiology (e.g., psychological factors" and CNS-based approaches (e.g., behavioral modification, centrally acting drugs) or occlusal splints.

Case study

A male patient visits his recently graduated dentist for some prosthodontic treatment. He tells the young dentist that on his hurried way to the dental office he started to feel some numbness and tingling sensation on the left side of his face and that he was having some trouble opening his mouth and making chewing movements and swallowing. The dentist notes that the patient is 65 years old, is somewhat obese, and has a history of cardiovascular disease. The dentist carries out sensory testing of the patient's face and mouth and finds that, compared to the right side of the face and mouth, the left orofacial region shows a loss of touch sensibility. The dentist also confirms that the patient has difficulty carrying out chewing movements, including opening the jaw, and he also has difficulty in bringing his upper and lower lips together. Given the dentist's knowledge of neuroanatomy and neurophysiology learned in dental school and the tests that indicated both touch and motor functions were affected, the dentist reaches a provisional diagnosis that the patient may have suffered a cardiovascular event, perhaps a stroke, that most likely affected either the right side of the sensorimotor cortex where the orofacial region is represented, or the left side of the brainstem, possibly involving the left trigeminal main sensory nucleus that relays touch information from the left orofacial region and the adjacent fifth and twelfth cranial nerve motor nuclei that supply the jaw and facial muscles on the left side. He arranges for the patient to be immediately taken to the local hospital which confirms the cortical stroke and promptly institutes therapeutic approaches that minimize the cortical damage, thereby allowing the patient over the next few weeks to regain most of his lost sensory and motor functions.

References

1. Avivi-Arber, L., Martin, R., Lee, J.C., & Sessle, B.J. (2011) Face sensorimotor cortex and its neuroplasticity related to orofacial sensorimotor functions. *Archives of Oral Biology,* 56, 1440–1465.

2. Chiang, C.Y., Dostrovsky, J.O., Iwata, K., & Sessle, B.J. (2011) Role of glia in orofacial pain. *Neuroscientist,* 17, 303–320.

3. Dubner, R., Sessle, B.J., & Storey, A. T. (1978) *The Neural Basis of Oral and Facial Function.* Plenum, New York.

4. Dubner, R., Ren, K., & Sessle, B.J. (2013) Sensory mechanisms of orofacial pain. In: *Treatment of TMDs: Bridging the Gap between Advances in Research and Clinical Patient Management* (eds. C. Greene & D. Laskin), pp. 3–16. Quintessence, Chicago.

5. Hargreaves, K.M. & Goodis, H.E. (eds.) (2002) *Seltzer and Bender's Dental Pulp,* p. 500. Quintessence, Chicago.

6. Jean, A. (2001) Brain stem control of swallowing: neuronal network and cellular mechanisms. *Physiological Reviews,* 81, 929–969.

7. Lam, D.K., Sessle, B.J., Cairns, B.E., & Hu, J.W. (2005) Neural mechanisms of temporomandibular joint and masticatory muscle pain: a possible role for peripheral glutamate receptor mechanisms. *Pain Research and Management,* 10, 145–152.

8. Lund, J.P. , Kolta, A., & Sessle, B.J. (2009) Trigeminal motor system. In: *Encyclopedia of Neuroscience,* Vol. 7 (ed. L. Squire), pp. 1167–1171. Academic Press, Oxford.

9. Martin, R.E. (2009). Neuroplasticity and swallowing. *Dysphagia,* 24, 218–229.

10. Melzack, R. & Wall, P.D. (1965) Pain mechanisms: a new theory. *Science,* 150, 971–979.

11. Meyer R.A., Ringkamp M., Campbell J.N., & Raja S.N. (2006) Peripheral mechanisms of cutaneous nociception. In: *Wall and Melzack's Textbook of Pain,* 5th edn. (eds. S.B. McMahon & M. Koltzenburg). Elsevier, Amsterdam.

12. Miles, T.S., Nauntofte, B., & Svensson, P. (2004) *Clinical Oral Physiology.* Quintessence, Copenhagen.

13. Sessle, B.J. (1981a) Pain. In: Oral Biology (eds. G. I. Roth & R. Calmes), pp. 3–28. Mosby, St.Louis.

14. Sessle, B.J. (1981b) Temperature, touch, taste, and olfaction. In: Oral Biology (eds. G. I. Roth & R. Calmes), pp. 29–50. Mosby, St.Louis.

15. Sessle, B.J. (2000) Acute and chronic craniofacial pain: brainstem mechanisms of nociceptive transmission and neuroplasticity, and their clinical correlates. *Critical Reviews in Oral Biology and Medicine,* 11, 57–91.

16. Sessle, B.J. (2006) Mechanisms of oral somatosensory and motor functions and their clinical correlates. *Journal of Oral Rehabilitation,* 33, 243–261.

17. Sessle, B.J. (2009) Orofacial motor control. In: *Encyclopedia of Neuroscience,* Vol. 7 (ed. L. Squire), pp. 303–308. Academic Press, Oxford.

18. Sessle, B.J., Lavigne, G., Lund, J.P., & Dubner R. (2008). *Orofacial Pain: from Basic Science to Clinical Management,* 2nd ed. Quintessence, Chicago.

Glossary

Active contractile component: the numerous individual striated (contractile) muscle fibers in a muscle.

Allodynia: a subject's perception of pain to a normally innocuous stimulus (e.g., tactile) applied to a peripheral tissue.

Central neural pattern generator: several groups of neurons in the CNS, the patterned output of which projects to motoneurons which, through their connections to muscles, produce cyclic patterned movements such as those that occur in chewing, swallowing, and locomotion.

Central sensitization: a neuroplastic change reflecting a prolonged increase in excitability of nociceptive neurons in the CNS following injury or inflammation of peripheral tissues.

Electromyogram (EMG) of a muscle: an electrophysiological recording of the electrical impulses that are generated in the muscle fibers by motor unit activity and associated with the muscle's contraction.

"Facultative" swallow muscles: muscles that show a variable participation during swallowing, i.e., they may or may not be active during every swallow.

Gate control theory of pain: a conceptual framework for considering the multifactorial nature of pain. It emphasizes the sensory interaction that occurs within the CNS between neural signals carried into the CNS by the large-diameter, low-threshold primary afferent fibers and those conveyed by the small-diameter, high-threshold afferent fibers; through this interaction the "gate" can be opened or closed for pain transmission through CNS nociceptive neurons (e.g., in the dorsal horn of the spinal cord gray matter). The theory also emphasizes descending central neural controls (e.g., emanating from higher brain centers) related to the cognitive, affective, and motivational dimensions of pain that through their influences on the nociceptive neurons can modulate the gate for pain.

Golgi tendon organ: a receptor (sense organ) that occurs in most muscles and/or their tendons and provides the CNS with sensory information about muscle tension produced during the muscle's contraction.

Hyperalgesia: a subject's exaggerated perceptual response to a noxious stimulus applied to a peripheral tissue.

Kinesthesia: a subject's conscious perception of position, e.g., of the jaw or a limb.

Mechanoreceptors: receptors (sense organs) that respond either transiently or throughout the application of a mechanical stimulus to a localized area of the body.

Motor unit: a single α-motoneuron and the several muscle fibers that it supplies by its α-efferent.

Muscle spindle: a stretch-sensitive receptor (sense organ) that occurs in most muscles and provides the CNS with sensory information about muscle length.

Nociceptive-specific neurons: neurons in the CNS that respond exclusively to noxious stimuli applied to peripheral tissues.

"Obligate" swallow muscles: muscles that are always active during every swallow.

Passive viscoelastic component: the tendons, ligaments, and fascia of a muscle.

Peripheral sensitization: the increased excitability of the peripheral endings of nociceptive primary afferent fibers that may occur at a peripheral injury or inflammation site.

Referral of pain: a clinical pain state where pain may be felt at the site of injury or pathology and also, or instead, at other distant sites.

Somatosensory cortex: that region of the cerebral cortex where the cortical neural processing begins that eventually leads to a subject's perception of a somatosensory (e.g., mechanical, thermal) stimulus applied to part of the subject's body.

Stereognosis: a subject's ability to recognize the form of objects, e.g., if placed in the subject's mouth or hand.

Tactile threshold: the lowest intensity of a mechanical stimulus applied to a subject (usually to the skin or mucosa) that evokes a sensation of touch in the subject.

Temporomandibular disorder (TMD): a term referring to a number of clinical conditions which involve the masticatory musculature and/or temporomandibular joint and associated structures; most of these conditions manifest pain in these areas.

Thermoreceptors: receptors (sense organs) that are activated by a small thermal change in either a cooling (cold receptors) or warming (warm receptors) direction.

Trigeminal ganglion: the anatomical site where the primary afferent cell bodies of most trigeminal afferent nerve fibers are located.

Two-point discrimination: the smallest distance between two points applied simultaneously with equal force to a subject's skin for which the subject can discern two separate points.

Wide-dynamic-range neurons: neurons in the CNS that respond to innocuous as well as noxious stimuli applied to peripheral tissues.

Chapter 13 Anatomy and Physiology of Speech Production

Janet E. Rovalino

Otolaryngology - Head and Neck Surgery, School of Medicine, University of Connecticut

Phonation and vocal tract modulations

There are multiple points of clinical intersection amongst the fields of dentistry and speech pathology. Interdisciplinary treatment often is required in the management of disorders of **articulation**, **resonance**, and swallowing caused by congenital cleft of the lip and palate, in speech disorders due to morphologic variations in the facial skeleton and its oral tissue, and in supplementation of dysarthric speech resulting from neuromuscular dysfunction using **adaptive technology** (i.e. palatal lifts or **obturators**). It is also important to consider oral health initiatives in patients living in long-term care facilities who have speech and swallowing difficulties, feeding problems in newborns with dentofacial disorders due to **fetal alcohol syndrome**, and dental and speech/swallowing needs in irradiated patients following treatment of oral and laryngeal cancer. The opportunity for collaboration amongst speech and dental personnel is vast.

> Head and neck cancer patients undergoing radiation therapy are at risk for dental difficulties. Patients should see their dentist before starting head and neck radiation therapy.

In order to provide optimum treatment of such cases of speech and language disorders, the dental professional needs a standing knowledge of speech production patterns, swallowing dynamics, vocal tract differences, and an understanding of the neural basis of language comprehension and production. It is important to appreciate the function of various parts of the speech system as it generates an acoustic output in both quantitative and qualitative terms. Judgments of inadequate **velopharyngeal closure**, dental consonant misarticulations, and weak articulatory contacts currently are able to be calculated and defined more accurately by the speech pathologist or dental professional. More specifically, the speech professional seeks to characterize, both objectively and perceptually, the manner in which aberrant function impacts speech and swallowing physiology. Thereafter, the speech pathologist's role is to provide therapeutic management to change/adjust function within the framework of the physiologic and physical abnormalities or while the system undergoes surgical and/or clinical management.

Within the field of speech pathology, there are multiple areas of specialty and subspecialty. Likewise, there are multiple clinical disorders requiring concentrated clinical knowledge, including swallowing disorders, resonance disorders, voice disorders, vocal tract disorders (i.e., disorders of articulation) and language-based disorders. This chapter will focus on speech and voice/vocal tract disorders, with initial discussion of the normally functioning speech system.

> A speech pathologist is the professional with specialized training who works on rehabilitation of disordered speech and swallowing.

Normal speech production is a highly regulated process and a sufficiently dynamic process requiring interchange amongst pulmonary, laryngeal, and vocal tract structures of the human body. The speech production mechanism depends on the respiratory system, a laryngeal vibration, a functioning set of

Fundamentals of Oral Histology and Physiology, First Edition. Arthur R. Hand and Marion E. Frank.
© 2014 John Wiley & Sons, Inc. Published 2014 by John Wiley & Sons, Inc.

resonating cavities (larynx, pharynx, oral cavity, and nasal cavity), and rapid movement of coarticulating organs or articulators (tongue, lips, teeth, alveolar ridge, hard palate, velum, and pharynx). Any change that affects the size, shape, movement, or timing of these organs will alter the acoustic output. The subsequent alteration can result in speech variation or disorder. These areas will be examined individually.

> Try gently lifting your voice box while saying /ah/ and notice the change in the sound you hear. This change in sound, a perceived elevation of pitch, is actually the result of shortening of the vocal tract and not a change in the vibrating frequency of the vocal folds.

Phonation

The initiation of human sound begins at the larynx. The vocal folds, two paired **thyroarytenoid muscles**, obstruct the airflow generated upwards from the lungs. These vocal folds are made of muscle and ligament, covered with mucosa, and stretch from the front of the larynx to the back of the larynx (Fig. 13.1). The space between the vocal folds is called the **glottis** and peak glottal area is usually between 0.05 and 0.2 cm² during voicing for adults. Vocal folds are typically 13 to 18 mm long in females and 17 to 23 mm long in males.

> At puberty the adolescent male's vocal folds grow rapidly in length and mass. During adolescence, male vocal folds double in length and pitch drops by one octave. The adolescent male's voice may exhibit pitch breaks during this rapid growth phase.

The vocal folds are attached posteriorly to two **arytenoid cartilages** which sit atop the cricoid cartilages. The arytenoid cartilages move in a complex pattern (simplistically, rocking, rotating, and sliding). With neural input, the arytenoids change position to cause the vocal folds to **adduct** (close) or **abduct** (open). Anteriorly the vocal folds are attached to a fixed point on the thyroid cartilage. The size of the open glottis is accordingly controlled by the arytenoids and by tension within the thyroarytenoid (vocal fold) muscles themselves. Contraction of the cricothyroid muscle (moving the cricoid cartilage further away from the thyroid cartilage) stretches the vocal folds, leading to their elongation, and serving as a pitch change mechanism for voicing.

The vocal folds regulate the inward–outward flow of air. With a wide glottis the vocal folds are relaxed and air flows freely with minimal hindrance. During voicing, however, the arytenoid cartilages move toward each other, causing the vocal folds to approximate or adduct. As the vocal folds approximate, they produce a partial closing of the glottis, and obstruct the airflow from the lungs. Tension from the thyroarytenoid muscles is added, and pressure below the adducted vocal folds increases. Eventually the compressed air beneath the vocal folds forces them apart. The vocal folds are then brought back together by two forces, the elasticity of the vocal folds and the Bernoulli effect (Fig. 13.2). **Bernoulli's principle** indicates that when pressure between the vocal folds drops, negative pressure is created, causing the vocal folds to become sucked inward. The entire process repeats itself for as long as the aerodynamic and muscular conditions for phonation are met. The resulting vibrations/oscillations generate quasi-periodic broad spectrum excitations (or puffs of vibrating air). Their quality is akin to a "buzz-like" sound. Sound generated by the larynx is referred to as the **sound source** and visualized in a **sound spectrum** (Fig. 13.3a). These excitations of air are propelled into the vocal tract.

The sound produced by the vocal folds, then, is the result of careful and coordinated use of air pressure produced by the respiratory system. Lung pressure during voicing is released

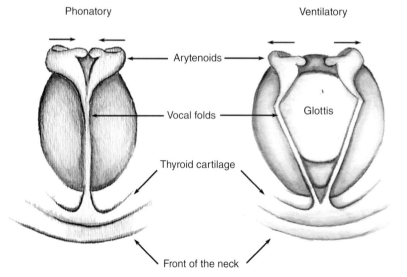

Figure 13.1   Schematic of the position of the vocal folds during phonation (vocal folds adducted) and during rest and breathing (vocal folds abducted). (Artwork courtesy of Hannah Plishtin, BA.)

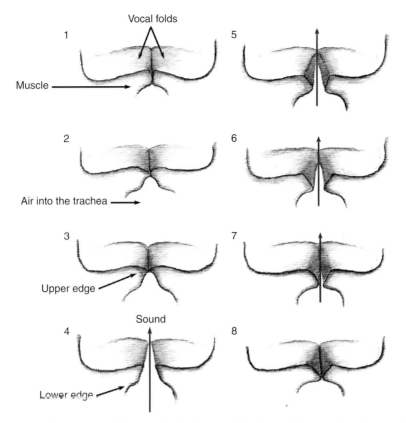

Figure 13.2   Schematic of the pattern of phonation: initial vocal fold adduction (1), column of transglottal airflow and air pressure opens bottom of vibrating vocal folds (2–3), column of air pressure moving upwards, opening the top of the vocal folds (4–6), the low pressure created by moving column of air produces Bernoulli effect initiating vocal fold closing (7), and vocal fold closing (8). (Artwork courtesy of Hannah Plishtin, BA.)

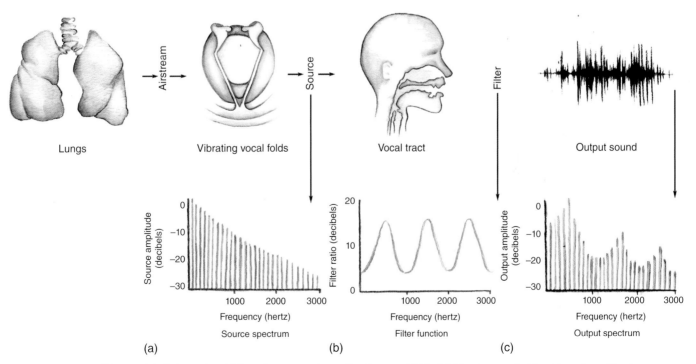

Figure 13.3   Source-filter model of phonation. (a) Sound spectrum from vibrating vocal folds. (b) Filter (or transfer) function of vocal tract. (c) Output spectrum showing final acoustic product radiated from the lips. (Artwork courtesy of Hannah Plishtin, BA.)

slowly. A steady subglottal pressure is maintained by activity of the respiratory muscles, including the intercostal, abdominal, and latissimus dorsi muscles. The speech pathologist is able to take measurements of air pressure across the vocal folds and then throughout the vocal tract, at areas of constriction. By studying patterns of air pressure in these regions and comparing it to available normative data, the degree of function or abnormality can be inferred. In a clinical speech laboratory, the easiest measurement to obtain and evaluate is the measure of intraoral pressure, using a small intraoral catheter. Measuring the pressure in the oral cavity, during the production of repetitive productions of /pa/, provides an indirect measure of pressure at the glottis, P_{subg} (Fig. 13.4). Abnormal findings may be indicative of a variety of issues, including **velopharyngeal insufficiency** and poor laryngeal closure, or it can suggest errors in degree, timing, or location of vocal tract constrictions.

The duration of one cycle of vocal fold vibration is called the pitch period, or **fundamental frequency** (typically measured in hertz, or cycles per second). The rate of vocal fold vibration is influenced by many factors. These factors include tension of the vocal folds, mass of the vocal folds, and the air pressure below the glottis. Vocal folds are capable of a variety of vibration rates ranging from 60 to 1000 Hz. Males have lower fundamental frequencies (typically phonating at 100–150 Hz) than females (who typically phonate at 180–220 Hz). The lower vibrating frequency of the vocal folds in males is due to the greater mass of male vocal folds.

Research has demonstrated that the average fundamental frequency of individuals who smoke is lower than that of control subjects who are nonsmokers. The resulting lower frequency of vibration of the vocal folds is a direct result of edema caused by the irritation from the inhaled smoke. This can result in the "yes sir" response which female smokers often receive when speaking over the telephone with unfamiliar listeners.

Vocal tract modulation

The vocal tract is defined structurally as the area existing from the superior surface of the vocal folds through to the lips and including coupling of the nasal passages. The vocal tract has an average length of 17 cm in a male and is shorter in length for females. Its shape is nonlinear. It consists of a set of cavities where sounds are resonated. The articulators of the vocal tract include the tongue, lips, teeth, alveolar ridge, hard palate, soft palate, and pharynx (Fig. 13.5). The vocal tract is considered to be a **filter** of the sounds (or source) produced by the larynx. Another way to understand this is to consider the source as the energy of the system being modified by the supralaryngeal vocal tract's filter which can either suppress the energy or amplify the energy. Furthermore, for vowels, the vocal folds produce a **harmonic**-rich signal that falls at or near resonance peaks in the vocal tract, which then enhances or amplifies them. Other harmonics are attenuated because they fall in areas beyond the resonant peaks.

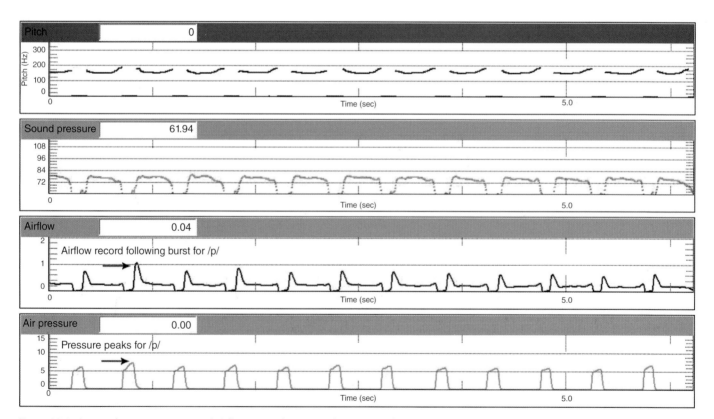

Figure 13.4   Intraoral pressures traces and airflow traces during rapid repetition of /pa/. Bottom tracing represents air pressure pulses for /p/. Third tracing shows speech airflow immediately following each pressure pulse. First and second tracings represent fundamental frequency and sound pressure levels, respectively. (Permission provided by Kay-Pentax Corporation for use of images from Phonatory Airflow System.)

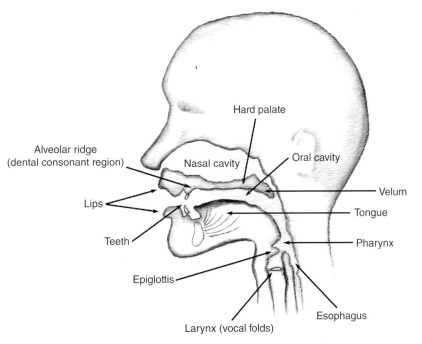

Figure 13.5 Schematic of larynx and vocal tract illustrating the larynx (sound source) and the vocal supralaryngeal structures (sound filter). (Art work courtesy of Hannah Plishtin, BA.)

The acoustic product of the filter is determined by the varying shape of its container(s). Any change in the acoustic output necessarily represents a change in the status of the speech organs. This can be visualized by use of **a frequency-amplitude spectrum**, also called a **transfer function**. The transfer function represents the acoustic response of the air in the vocal tract cavities. An **amplitude spectrum**, where the vertical axis represents amplitude and the horizontal axis represents frequency, is commonly used by speech pathologists (Fig. 13.3b).

The final output of the combined interaction of the source and the filter is called the spectrum and is visualized in spectrograms (Fig. 13.3c). The spectrogram allows the investigator to surmise considerable information about speech production. The frequency of a signal is drawn on the ordinate, and time is represented on the abscissa. Amplitude of the signal is indicated by the darkness of the signal. The closely spaced vertical striations represent the energy pattern resulting from the individual glottal pulses. There are points in time where the major excitation of the air in the supralaryngeal vocal tract occurs. These **resonant frequencies**, in speech science context, are referred to as **formant frequencies** or simply as formants. For vowels, due to changing position of the articulators, different spectrograms are produced, which correspond to the difference in the shape of the resonant cavities. For vowels, the major contributor to the formation of resonating cavities is the tongue. Thus each vocal tract shape is characterized by a collection of formants.

> Trained vocalists, especially male singers, deliver a clear formant around 3000 Hz. This formant is absent in the spectra of untrained singers. The increase in energy at 3000 Hz allows singers to be heard over an orchestra of many instruments, which have formants closer to 500 Hz.

Articulation

In vowel productions a near-periodic sound source is conveyed into the vocal tract. For articulation of vowels, the upper vocal tract is chiefly modified by tongue positioning, with additional influence from lip rounding. Studies assessing the formant characteristics of vowels (chiefly formant 1 and formant 2) have typically evaluated the mid-portion of a vowel in a standard phonetic context, or have utilized simple vowel prolongations. In studies which examined the formant frequencies of vowels for a variety of age groups, plotting the second formant against the first formant has allowed investigators to outline the zone in which each of the vowels typically lie (Fig. 13.6). Further research produced isovowel lines which identified the regular relationship among the formant locations for men, women, and children. Data from these investigations illustrated the "life history" of the vocal tract, helping to explain vocal tract development and growth across the lifespan. Deviations from these "plots" are helpful in identifying and describing disorders of the vocal tract, in this case in the production of vowels, the simplest speech unit. A note of caution must be made for the fact that vowels are not static signals, but are modified by their acoustic surroundings. Vowels reflect the previous speech sound's **acoustics** and also merge into the following sound's acoustic makeup.

Besides vowels, the vocal tract is responsible for the production of **consonants**. Consonants can be formed from a periodic glottal tone, an aperiodic turbulent noise, or a combination of the two (Table 13.1a). The tighter vocal tract constriction needed for the consonants results in less radiated sound energy than vowels. Consonants, like vowels, initiate as they transition from the acoustic characteristics of the preceding sounds and then

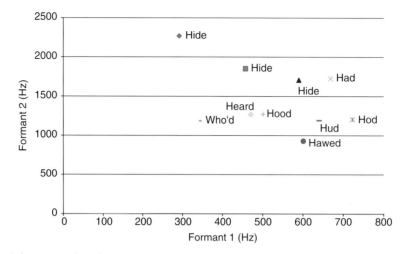

Figure 13.6   Isovowel chart with frequency of the first formant (F1) plotted against the second formant (F2) for several vowels. This chart represents ten different vowels spoken by a single adult male, who has normal speech patterns; spoken in the standard phonetic context "h_d."

Table 13.1a   Classification of consonantal sounds

Bilabial	[p, b, m]	Lips touch each other
Labiodental	[v,f]	Upper teeth touch lower lip
Dental	[ð,θ]	Tongue touches upper teeth
Alveolar	[d,t,n,l,s,z]	Tongue tip touches alveolar ridge
Palato-alveolar	[ʃ,3]	Tongue blade touches palato-alveolar region
Velar	[k,g]	Back of tongue touches velum
Glottal	[h]	Vocal folds approximate

Table 13.1b   Manner of articulation for consonants

Plosive/Stop	Complete obstruction within vocal tract. Air pressure builds behind obstruction and is then released (i.e., [p,d])
Fricative	Narrowing within the vocal tract, causing airflow to become turbulent as it passes (i.e., [f,z])
Affricative	Sequential obstruction and then narrowing of the vocal tract (i.e., [ch])
Nasal	Air passes into the nasal cavity (i.e., [m,n])
Approximant	Narrowing in the vocal tract, however narrowing is insufficient to cause turbulence (i.e.,[j,w])
Lateral approximant	Air flows lateral to the tongue (i.e., [l])

adjust again to accommodate to acoustic characteristics required in the subsequent sound(s). This is called **coarticulation**.

Plosives and **fricatives** are two categories of speech sounds (Table 13.1b). Plosives occur when the vocal tract is completely occluded by the articulators. This complete obstruction of airflow occurs in sounds such as /p/,/b/, /t/, /d/, /k/ and /g/. Pressure increases behind the obstruction or point of articulation in the

oral cavity, and sound is subsequently emitted when the obstruction is released. The /p/, /t/, and /d/ are referred to as voiceless plosives, as they do not require vocal fold vibration at initiation. They have a more intense burst, followed by significant **aspiration**. The glottal pulse (for the next sound) begins thereafter. The timespan between the two events is referred to as **voice onset time** and reflects articulator-laryngeal coordination. With voiced plosives (i.e., /b/, /d/ and /g/), glottal pulsing begins with the plosive itself. The spectrogram clearly illustrates the timing of these events (Fig. 13.7).

Fricative sounds require a tongue constriction in the back, center, or front of the oral tract. Constriction using the teeth or lips is possible (i.e., an /f/or /ʃ/as in the initial sound in "shoe"). The constriction separates the oral tract into front and back cavities. The glottal airflow is then rushed through the narrowed port with the tongue helping to channel the air. The spectrum is characterized as "noisy" because there is evidence of both noise and harmonics. Fricatives include the following sounds: /s/, /z/, / ʃ /as in "shoe," /f/, /v/and /θ/ as in the last sound in "with." Fine adjustments in the articulators are required when these are being produced. These sounds are mastered by children at a developmentally later time juncture than plosives. These sounds are also frequently more misarticulated than the plosive sounds.

Other sound categories include **nasals** and **affricates**. In nasal sounds, the sound source is quasi-periodic, emanating from the vocal folds. The vocal tract adjusts to lower the velum, preventing large airflow through the oral cavity. Sound is predominantly radiated from the nostrils for the three nasals: /m/, /n/, and / ŋ/ as in the last sound of "wrong."

Speakers of the French language nasalize vowels.

Affricates are consonant plosive-fricative combinations. This means that the sound rapidly transitions from the plosive to the fricative articulation. The fricative is preceded by a complete constriction

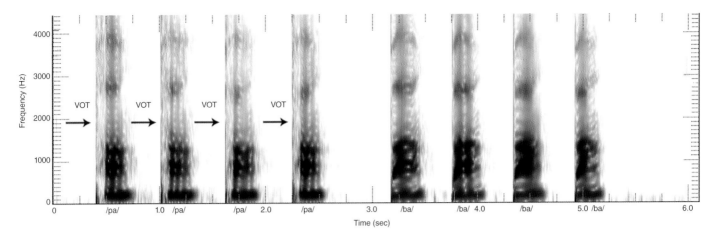

Figure 13.7 Voice onset time. Four repetitions of /pa/ and then /ba/. For /pa/ voicing begins after the oral closure for /p/ is released. The vertical red striation indicates the times it takes for voicing to begin. For /ba/ voicing begins at the same time that the plosive /b/ begins, thus there is an immediate onset of voice. (Permission provided by Kay Pentax Corporation for use of images from Computerized Speech Lab.)

of the oral cavity, formed at the same place as the plosive. Examples of affricates include the /tʃ/ in "chew" and the /dʒ/ as in "just."

Clinical correlations

Important associations among the fields of speech pathology and dental practice occur for management of the individual with cleft lip and palate, in management of speech difficulties in individuals with morphologic variation of the facial skeleton, and in management of individuals with speech and resonance disturbances as a result of neurologic dysfunction. The pediatric dentist, examining the child in early childhood, is an important partner in early identification of children with speech problems. Dental and occlusal difficulties are more likely to be causative problems in children exhibiting speech difficulties, under the following conditions: (1) when they occur in combination rather than singly; (2) when they are present during the years of speech development; and (3) when they influence the spatial relationship between the tip of the tongue and the incisors. An abnormal space between the maxillary and mandibular teeth can result in lateral emission of the oral air stream. Children with this dental difference may try altering placement of their articulators to prevent air escape. Appropriate intervention includes correction of the aberrant structure, followed by use of speech therapy to correct inadequate function. Research has shown that if the anterior opening for /s/ is greater than 10 mm² intraoral pressure is likely decreased and the frication generated by turbulence in the airway is accordingly diminished. This results in distortion of the /s/. These are relatively common types of speech disorders in children.

Cleft palate

Cleft palate is a congenital anomaly resulting in a structural defect of the palate (Fig. 13.8). It is observed in approximately one of 500 to 750 live births. Infants with cleft palate exhibit difficulties which may include poor nutritive sucking due to an inability to create negative intraoral pressure. Liquids escape into nasal passages. This often is managed by use of special

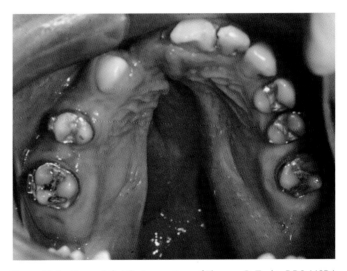

Figure 13.8 Open cleft. (Photo courtesy of Thomas D. Taylor DDS, MSD.)

nipples, special bottles, and feeding plates. Speech problems resulting from cleft palate include hypernasality, nasal emission, and speech errors on plosive consonants requiring high intraoral air pressure. Hypernasality in these cases can result from velopharyngeal insufficiency, oronasal fistulae, or compensatory and learned speech patterns attempting to manage the poor potential for creation of appropriate oral pressures. Posterior articulatory placement of portions of the tongue is a typical error pattern for speech (i.e., /t/→[k] where the alveolar plosive is replaced by a velar plosive). Glottal plosives, pharyngeal fricatives, and posterior nasal fricatives and pharyngeal plosives are typical patterns in cleft palate speakers. Palatal obturators are specially designed appliances which can be constructed for individuals with opens clefts or oronasal fistulae to obstruct the palatal defect (Fig. 13.9).

Facial skeleton variation

Multiple studies have attempted to relate dental malocclusions to misarticulations in speech. A 2007 literature survey of 18 studies (1996–2006) addressed the following considerations.

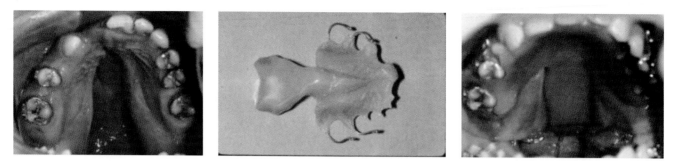

Figure 13.9   The construction and placement of an obturator. (Photos courtesy of Thomas D. Taylor, DDS, MSD.)

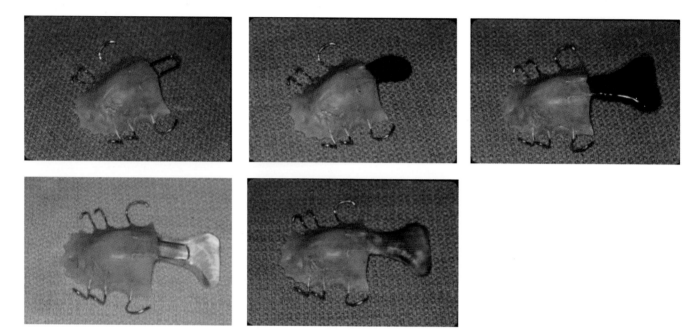

Figure 13.10   Stages of construction of a palatal lift. (Photos courtesy of Thomas D. Taylor, DDS, MSD.)

- The association between malocclusion and speech among individuals before surgical intervention.
- The effect of combined orthodontics and orthognathic surgery on speech.
- The effect of type and degree of surgical movements upon speech.

Although results were limited, it was found that in a majority of the research the most frequent difference observed in speech occurred for consonant articulation of fricatives (before surgery). Similarly, findings showed a trend indicating that individuals with vertical maxillary excess and Class III malocclusions produced a greater average number of articulation errors compared with Class II occlusions or asymmetries. Interestingly, one of the 18 studies identified voice disorders (sound source) to be more prevalent with closed-bite presentations. After surgery, in the majority of cases reviewed, articulation errors were either reduced or eliminated. Four of the 18 studies, however, reported very little change. Finally, with respect to maxillary surgery, three studies found that maxillary repositioning did not result in hypernasal speech or velopharyngeal dysfunction, although this was felt to be a risk of the procedure.

Neurological dysfunction

Treatment of the **dysarthrias** (defined as a motor speech disorder caused by neurological insult), typically requires assessment and management of difficulties of both speech production and resonance. For example, flaccid dysarthria often has symptoms of imprecision in speech patterns (i.e., poorer generation of air pressure) and velopharyngeal insufficiency. Motor movements of the articulators are slowed.

> Alternate motion rates (AMRs) are measured to see how fast an individual can move their articulators while maintaining rhythm. For example, an adult should repeat the syllable "pa" at a rate of 6.0 times per second.

Speech therapy is the main rehabilitative intervention in these cases. A palatal lift (Fig. 13.10), designed in conjunction with the prosthodontist, assists the patient in mechanically lessening nasal air escape by lifting the flaccid velum. Swallowing intervention, also provided by the speech pathologist, is also often required by this group of patients, and the palatal lift can prevent backflow into the nasal cavity.

Case study 1

A 9-year-old male was referred to the Center for Speech and Voice of the University of Connecticut Health Center by his pediatrician and pediatric neurologist. This child had been receiving speech therapy for many years for delayed development in speech and language skills. He had significant difficulty with development of oral skills in early childhood, with findings of sensory defensiveness for textured foods and multiple gastrointestinal difficulties (long history of diarrhea, gastroesophageal reflux, and multiple food allergies). His neurologist had diagnosed "low amplitude movements of the face, pectoralis muscle, anterior abdominal wall, lumbar paraspinal region, arms and fingers."

At the age of 2 years and 11 months, during articulation testing, the patient had a total of 52 substitutions and omission errors which significantly affected speech intelligibility. Patterns noted within speech included final consonant deletion, and **cluster reduction**. The patient's language skills at this time were in the average range. By the time the patient was 5 years and 11 months, and following three years of speech therapy, he continued to have final /r/ deletion, dialectal substitution of /f/ for /θ/, and cluster simplification and continued to be difficult to understand. His speech production was considered to be "choppy." By the time the patient was 8 years and five months old, his speech sound production patterns were much improved, but questions remained about speech fluency and reports indicated "speech **prosody** is choppy and appeared labored."

During our assessment, the patient was observed to have difficulty completing tasks of alternating movements within speech (i.e., rapidly producing /pataka/). These findings were suggestive of **verbal praxis** difficulties. Likewise individual production of repeated movements (i.e., /papapa/) were slower than normative rates.

> Praxis difficulties can also take the form of spoonerisms, where "Mall Cop" becomes "call mop" or "know your blows" is substituted for "blow your nose."

An analysis of the phonatory frequencies (in hertz) for vowel productions was conducted following the Peterson and Barney protocol. The F1 and F2 formant coordinates were placed on a graph into a vowel chart, where the horizontal dimension represented frequency of the first formant and the vertical axis represents frequency of the second formant. The first formant demonstrated influence of tongue body height, while the second formant represented influence of tongue body frontness or backness. The patient was asked to produce each vowel within a 'h_d' format (i.e., hod, hid, head, heed) (Fig. 13.11). During his productions a great deal of variability in performance was demonstrated by the movement of each individual vowel's isoline. For example, F1 variability was noted and achieved the following frequencies across five trials, for the vowel /ɔ/ as in hod: 574 Hz, 745 Hz, 901 Hz, 1013 Hz, and 1110 Hz (norm for children = 724 Hz). This same pattern was noted across all vowels in all trials. The findings were felt to be representative of either tongue **myoclonus** or **choreiform** movements and/or an **apraxia** of vocal tract movements.

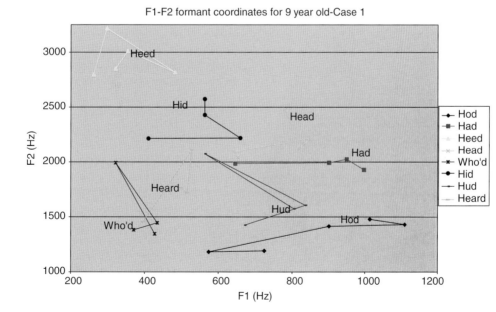

Figure 13.11   F1/F2 formant plotting of vowels: Case Study 1 (9-year-old male subject).

Case study 2

A 19-year-old male was seen in the Voice and Speech Clinic for speech evaluation and treatment for a significant dysarthria, approximately eight months following a bilateral brainstem stroke. He was hospitalized in intensive care for three weeks after the stroke. Prior to that time, he had been in his usual state of good health and had had no significant medical problems. The patient left intensive care and was transferred to a rehabilitation hospital where he underwent intensive speech therapy, physical therapy, and occupational therapy. The speech therapist at the rehabilitation center referred the patient to the Voice and Speech Clinic for specific management of hypernasal speech patterns and for assessment of candidacy for use of a palatal lift.

Upon initial assessment, the patient was observed to have a mild voice disorder, a severe resonance disorder, and a moderate motor speech disorder. His findings were felt to be consistent with a flaccid dysarthria secondary to neurological insult.

> Speech characteristics of flaccid dysarthria include paralysis, weakness, hypertonicity, and atrophy of the involved speech musculature.

Examination of the patient's vocal folds revealed fair glottal competence for voicing, and examination of the velopharyngeal mechanism revealed poor velopharyngeal closure. For motor speech assessment, the patient had fair to poor lingual and labial range of motion and strength. Overall findings suggested a significant impairment in communication function.

Initial intervention entailed design of a working palatal lift to facilitate lessening of hypernasal speech patterns. This was devised by the prosthodontist, and adjustments to the palatal lift were made based upon measurements of nasal airflow with the palatal lift in place. When sufficient lessening of nasal air escape on non-nasal phonemes was accomplished (yet still allowing for some nasal resonance for /m/ /n/ and /ŋ/), the palatal lift was finalized. Speech therapy sessions concentrated thereafter on tolerance of the palatal lift and on improving production of several phonemes requiring high pressure (i.e., plosives). The patient's speech intelligibility improved substantially from the time of the initial assessment to a point several months later with use of the palatal lift.

References

1. Broad, K.J. (1976) Toward defining acoustic phonetic equivalence for vowels. *Phonetica*, 33, 401–424.
2. Church, M.W., Eldis, F., Blakely, B.W., et al. (1997) Hearing, language, speech, vestibular, and dentofacial disorders in fetal alcohol syndrome. *Alcoholism, Clinical and Experimental Research*, 21, 227–237.
3. Eguchi, S, & Hirsh I.J. (1969) Development of speech sounds in children. *Acta Otolaryngologica*, Suppl., 257, 5–43.
4. Fitch, J.L. & Holbrook, A. (1970). Modal fundamental frequency of young adults. *Archives of Otolaryngology*, 92, 379–382.
5. Hassan, T., Naini, F., & Gill, D., (2007). The effects of orthognathic surgery on speech: a review. *American Association of Oral and Maxillofacial Surgeons*, 65, 2536–2543.
6. Hollien, H. & Shipp, T. (1972) Speaking fundamental frequency and chronological age in males. *Journal of Speech and Hearing Research*, 15, 155–159.
7. Petersen, G.E. & Barney, H.L. (1952) Control methods used in a study of the vowels. *Journal of the Acoustical Society of America*, 24, 175–184.
8. Peterson-Falzone, S.J., Hardin-Jones, M.A., & Karnell, M.P. (2001) *Cleft Palate Speech*, pp. 275. Mosby, St. Louis.
9. Stevens, K.N., Kasowski, S., & Fant, G. (1953) An electrical analog of the vocal tract. *Journal of the Acoustical Society of America*, 25, 734–742.
10. Trost, J.E. (1981) Addition to the classical description of the speech of persons with cleft palate. *Cleft Palate Journal*, 18, 193–203.

Glossary

Abduct: Draw away from.

Acoustics: A branch of physics that studies sounds produced by a mechanical wave.

Acoustic Filter: A function of the supralaryngeal vocal tract, which serves to reject sound in a particular range of frequencies while passing sound in another range of frequencies.

Adaptive technology: Hardware or software solutions for people with disabilities.

Adduct: Draw towards or bring together.

Affricate: A consonant that begins as a plosive (such as [t] or [d]) and finishes as a fricative (such as [s] or[z]), as in the sounds that begin the words "chirp" or "just."

Amplitude spectrum: A representation of vibratory events where the vertical axis represents the amplitude of the signal and the horizontal axis represents the component frequencies.

Apraxia: The failure to appropriately execute or perform learned and purposeful movements.

Articulation: How speech organs interact to make contact and produce sounds.

Arytenoid cartilages: A pair of small three-sided pyramidal-shaped cartilages that form part of the larynx, to which the vocal folds are attached.

Aspiration: Audible breath that accompanies or comprises a speech sound.

Bernoulli principle: A physical principle formulated by Daniel Bernoulli stating that as the speed of a moving fluid (liquid or gas) increases, the pressure within the fluid decreases.

Choreiform: Occasional jerking or writhing movements.

Cluster reduction: When a consonant cluster of two or three consonants occurring in a sequence in a word (like "sp" in spider), is reduced to a single consonant through omission (pider).

Coarticulation: A description of how a conceptually isolated speech sound is influenced by, and becomes more like, a preceding or following speech sound.

Consonants: A speech sound that is articulated with complete or partial closure of the vocal tract.

Dysarthria: Difficulty producing words because of problems with the muscles that help one to speak.

Fetal alcohol syndrome: The pattern of mental and physical defects that can develop in a fetus due to high levels of alcohol consumption during pregnancy.

Formant frequencies/resonant frequencies: A formant is a concentration of acoustic energy around a particular frequency in the speech wave. Formants occur at roughly 1000-Hz intervals. Each formant corresponds to a resonance in the vocal tract.

Frequency amplitude spectrum/filter function/transfer function: The frequency response of the vocal tract which is dependent on the vocal tract shape.

Fricative: A consonant that is produced by forcing air through a narrow channel by placing two articulators close together.

Fundamental frequency: The lowest resonant frequency of a vibrating object is called its fundamental frequency.

Glottis: The opening in the larynx that exists anteriorly (to the front) between the vocal folds and posteriorly (to the back) between the arytenoid cartilages. The part of the glottis between the vocal folds is known as the membranous glottis and the part of the glottis between the arytenoid cartilages is known as the cartilaginous glottis.

Harmonic: A series of vibration frequencies in which each vibration frequency is a multiple of the same basic or reference frequency.

Myoclonus: A brief or involuntary twitching of a muscle or a group of muscles.

Nasal: A consonant produced with a lowered velum, or soft palate, allowing the air to pass through the nasal cavity (as in "m" or "n").

Obturator: A prosthesis that totally occludes an opening, as in the opening of the palate in cases of cleft palate.

Plosives: A consonant produced when the vocal tract is blocked so that all airflow is stopped.

Prosody: The rhythm, stress, and intonation used in speech.

Resonance: A quality of sound imparted to voiced sounds which is the result of vibration in anatomical chambers (as in the mouth or nasal cavity)

Sound source: The conversion of aerodynamic energy into acoustic energy which yields a waveform. The airflow through a vibrating larynx yields this waveform.

Sound spectrum: A representation of a sound in terms of the amount of vibration at each individual frequency. It typically is represented by a graph of pressure as a function of frequency. The power or pressure is usually measured in decibels and the frequency is measured in vibrations per second (or hertz, Hz) or thousands of vibrations per second (kilohertz, kHz).

Thyroarytenoid muscle: A strong elastic muscle band passing on either side from the angle of the thyroid cartilage to the anterior angle of the base of the arytenoid cartilage. It is covered with thin mucous membrane and forms the true vocal fold.

Transfer function: The supralaryngeal vocal tract, consisting of both the oral and nasal airways, serves as an acoustic filter that suppresses the passage of sound energy at certain frequencies while allowing its passage at other frequencies. The detailed shape of the filter (transfer) function is determined by the entire vocal tract, which acts as an acoustically resonant system.

Velopharyngeal closure: Closing off of the nasal airway from the oropharyngeal region by the elevation of the soft palate and contraction of the posterior and lateral pharyngeal walls.

Velopharyngeal insufficiency: The inability of the velopharyngeal sphincter to sufficiently close off and separate the nasal cavity from the oral and pharyngeal cavities during speech.

Verbal praxis: Impaired control of proper sequencing of muscles used in speech (tongue, lips, jaw muscles, vocal folds).

Voice onset time: The length of time that passes between the release of a stop consonant and the onset of the vibration of the vocal folds.

Index

Note: page numbers in *italics* indicate figures; page numbers in **bold** indicate tables; page numbers followed by a 'b' indicate text boxes.

Fundamentals of Oral Histology and Physiology, First Edition. Arthur R. Hand and Marion E. Frank.
© 2014 John Wiley & Sons, Inc. Published 2014 by John Wiley & Sons, Inc.